ENDOSCOPIC SURGERY

Endoscopic Surgery

RODNEY A. WHITE, M.D.
Associate Professor of Surgery
UCLA School of Medicine
Chief, Vascular Surgery
Harbor-UCLA Medical Center
Torrance, California

STANLEY R. KLEIN, M.D.
Associate Professor of Surgery
UCLA School of Medicine
General and Vascular Surgery
Harbor-UCLA Medical Center
Torrance, California

Mosby
Year Book

St. Louis Baltimore Boston Chicago London Philadelphia Sydney Toronto

Mosby
Year Book
Dedicated to Publishing Excellence

Sponsoring Editor: Nancy E. Chorpenning
Associate Managing Editor, Manuscript Services: Deborah Thorp
Production Project Coordinator: Karen Halm
Proofroom Manager: Barbara Kelly

A Year Book Medical Publishers imprint of Mosby-Year Book, Inc.

Mosby-Year Book, Inc.
11830 Westline Industrial Drive
St. Louis, MO 63146

1 2 3 4 5 6 7 8 9 0 CL WA WA 95 94 93 92 91

Library of Congress Cataloging-in-Publication Data
Endoscopic surgery / [edited by] Rodney A. White, Stanley R. Klein.
p. cm.
Includes bibliographical references and index.
ISBN 0-8016-9010-2
1. Endoscopic surgery. I. White, Rodney A. II. Klein, Stanley R.
[DNLM: 1. Endoscopy. 2. Surgery, Operative. WO 500 E565]
RD33.53.E53 1991
617′.05—dc20
DNLM/DLC 91-15459
for Library of Congress CIP

This book is dedicated to our wives, Joan Wright, M.D., and Deanna White, and to our families. In addition, we would like to express our gratitude for the ongoing encouragement and support of David State, M.D., to the development of our academic careers. We also dedicate this book to him.

CONTRIBUTORS

Fred Bongard, M.D.
Assistant Professor of Surgery
UCLA School of Medicine
Director of Surgical Critical Care
Harbor-UCLA Medical Center
Torrance, California

Douglas Cavaye, M.D.
Research Associate
Harbor-UCLA Medical Center
Torrance, California

David E. Fleischer, M.D.
Professor of Medicine
Chief, Endoscopy
Georgetown University Hospital
Washington, D.C.

John E. Gunning, M.D.
Professor and Associate Chairman
Department of Obstetrics and Gynecology
Harbor-UCLA Medical Center
Torrance, California

Stanley R. Klein, M.D.
Associate Professor of Surgery
UCLA School of Medicine
General and Vascular Surgery
Harbor-UCLA Medical Center
Torrance, California

George Kopchok
Biomedical Engineer
Supervisor, Surgical Research Laboratory
Harbor-UCLA Medical Center
Torrance, California

Se-Yuan Liu, M.D.
Critical Care Fellow
Harbor-UCLA Medical Center
Torrance, California

Lindsay Machan, M.D.
Interventional Radiologist
University of British Columbia
Vancouver, Canada

Cuong C. Nguyen, M.D.
Assistant Professor in Medicine
Division of Gastroenterology
Department of Medicine
Georgetown University Medical Center
Washington, D.C.

Anthony Nobles, Ph.D.
Nobles-Lai Engineering
Santa Ana, California

Bruce A. Rosenzweig, M.D.
Clinical Instructor
Department of Obstetrics and Gynecology
Harbor-UCLA Medical Center
Torrance, California

Marwan R. Tabbara, M.D.
Clinical Assistant Professor of Surgery
UCLA School of Medicine
Staff Surgeon
Harbor-UCLA Medical Center
Torrance, California

Richard C. Waugh, M.D.
Department of Radiology
Royal Prince Alfred Hospital
Camperdown, Australia

Geoffrey H. White, M.D.
Department of Vascular Surgery
Royal Prince Alfred Hospital
Camperdown, Australia

Rodney A. White, M.D.
Associate Professor of Surgery
UCLA School of Medicine
Chief, Vascular Surgery
Harbor-UCLA Medical Center
Torrance, California

Samuel E. Wilson, M.D.
Professor and Chairman
Department of Surgery
Harbor-UCLA Medical Center
Torrance, California

Miguel Velez, M.D.
Clinical Attending Staff
Harbor-UCLA Medical Center
Torrance, California

PREFACE

Endoscopic surgical principles and techniques are established methods of therapy in medical subspecialties, including gynecology, urology, and gastroenterology. Technologic advances in imaging and miniaturization of ablation, dissection, and coagulation devices have stimulated rapid adaptation of the methods to other disciplines, such as laparoscopic general or endovascular surgery. Continuing evolution of the technology, in particular, miniaturization of devices, is enabling catheter-based interrogation and therapy of small tubular structures such as the lacrimal or salivary ducts, and in confined spaces with difficult access, such as intracranial and spinal cord locations.

This book reviews in detail the development and principles of endoscopic surgery, emphasizing the intra-abdominal general surgical and endoscopic applications. Currently developing procedures and future perspectives are highlighted. The focus of the initial chapters is to review extensively the information regarding instrumentation, essentials of device fabrication such as fiberoptic transmission and imaging, pertinent safety considerations, and recommended credentialing guidelines.

The book emphasizes the multispecialty interest and perspective for use and development of the techniques, and provides an interesting comparison of the benefits derived from various approaches. An additional focus of the text is to identify developing procedures and technologies and to demonstrate the potential directions in the field.

Rodney A. White, M.D.
Stanley R. Klein, M.D.

ACKNOWLEDGMENTS

We thank the contributors for their timely assistance in the preparation of this book. Special thanks are given to Gloria Stevens and Teresa Ossea, who provided expert manuscript preparation and word processing. Recognition is also given our colleagues, research associates, and support personnel at Harbor-UCLA Medical Center who provided help and encouragement. Special recognition is extended to Robert Nejdl, M.D., and Gary Belzberg, M.D., Kaiser-Permanente, Harbor City, California, for their invaluable contributions to the development of this technology and for providing material for several chapters. We also thank Karen Halm, Deborah Thorp, Karyn Fell, and Nancy Chorpenning of Mosby-Year Book, Inc., for their help and support.

Rodney A. White, M.D.
Stanley R. Klein, M.D.

CONTENTS

PART I

Introduction

Chapter 1

Evolution of Endoscopic Surgery

John E. Gunning, M.D.

Bruce A. Rosenzweig, M.D.

The evolution of operative endoscopy would be incomplete without due credit to the development of endoscopes, which make it all possible. Man's innate curiosity to view the inside of body cavities or canals dates back to the time of Hippocrates II (460–375 B.C.)[1] who mentions examination of the rectum by looking with a rectal speculum to see where the rectum is affected. The Babylonian Talmud refers to an instrument described in the thesis *Niddah* (65 B.C.) that is intended to distinguish between vaginal and uterine bleeding. This probably represents the oldest form of vaginal speculum and therefore the earliest incidence of endoscopy in gynecologic annals.[1] Archigenes of Apamea in Syria (95–117 A.D.) and Soranus of Ephesus (98–108 A.D.) both mentioned in their writings vaginal speculums.[1] Abulkasim (1012–1013 A.D.), an Arab, used a glass mirror to reflect light into the vaginal cavity.[1] He was thus the first to use reflected light for the purposes of illuminating and observation of the interior of a body orifice. The first endoscopic light should be credited to Tulio Caesare Aranzi who in 1585 wrote of using solar rays entering through a hole in a window shutter and brought to a focus through a spherical glass flask filled with water and projected into the nasal cavity.[1]

Bozzani (1805 A.D.) of Frankfurt was the first to visualize the interior of the urethra, which he visualized in a human by using candlelight and a cumbersome tube as an endoscope.[2] Segalas (1826) of France refined the technique of urethroscopy by adding a cannula to the endoscopic tube as an obturator to facilitate introduction and a system of mirrors to reflect light into the cavity.[2] At about the same time Fisher of Boston described an instrument to inspect the vagina and extended its use to view the urethra.[2] Desormeaux (1835) is credited with being the father of cystoscopy when he developed the first servicable urethroscope and cystoscope by using mirrors to reflect light of a kerosene lamp.[2] In July 1869, Commander Pantaleoni of England described the use of a sponge tent by the Sims' method to dilate the cervix. Twenty-four hours later he introduced his modification of the Desormeaux endoscope into the cavity of the uterus and cauterized a hemorrhagic necrotic growth with nitrate of silver.[3] His is the first description of endoscopic visualization of the endometrial cavity and use of the endoscopic tube as a channel to treat an abnormality and thus the birth of hysteroscopy in 1869.

Nitze (1877) added a lens system to the endoscopic tube that magnified the area being illuminated, and this lens system is the forerunner of the optical system of modern cystoscopy and all other endoscopes.[2] Edison (1880) invented the incandescent lamp, and Newman (1883) describes an instrument using the incandescent lamp as a light source.[2] Dittel, in 1887, placed a small incandescent lamp bulb at the tip of the break of the cystoscope.[2] Boisseau de Rocher (1889) separated the ocular part of the cystoscope from the sheath, thus allowing the use of multiple telescopes providing greater latitude of observation and making manipulation through the sheath possible.[2] It was also in 1889 that Poirer, using Boisseau de Rocher's instrument, successfully catheterized both ureters in a living subject.[2]

At the close of the 19th century cystoscopy and other open-cavity endoscopic procedures such as proctoscopy, laryngoscopy, and esophagoscopy were well established and in daily use in most medical centers. Ott, a famous Petrograd gynecologist, was the first to introduce endoscopic inspection of the abdominal cavity. In this "ventroscopy" procedure he inspected the abdominal cavity with the help of a head mirror and a speculum introduced through a small anterior abdominal wall incision. He published articles on the clinical use of this technique in 1901, 1902, and 1903.[4] A few months later in the same year at the 73rd Congress of German Naturalists and Physicians, Kelling, a surgeon from Dresden, demonstrated its use on a living dog into whose abdomen he had inserted a cystoscope for the purpose of examining the abdominal viscera.[4] He called the procedure "coelioscopy," which he described in his paper published in January 1902.

In 1910 Jacobaues of Stockholm published two cases of visceral exploration: one abdominal and one thoracic. He used a cystoscope and trocar, as had Kelling, and called his method "thoraco-laparoscopy."[5] His method was less advanced than that reported by Kelling in that Kelling had used a separate needle to produce a pneumoperitoneum with filtered air. Jacobaeus used no separate pneumoperitoneum needle but introduced air by means of the trocar used for the introduction of the cystoscope. On the other hand, he made a forward step by using his method in human beings and stressed its harmlessness when applied to patients suffering from ascites.[4] In the meantime Kelling had perfected the technical aspects of the pneumoperitoneum procedure. He failed to publish his work or to transfer its use to humans. However, he deserves the credit of introducing closed-cavity endoscopy.[6] In 1911 Bernheim, an assistant surgeon at Johns Hopkins, published in the *Annals of Surgery* an article entitled "Organoscopy."[7] He described two cases where a proctoscope was passed through a small abdominal incision by using reflected light. By 1912 Jacobaeus had reported on 115 examinations in 69 patients, 42 abdominal and 27 thoracic.[6] He described the liver changes in cirrhosis, metastatic cancer, lues, and tuberculous peritonitis and predicted a great future for laparoscopy.

Nordentoft and his brother of Copenhagen in 1912 designed an instrument that they called a "trocar-endoscope."[6] In principle their method was identical to that of Kelling, Jacobaeus, and Bernheim. They are the first to report viewing the female pelvis in a cadaver that had been placed in the deep Trendelenburg position with an inflated abdominal cavity. The credit of using the Trendelenburg position belongs to them.

In 1912 at the monthly session of the Society of Internal Medicine and Pediatrics in Vienna, Tedesko told of his experiences with laparoscopy as practiced by Jacobaeus on patients with ascites.[6] The discussion that followed indicated that the method had already been put to trial and had been retained by some of the clinicians in Vienna.

Meirelles of South America, in 1913, published a discussion on laparoscopy. This paper is mentioned in most bibliographies on the subject matter; however, the original paper has been lost.[6]

In 1914 Roccavilla of Italy described a modified method of Kelling and Jacobaeus.[5] He designed an instrument that permitted the source of light to remain outside the abdomen: a strong beam of light was directed by reflection into the trocar tube.

Orndoff of Chicago, in 1920, published extensive experiences using laparoscopic techniques in conjunction with roentgenographic screening.[8] He denied knowing of the experiences of others and was the first to devise a sharp pyramid point, which he used on his trocar.

Zollikofer of Switzerland, in 1924, felt that laparoscopy offered its best diagnostic services in the afflictions of the liver.[6] He introduced the use of carbon dioxide as the gas of choice for insufflation because it is easily and quickly absorbed. In 1924, Stone of Kansas, without knowledge of the work in Europe, used a nasopharyngoscope introduced in the abdominal cavity of dogs.[9] He later learned that a similar method had been developed and used in Europe for some years. His technique described the fitting of the outer portion of the trocar with a rubber gasket that prevented the leakage of gas. Steiner of Atlanta, Georgia, published "Abdominoscopy" in 1924, a paper that refers to a new method of examination.[10] He stated that he was unable to find any papers dealing with the subject, either experimental or theoretical. He felt he had discovered an entirely new diagnostic method that had never been tried before either on the living or a cadaver. His method varied little from that originally developed by Kelling.

Nadeau and Kampmeire of Chicago, in 1925, published a paper titled "Endoscopy of the Abdomen."[6] This scholarly presentation is an extensive review of the literature representing the works of 22 investigators. In spite of numerous reports and frequent usage in the European countries the author states that "the method was seldom used."

Kalk, a brilliant German, was a most outstanding exponent and promotor of peritoneoscopy. He devised a new system of lenses that produced a foroblique (135 degrees) viewing system. He used a pneumoperitoneum needle. In 1929 Kalk reported his experiences with 100 laparoscopic examinations and described his own instrument and technique.[4] His brilliant instrument led to the widespread adoption of the method in many countries. He can probably be referred to as the Father of Modern Laparoscopy, and it is to his credit that it became possible to study and to make an accurate pathologic diagnosis of internal organs. Probably the first operative procedure to be performed by utilizing endoscopic visualization and the first to utilize a second puncture should be credited to Kalk. An eloquent testimony for successfully performing directed liver puncture is the relevant passage in Kalk's book (Kalk and Wildhirt, 1962); 4,000 liver biopsy procedures are described without any serious complication. Kalk published 21 papers between 1929 and 1959, most dealing with liver and gallbladder disease.[4]

Operative procedures combined with endoscopy was reported in 1933 by Fervers, who burned abdominal adhesions and excised biopsy tissue under direct visualization.[4] Ruddock, an American, perfected his own peritoneoscope, pneumoperitoneum needle, and trocar and described ancillary biopsy instruments. Ruddock's peritoneoscope was modified after the McCarthy cystoscope. He utilized air for the pneumoperitoneum and local anesthesia. In 1934 he published his work reporting an initial series of 200 cases.[11] Besides his original paper, Ruddock published his results in over 2,500 cases. Hope, a contemporary of Ruddock, suggested the use of peritoneoscopy in the differential diagnosis of ectopic pregnancy. He reported on ten cases, several of which were from the service of Ruddock.[12]

In 1937, Anderson of Texas reported using peritoneoscopy on a few cases.[13] He states in his paper:

> This work should be of special interest and value to the gynecologist as it allows ocular examination of intrapelvic reproductive organs and will help to decide the location and the variety of many masses found on bimanual palpation. Sterilization of the female using my special electrode and endothermic coagulation can be performed."

He does not mention having done this; however, he should receive credit for the first thought on the matter. Powers and Barnes of the University of Michigan in 1941 published a paper on their experience and histology of tubes fulgurated by using high-frequency, high-voltage pulsating current through a modified Ruddock peritoneoscope.[14] In America aside from a few exponents, namely, Ruddock, Benedict, and Beling, peritoneoscopy was not accepted as a diagnostic tool.[11, 15–17] However, in the European countries under the influence of Kalk many clinics and physicians used the technique extensively.

In 1952 a new apparatus developed by Fourestier, Gladu, and Valmiere revolutionized endoscopic techniques.[18] They developed a method of transmitting an intense light along a quartz rod from the proximal to the distal end of the telescope. Previous sources of light consisted of lamps introduced into the cavity. This immediately removed the dangers of accidents due to electrical faults and heat and allowed intense light to be concentrated so that photographs could be taken. Endoscopic color films were produced, and in 1959 a closed-circuit television program was first produced by using the apparatus of Fourestier, Gladu, and Valmiere.[5] Frangenheim in 1957 stressed general anesthesia, extreme caution in introducing the pneumoperitoneum, and avoidance of puncture through previous laparotomy scars. He further refined the optical instruments, and the laparoscope of Frangenheim is one of the standard optical instruments available today. Frangenheim published the first textbook on gynecologic laparoscopy in 1959.

In spite of these great advances in technique and safety very few clinicians in England and America were impressed by the procedure. In England, Handley, a general surgeon, described his experiences with peritoneoscopy and together with Nurick, in 1956, reported a series of 136 cases.[19, 20] They were primarily interested in the liver, peritoneum, omentum, gallbladder, and stomach. They emphasized the ease with which the female organs could be studied. In 1962 Palmer of France used unipolar electrosurgery on the fallopian tube to effect permanent sterilization.[18] The first International Symposium of Gynecological Endoscopy took place in Italy in 1964. In 1967 Steptoe of England published what he prefaces as the first book in the English language on laparoscopy.[18] Publications in America By Fear[21] and by Cohen[22] in 1968 stimulated great interest in gynecologic laparoscopy.

It is very interesting to speculate why, with great advances in lighting and optics, laparoscopy was not used in America from the era of Ruddock (1930s) until almost the 1970s when it attracted the attention of gynecologists with great vigor. This can probably be attributed to their fascination and concentration on culdoscopy under the influence of Albert Decker of New York City.

Siegler and Berenyi's report in 1969 included 44 patients who had permanent tubal sterilization via laparoscopy.[23] In 1970, Peterson and Behrman published the results of 538 laparoscopies,[24] and Cohen published a textbook.[5] Since laparoscopy was, so to speak, reintroduced into the United States in 1968 and with the improvement in lighting techniques utilizing fiber optics,[25] the widespread and extensive use of laparoscopy in the United States has been phenomenal.

A new organization, the American Association of Gynecological Laparoscopists, held its first annual meeting in 1972 with an attendance of over 600.[26] By March 1973, the association had received well over 500 applications for membership.[26] Their first International Congress of Gynecological Laparoscopy was held in New Orleans in November 1973. Laparoscopic sterilization quickly became the method of choice worldwide.

To attempt to chronical the modern advances in laparoscopic surgery would be difficult at best. Even the appropriate terminology "operative laparoscopy" or "pelviscopy" has not been agreed upon. There have been, however, several major advances in laparoscopic surgery that are worthy of mention.

Steptoe and Edwards (1970) described the use of the laparoscope in oocyte retrieval, which pioneered the technology of in vitro fertilization.[27] Shapiro and Adler (1973) described the first case of an ectopic pregnancy removed via the laparoscope.[28] The tubal segment containing the ectopic gestation was completely excised, and bleeding points were endocoagulated.

Kurt Semm described techniques most commonly associated with operative laparoscopy. His endocoagulator allowed a safe means of controlling blood loss when performing laparoscopic surgery to treat endometriosis, pelvic adhesions, and removal of ovarian cysts and when performing salpingostomies.[29] His loop-ligation applicator and morcellation forceps enabled him to describe techniques for ovarectomy, adnectomy, and myomectomy.[30] He has truly pioneered the modern techniques of operative laparoscopy.

In the late 1970s several investigators described laparoscopic techniques to treat infertility via the laparoscope. Gomel treated pelvic adhesions and tubal occlusion with salpingolysis,[31] sharp adhesiolysis, and neosalpingostomy,[32] while Mettler et al. used endocoagulation for pelvic endometriosis and ovariolysis-salpingolysis for pelvic adhesions.[33]

Techniques for managing ectopic pregnancies via the laparoscope also advanced rapidly. Soderstrom (1975) used a snare loop to excise an ectopic pregnancy,[34] while Bruhat et al. were the first to describe a laparoscopic linear salpingostomy with tubal aspiration.[35] In the early 1980s the laser was added to the surgical armamentarium. Bruhat (1980), Tadir (1981), and Daniell et al. (1982) initially described the use of the carbon dioxide laser.[36–38] Keye et al. (1983) used an argon laser to treat pelvic endometriosis,[39] and Lomano (1985) described photocoagulation of pelvic endometriosis with Nd:YAG laser therapy.[40]

Laparoscopy has also been used to treat traditional surgical conditions. Semm (1983) performed the first appendectomy through a laparoscope.[41] The first cholecystectomy (with or without laser technology) was described in 1989.[42–44] The laparoscopy has recently been used to perform some rather unconventional laparoscopic procedures. Letterie et al. (1988) treated prolapsed fallopian tubes with a combined laparoscopic-vaginal approach.[45] Nezhat et al. (1989) removed a dermoid cyst via the laparoscope.[46] Reich et al. described a laparoscopic hysterectomy[47] and the management of stage I ovarian cancer[48] through the laparoscope. Finally, chronic pelvic pain can be treated either by laparoscopic uterine ablation[49] or laparoscopic presacral neurectomy.[50]

What has been witnessed has been a remarkable advancement of laparoscopic surgical techniques in recent years. What once were considered primarily open abdominal procedures are being performed partially or exclusively through the laparoscope. There are many advocates of these advances in laparoscopic technology. The patient avoids a large abdominal incision, and the hospital stay is shortened, as is postoperative convalescence, which decreases medical cost. However, these techniques are time-consuming and require a larger expediture of time and money for equipment and training. What is evident is that laparoscopic procedures are here to stay, but it is doubtful whether the laparoscope will ever completely replace the scapel.

REFERENCES

1. Semm K: in Borow LS (ed): *Atlas of Gynecologic Laparoscopy and Hysterectomy.* Philadelphia, WB Saunders Co, 1977.
2. Belt AE, Charnock DA: The history of the cystoscope, in Cabot H (ed): *Modern Urology.* Philadelphia, Lea & Febiger, 1936, p 15.
3. Pantaleoni DC: On endoscopic examination of the cavity of the womb. *The Medical Press and Circular* July 14, 1869, pp 26–27.
4. Wittman I: *Peritoneoscopy.* Budapest, Publishing House of the Hungarian Academy of Sciences, 1966, pp 3–5.
5. Cohen MR: *Laparoscopy, Culdoscopy and Gynecology.* Philadelphia, WB Saunders Co, 1970, pp 1–12.
6. Nadeau OE, Kampmeier OF: Endoscopy of the abdomen: Abdominoscopy. A preliminary study, including a summary of the literature and description of the technique. *Surg Gynecol Obstet* 1925; 41:259.
7. Bernheim BM: Organoscopy. *Ann Surg* 1911; 53:764.
8. Orndorf RH: The peritoneoscope in diagnosis of diseases of the abdomen. *J Radiol* 1920; 1:307.
9. Stone ZE: Intra-abdominal examination with the aid of the peritoneoscope. *J Kans Med Soc* 1924; 24:63.
10. Steiner OP: Abdominoscopy. *Surg Gynecol Obstet* 1924; 38:266.
11. Ruddock JC: Peritoneoscopy. *West J Surg* 1934; 42:392.
12. Hope RB: Differential diagnosis of ectopic gestation by peritoneoscopy. *Surg Gynecol Obstet* 1937; 64:229.
13. Anderson ET: Peritoneoscopy. *Am J Surg* 1937; 35:136.
14. Powers FH, Barnes AC: Sterilization by means of peritoneoscopy tubal fulguration. *Am J Obstet Gynecol* 1941; 41:1038.
15. Beling CA: Selection of cases for peritoneoscopy. *Arch Surg* 1941; 42:872.
16. Benedict EB: Peritoneoscopy. *N Engl J Med* 1938; 218:713.
17. Ruddock JC: Peritoneoscopy. *Surg Gynecol Obstet* 1937; 65:623.
18. Steptoe PC: *Laparoscopy in Gynaecology.* Edinburgh, E & S Livingston Ltd, 1967, pp 1–3.
19. Handley RS: Peritoneoscopy. *Postgrad Med J* 1955; 31:81.
20. Handley RS, Nurick AW: Peritoneoscopy: Evaluation and report of 136 cases. *Br Med J* 1956; 2:1211.
21. Fear R: Laparoscopy: A valuable aid in gynecological diagnosis. *Obstet Gynecol* 1968; 31:297.
22. Cohen MR: Culdoscopy vs. peritoneoscopy. *Obstet Gynecol* 1968; 31:310.
23. Siegler AM, Berenyi KJ: Laparoscopy in gynecology. *Obstet Gynecol* 1969; 34:572.
24. Peterson EP, Behrman SJ: Laparoscopy of the infertile patient. *Obstet Gynecol* 1970; 36:363.
25. Balin H, Wan LS, Israel SL: Recent advances in pelvic endoscopy. *Obstet Gynecol* 1966; 27:30.
26. Phillips JM: Personal communication, 1974.
27. Steptoe PC, Edwards RG: Laparoscopic recovery of preovulatory human oocytes after priming of ovaries with gonadotrophins. *Lancet* 1970; 1:7649.
28. Shapiro HI, Adler DM: Excision of an ectopic pregnancy through the laparoscope. *Am J Obstet Gynecol* 1973; 117:290.
29. Semm K: Endocoagulator: New possibilities for tubal surgery via pelviscopy. *Excerpta Medica* 1974; 370:242.

30. Semm K: Tissue-puncher and loop-ligation—New aids for surgical-therapeutic pelviscopy (laparoscopy) = endoscopic intraabdominal surgery. *Endoscopy* 1987; 10:19.
31. Gomel V: Laparoscopic tubal surgery in infertility. *Obstet Gynecol* 1975; 46:47.
32. Gomel V: Salpingostomy by laparoscopy. *J Reprod Med* 1977; 18:265.
33. Mettler L, Giesel H, Semm K: Treatment of female infertility due to tubal obstruction by operative laparoscopy. *Fertil Steril* 1979; 32:384.
34. Soderstrom RM: Unusual uses of laparoscopy. *J Reprod Med* 1975; 15:77.
35. Bruhat MA, Manhes H, Mage G, et al: Treatment of ectopic pregnancy by means of laparoscopy. *Fertil Steril* 1980; 33:411.
36. Feste JR: Laser laparoscopy. A new modality. *J Reprod Med* 1985; 30:413.
37. Daniell JF, Brown DH. Carbon dioxide laser laparoscopy: Initial experience in experimental animals and humans. *Obstet Gynecol* 1982; 59:761.
38. Daniell JF, Pattaway DE: Use of the CO_2 laser in laparoscopic surgery. Initial experience with second puncture technique. *Infertility* 1982; 5:15.
39. Keye WR, Matson GA, Dixon J: The use of the argon laser in the treatment of experimental endometriosis. *Fertil Steril* 1983; 39:26.
40. Lomano JM: Photocoagulation of early pelvic endometriosis with the Nd:YAG laser through the laparoscope. *J Reprod Med* 1985; 30:77.
41. Semm K: Endoscopic appendectomy. *Endoscopy* 1983; 15:59.
42. Reddick EJ, Olsen DO: Laparoscopic laser cholecystectomy: A comparison with mini-lap cholecystectomy. *Surg Endosc* 1989; 3:131.
43. Rubio PA, Rowe G, Feste JR: Endoscopic laser cholecystectomy. *Houston Med* 1989; 5:124.
44. Dubois F, Kard P, Barthelot G, et al: Coelioscopic cholecystectomy: Preliminary report of 36 cases. *Ann Surg* 1990; 211:60.
45. Letterie GS, Byron J, Salminen ER, et al: Laparoscopic management of fallopian tube prolapse. *Obstet Gynecol* 1988; 72:508.
46. Nezhat C, Winer WK, Nezhat F: Laparoscopic removal of dermoid cysts. *Obstet Gynecol* 1989; 73:278.
47. Reich H, DeCaprio J, McGlynn F: Laparoscopic hysterectomy. *J Gynecol Surg* 1989; 5:213.
48. Reich H, McGlynn F, Wilkie W: Laparoscopic management of Stage I ovarian cancer. *J Reprod Med* 1990; 35:601.
49. Lichten EM, Bombard J: Surgical treatment of primary dysmenorrhea with laparoscopic uterine nerve ablation. *J Reprod Med* 1987; 32:37.
50. Perez JJ: Laparoscopic presacral neurectomy: Results of the first 25 cases. *J Reprod Med* 1990; 35–625.

PART II

Principles of Endoscopic Surgery

Chapter 2

Facilities, Instrumentation, and Equipment for Endoscopic Surgery

Stanley R. Klein, M.D.

The popularity of laparoscopy for diagnostic and therapeutic procedures is due mainly to technological advances made over the last few decades.[1] Much like a craftsman in any endeavor, the surgeon must master the tools he utilizes. Complete understanding of the advantages, limitations, and common pitfalls of each device may prove pivotal to a successful outcome of any procedure. In a rapidly evolving and changing field, it is imperative that the surgeon consider adapting and modifying his practice as new technology is introduced to optimize patient gain and minimize inherent procedure risk.

The purpose of this chapter is to familiarize the reader with the endoscopes, equipment, and other unique ancillary instruments necessary to perform endoscopic surgical procedures. While we have no intention to promote any specific manufacturer's equipment, it is our purpose to clearly state the instruments we prefer and currently employ. In some cases specific instruments are unique to a single manufacturer; usually similar instruments are produced by several companies. In addition, by the time the reader has completed this chapter, he will have an understanding of what instruments are on the horizon and have an idea of how to select contemporary instrumentation and equipment that is most cost-effective.

FACILITIES AND EQUIPMENT ORGANIZATION

Endoscopic surgery is best performed in a room large enough to accommodate several tables and carts to position essential equipment. Both ambulatory surgical facilities and conventional operating rooms have proved satisfactory for performing endoscopic surgical procedures.[2–4] The selection of the type of facility is governed primarily by the patient, surgeon's experience, and community availability and is not limited by the equipment and/or instrumentation (Table 2–1).[5,6]

Surgeons are no longer taking turns at the laparoscope for direct visualization of a surgical procedure; instead, they simultaneously visualize the operation on a video monitor. The orga-

TABLE 2–1.

Factors Influencing the Selection of a Facility for Endoscopic/Laparoscopic Surgery

	Surgical Environment	
Factors Affecting Choice	Inpatient	Ambulatory
Patient age	≥60	≤60
Complicating chronic illness	+	−
Case variables		
Difficulty	↑	↓
Length	↑	↓
Complications	+	−
Surgeon experience	Minimal	Advanced
Adequate home supervision	−	+

nization of the operating room is dependant upon the nature of the procedure and the surgeon's position at the operating table.[7,8] Options for organizing the operating room setup for laparoscopic cholecystectomy are shown in Figure 2–1. Room organization may be different when lower abdominal surgery (e.g., hernioplasty) is performed, the monitor being placed at the foot of the operating table rather than at the head of the table as it is during most procedures.[9]

Various structures are visualized during intra-abdominal procedures with the patient in different positions. The pelvic organs are best approached and completely visualized with the patient in the Trendelenburg position, whereas the upper abdominal structures require the patient to be in the Fowler (head up) position with varying degrees of right or left lateral decubitus to enhance visualization of specific organs. An electric operating table facilitates positioning expediently with the least amount of effort (Fig 2–2). In addition, appropriate facilities to obtain intraoperative contrast studies (e.g., cholangiography) are an essential component. If fluoroscopic x-ray equipment or ultrasonography is to be utilized during procedures, provisions for space to accommodate the devices should be made prior to the operation.

Most components of an endoscopic surgical setup are easily organized on a mobile cart with shelves and storage for all specialized equipment, including photography supplies. This reduces the incidence of damage to delicate instruments and ensures easy access for use and maintenance.

Numerous equipment storage carts are available. One that is totally self-contained and por-

FIG 2–1 (opposite).
A and **B,** our preference for endoscopic abdominal surgery is to have the patient's left arm at his side to allow unobstructed movement of the surgeon from this position. The patient's right arm is on an arm board and is extended to accommodate an intravenous line and access for the anesthesiologist's monitoring equipment. Nonsterile devices (light source, insufflation equipment, monitor, etc.) are visible at the head of the patient. In this setup both surgeon and assistant use a single video monitor. A circulating nurse manages the equipment; the scrub nurse stands next to the surgeon's assistant. The assistant surgeon manipulates the laparoscopic-camera unit and actively participates in the operative procedure. **C,** an alternative setup where the surgeon and assistant each view a separate monitor. **D,** a convenient arrangement of the sterile instruments. (Figures B and C, courtesy of Robert J. Nejdl, M.D.)

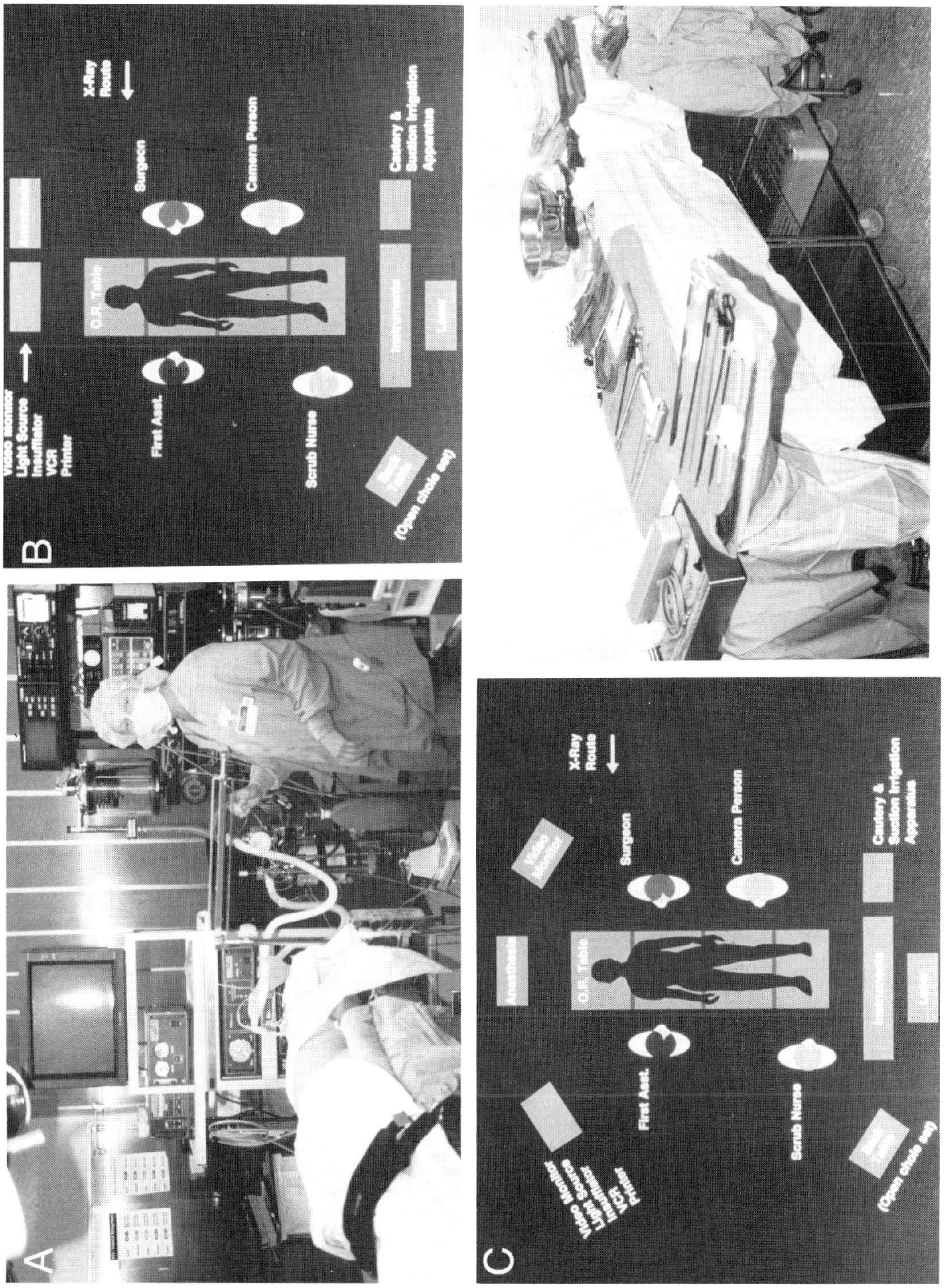
A
B
Video Monitor
Light Source
Insufflator
VCR
Printer
Anesthesia
First Asst.
O.R. Table
Surgeon
Camera Person
X-Ray Route
Scrub Nurse
Instruments
Laser
Cautery & Suction Irrigation Apparatus
(Open chole set)
C
Video Monitor
Light Source
Insufflator
VCR
Printer
Video Monitor
Anesthesia
First Asst.
O.R. Table
Surgeon
Camera Person
X-Ray Route
Scrub Nurse
Instruments
Laser
Cautery & Suction Irrigation Apparatus
(Open chole set)

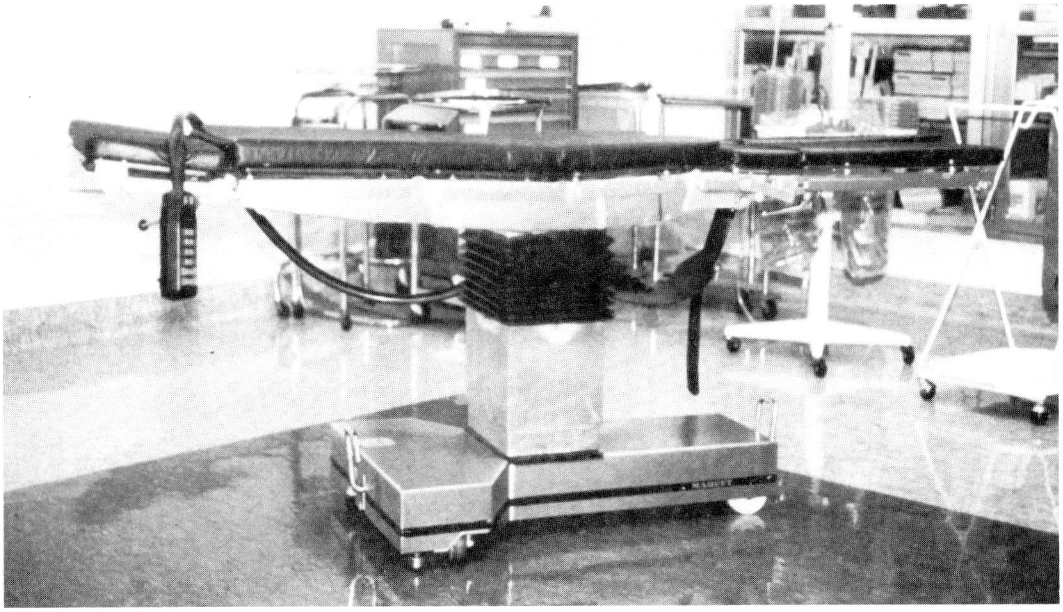

FIG 2–2.
Electrically powered operating tables are desirable to attain optimal patient positioning and intraoperative x-ray studies.

table and provides ample space for all equipment is shown in Figure 2–3. It has recessed power outlets and drawers that are lined to protect the instruments. A conventional tool cart may be modified to provide additional portable storage space for the laparoscope and ancillary instrumentation. When purchasing a storage cart, it is best to provide extra space for future equipment needs. It is important that the video screen be positioned so that it is easily visible by all personnel. Many manufacturers have designed storage carts that accommodate the devices they sell.

NONOPTICAL EQUIPMENT

Several types of nonoptical equipment are essential for endoscopic surgery. These instruments include (1) devices for induction of pneumoperitoneum, (2) cannulas and trocars for introduction of the laparoscope and ancillary surgical instruments, (3) hemostatic and dissection devices including lasers or electrocautery, and (4) irrigation-aspiration systems to maintain a meticulous surgical field. In addition, surgical instruments that have been designed for specific functions should be carefully selected prior to each procedure.[6, 7, 10, 11] Proper preparation is a major consideration to assure a gratifying result.

Equipment for Establishment of Pneumoperitoneum

The separation of intracavitary organs from the body wall by the introduction of gas (in the abdomen this is called a pneumoperitoneum) is fundamental for successful visualization of or-

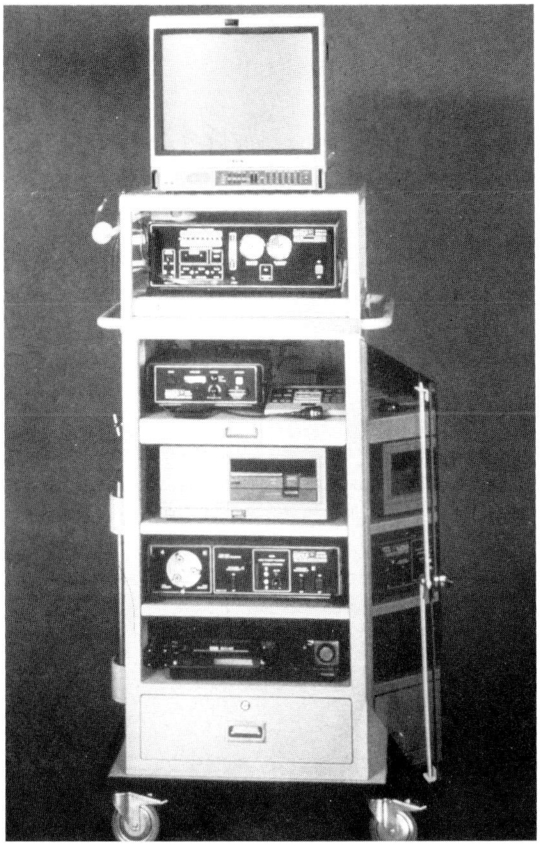

FIG 2–3.
Self-contained endoscopic storage unit.

gans and structures during endoscopic surgical procedures. A variety of gases (carbon dioxide, nitrous oxide, room air) and routes of insufflation (transabdominal, via the posterior vaginal fornix) have been advocated, each having specific advantages and liabilities.[12, 13]

Insufflation Needles

The Veress needle and the Foures-Kuss needle are available to facilitate the creation of pneumopentoneum.[9]

Veress Needle*.—The Veress needle was initially used for the induction of a pneumothorax in tuberculous lungs.[14] This device is now used almost exclusively in abdominal endoscopic procedures to produce a pneumoperitoneum (Fig 2–4).

The Veress cannula is a clever double-barreled device consisting of an inner, blunt-shaped, spring-action stylet and an outer, sharply beveled needle. The outer needle perforates the fascial planes, and the blunt-ended, inner stylet protrudes following advancement of the needle through resistant tissues to push aside any freely mobile intra-abdominal structures (e.g.,

*The name is often misspelled as "Verres."

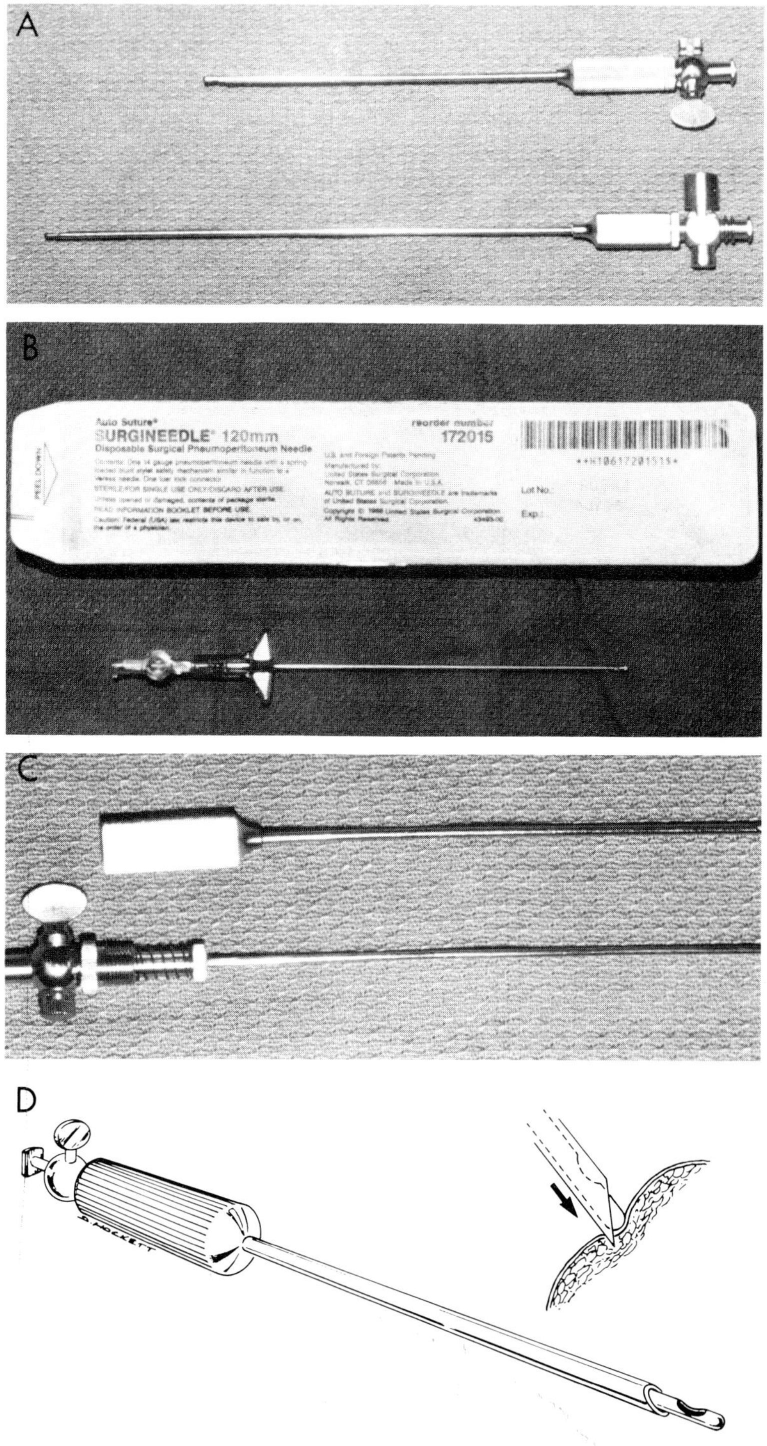

FIG 2–4.
Veress needles are available in reusable **(A)** and disposable **(B)** formats. **C,** a disassembled unit reveals the inner spring-action stylet *(below)* and outer sleeve *(above)*. **D,** the Veress needle mechanism during tissue penetration.

bowel). Upon introduction, the needle is held by the outer sheath component to allow free movement of the inner stylet as the device penetrates different tissue layers. In addition, grasping the outer sheath at a distance from the tip equal to the thickness of the abdominal wall prevents excessive insertion and risk of injury. During passage of the Veress needle through the abdominal wall, two "pops" can generally be appreciated: the first occurs as the abdominal wall fascia is traversed, and the second is produced by passage of the device through the peritoneum.

The Veress needle is manufactured in both reusable and disposable forms in several diameters and lengths. The external diameter of the most commonly used needle is 2.1 mm (14 gauge); needles with 1.7-mm and 2.5-mm outer dimensions are also available. Knowledge of the type of needle used is essential to enable accurate interpretation of the intra-abdominal pressure measured during gas insufflation. A smaller–internal diameter needle has increased resistance to gas flow and produces an increased recording of intra-abdominal pressure while gas is being introduced. In contrast, larger-bore needles produce the opposite effect. Veress needles that have two ports (one for the introduction of gas and one for pressure recording) enable the operator to measure intraperitoneal pressures accurately during insufflation.

When the usual infraumbilical site of insertion of the Veress needle is used, a standard 80-mm-length device is sufficient to traverse all the abdominal layers in the majority of cases. The abdominal wall seldom exceeds 1 to 2 cm in depth in this region, although longer needles are available for obese patients. As will be discussed in more detail in Chapter 5, failure to enter the peritoneal cavity is usually caused by improper technique of needle insertion rather than inadequate needle length. To confirm the correct placement of the needle in the peritoneal cavity following introduction, several confirmatory tests can be performed (see Chapter 5). In all cases, it is important to carefully observe the abdomen during insufflation. Asymmetric distension or pressures above 15 mm Hg suggest that the needle is not in the proper position. In these situations, the needle should be removed and reinserted.

Foures-Kuss Needle.—This needle was developed and is currently manufactured in Europe. The device is 65 mm long and 1.5 mm in diameter and has a sharp-tipped removable inner core surrounded by an outer sleeve with lateral holes. Once the needle has been inserted into the peritoneal cavity, the inner core is retrieved, and the outer sleeve is connected to the insufflator. The advantages of this needle are its thin profile and the ability to insufflate through the lateral holes when the tip is impacted in tissue (i.e., the omentum). This device is not widely used in the United States at the present time.

Insufflation Devices

Pneumoperitoneum was originally obtained by injecting room air by hand into the peritoneal cavity.[9, 15] This procedure is now easily accomplished by using instruments that introduce the gas and simultaneously monitor the rate of flow, the volume delivered, and the intra-abdominal pressure. These parameters are displayed on a panel to enable safe, expedient insufflation (Fig 2–5). In accordance with current safety guidelines, gas should be instilled at no greater than 1 L/min at a low flow rate. In order to perform endoscopic surgery, the insufflator should also be capable of delivering flows of 6 to 10 L/min.[6, 11] The high-flow feature facilitates preservation of the surgical field during the exchange of surgical instruments and during aspiration of blood or irrigation fluid from the field. The ability to accurately control flow rate and yet prevent excess insufflation pressure is a critical safety feature for insufflation devices.

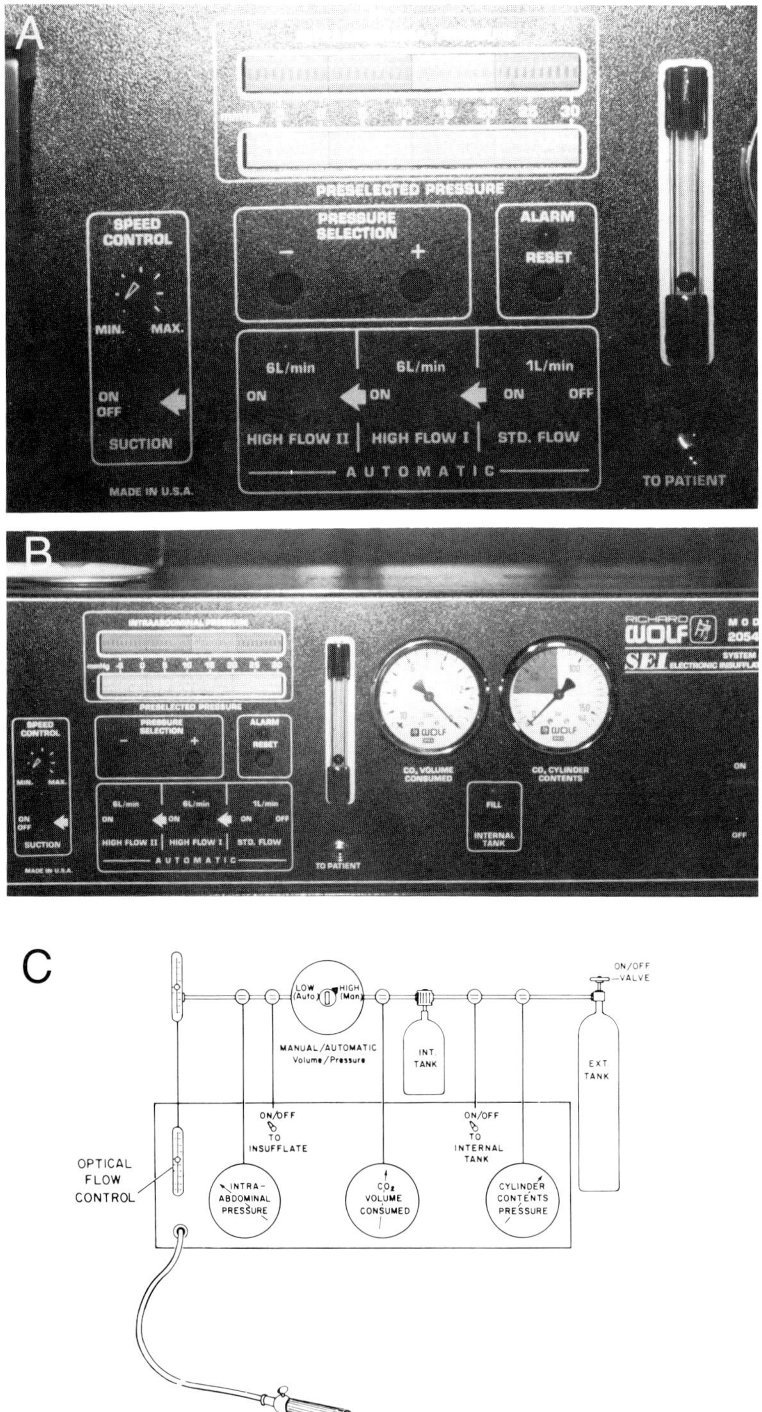

FIG 2–5.

Insufflation apparatus. There are visual displays **(A** and **B)** of the rate of gas flow, volume of gas delivered, intraperitoneal pressure, and amount of gas in reserve. Controls for manual or automatic insufflation and refill of insufflator gas tank are also present. **C,** a schematic of the gas flow and controls of a insufflation device.

Gas Flow.—The initial flow of gas should be set at 1 L/min. A flow control (usually a floating plastic ball) indicates the flow rate. Low flow rates should be maintained until it is confirmed that pneumoperitoneum is being safely achieved via the insufflation needle. An on-off control is essential to allow the operator to interrupt and restart the gas insufflation at any interval during the procedure. A separate switch is used to control the passage of gas from the reserve tank into the storage gas cylinder within the apparatus. An indicator to record the amount of gas or pressure available in the reserve cylinder is also required to ensure that a sufficient amount of gas is available to complete the procedure.

Pressure Monitoring.—The intraperitoneal pressure (more specifically, the pressure of the gas pocket in the region of the tip of Veress needle) should be displayed for constant monitoring during insufflation. If the insufflation apparatus measures this pressure through the inflow gas channel, flow of gas should be discontinued when observing the pressure to obtain the true intraperitoneal value. Otherwise, a falsely elevated pressure is recorded because the pressure measured is the sum of the intraperitoneal pressure plus the resistance to gas flow.[15]

Volume of Gas Insufflated.—The total volume of gas delivered by the apparatus is monitored to ensure safe insufflation. This volume is usually less than the amount that is in the abdomen once the procedure is initiated because of leakage of gas during instrument manipulation and other maneuvers.

Shutoff Valves.—Safety valves that can be rapidly closed to interrupt the flow of gas are an indispensable safety feature. Additional flow control valves are located on the Veress needle and on the laparoscopic cannula. These controls permit the surgeon to regulate the flow of gas into the patient's abdomen as needed. Most insufflation equipment is also designed to automatically stop the flow of gas when a pre-established pressure limit is exceeded.

Automatic Insufflation Features.—Some insufflation systems have mechanisms to replace the amount of gas that leaks from the abdomen during the procedure. It is imperative that an operating team monitor the servocontrol function to ensure that excess intraperitoneal or thoracic pressure is avoided. This consideration is particularly important in children, where the introduction of small volumes of additional gas may create significant increments in intracavitary pressure.[15]

A variety of different gases, ranging from room air to pure oxygen, have been used to distend the peritoneal cavity.[9, 15] Each gas has its own particular physical properties and features, and this may make it preferable for one type of procedure or contraindicate it for others. Knowledge of the potential problems inherent with each distending gas is essential. For example, absorption of carbon dioxide may have respiratory and cardiovascular effects that can influence patient management. These considerations are covered in detail in Chapter 9.

Cannulas and Trocars

A cannula is a hollow tube with a valve mechanism that is placed into a body cavity by passing a cutting-tipped rod (trocar) through the lumen in the cannula. Following penetration of the body wall, the trocar is removed, and the cannula lumen may be used to introduce other surgical devices. Both cannulas and trocars are manufactured in reusable and disposable versions, each type having advantages (Fig 2–6).

Reusable cannulas are available in diameters from 3 to 12 mm. Concentric reducing cylinders can be used to diminish the internal diameter of the reusable cannula to enable placement of smaller-diameter instrumentation and prevent leakage of insufflated gas. The internal diameters of available disposable cannulas are adjusted by silicon reducing gaskets that are attached at the entry orifice (Fig 2–7). Disposable nonmetallic cannulas permit unobstructed intraoperative x-ray contrast studies such as cholangiography because they avert images in the field produced by metallic devices.

Cannulas are equipped with one of two types of valves to prevent a loss of insufflation gas.

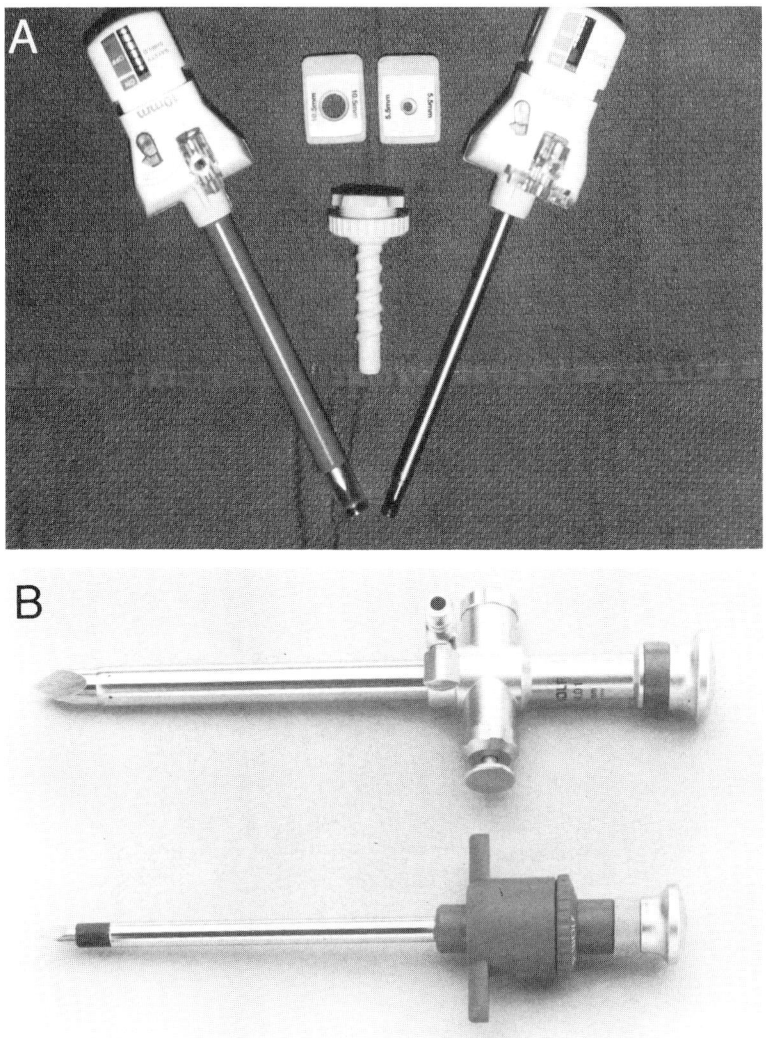

FIG 2–6.
A, disposable Surgiport trocars and cannulas displayed with an abdominal wall fixator and reducers. **B,** reusable trocars and cannulas. (Note the Luer-lock gas line connector on the side of the cannulas for CO_2 insufflation.)

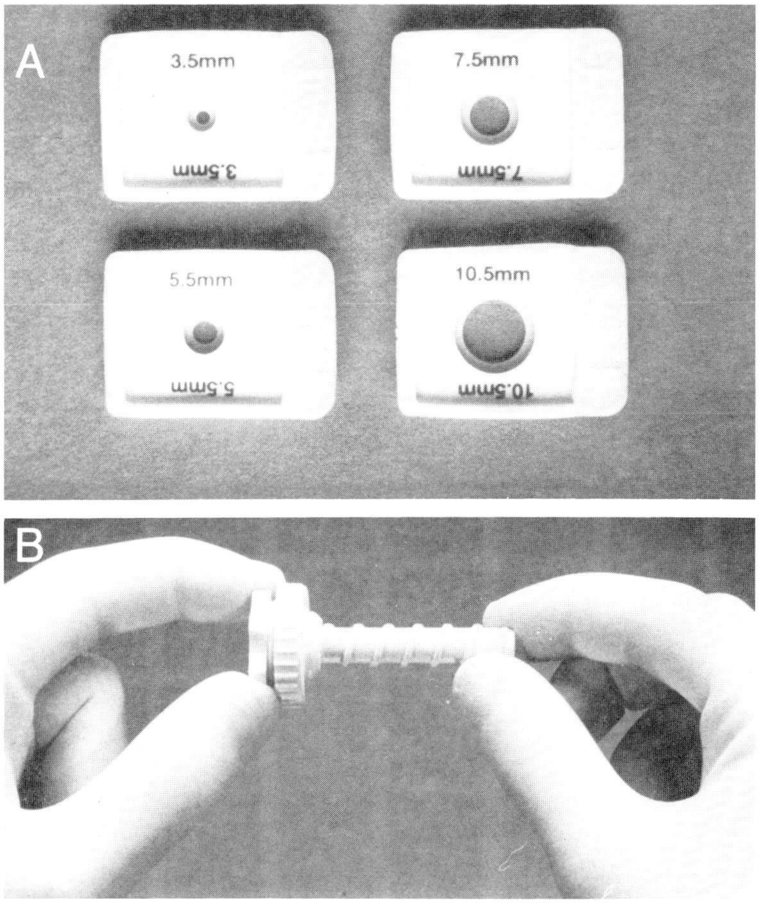

FIG 2–7.
A, reducing silicon gasket that enables a larger cannula to accommodate smaller-diameter laparoscopes and instruments without a loss of gas. **B,** optional abdominal wall fixator that assists in tethering the cannula during manipulation.

Trumpet valves are depressed by means of an external plunger permitting passage of laparoscopic endoscopes and instruments. Trapdoor or flap valves automatically open when a laparoscope or other instruments are passed through the lumen of the cannula. Both type of valves work equally well, but regular maintenance in reusable cannulas is required to ensure uninhibited movement. Available disposable cannulas use the trapdoor-type valve to obtain a gas seal. Virtually all available cannulas are fitted with a side Luer-lock connector for attachment of gas tubing from the insufflator. Additional gas may be insufflated directly through the cannula Luer-lock during the procedure in order to maintain the operative field.

If a reusable cannula is dropped, the tip may become bent, and the laparoscope will not pass smoothly through this damaged sheath. The cannula should be repaired immediately since very minor distortions in the shape of the cannula may result in scratching and damage to the laparoscope.

To enable penetration of the abdominal wall, a cannula has a slightly tapered end that fits snugly around the trocar. Trocar tips have either a pyramidal or conical shape (Fig 2–8).

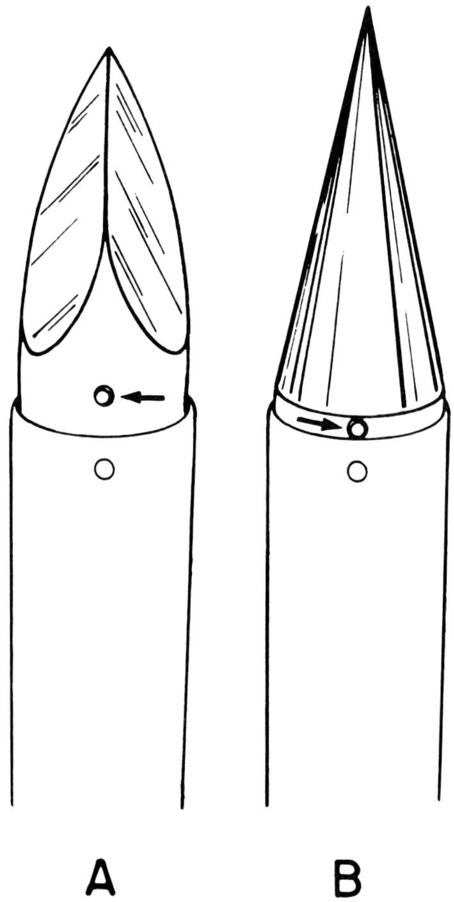

FIG 2–8.
Pyramidal **(A)** and conical **(B)** trocar tips. Both designs possess an internal gas escape channel noted by the *arrow*.

There is debate, even among experienced laparoscopists, as to which tip is better.[9, 10] We believe that the pyramidal tip is preferable. Because of its three sharp edges, less force is required to pass the trocar through various tissue layers into the abdominal cavity. Trocar tips must be kept sharp; thus, reusable devices may require frequent maintenance. Dull trocars and conical-tip trocars require greater force to penetrate the abdominal wall. The greater the force, the greater the risk of sudden, uncontrolled entry and damage to the viscera.

Disposable trocars have an additional safety feature; the obturators have a spring-loaded plastic safety shield that retracts during insertion through the abdominal wall (Fig 2–9). Once the obturator passes through the peritoneum, the plastic safety shield snaps forward to prevent injury to underlying organs. Most trocars also have a hollow lumen with openings at the tip as well as at the top of the instrument. This permits a rush of gas to occur when the peritoneal cavity is penetrated by the trocar. At this point the surgeon need not pass the instrument any more deeply, thus reducing the risk of visceral damage.

It is also possible to place a cannula by direct visualization of the peritoneal cavity, i.e., the "open" technique. This requires special instrumentation.[16] The Hasson cannula and trocar are designed to be inserted into the peritoneal cavity under direct vision. The indication for such an approach is usually in the setting of prior surgery when viscera might be adherent to the

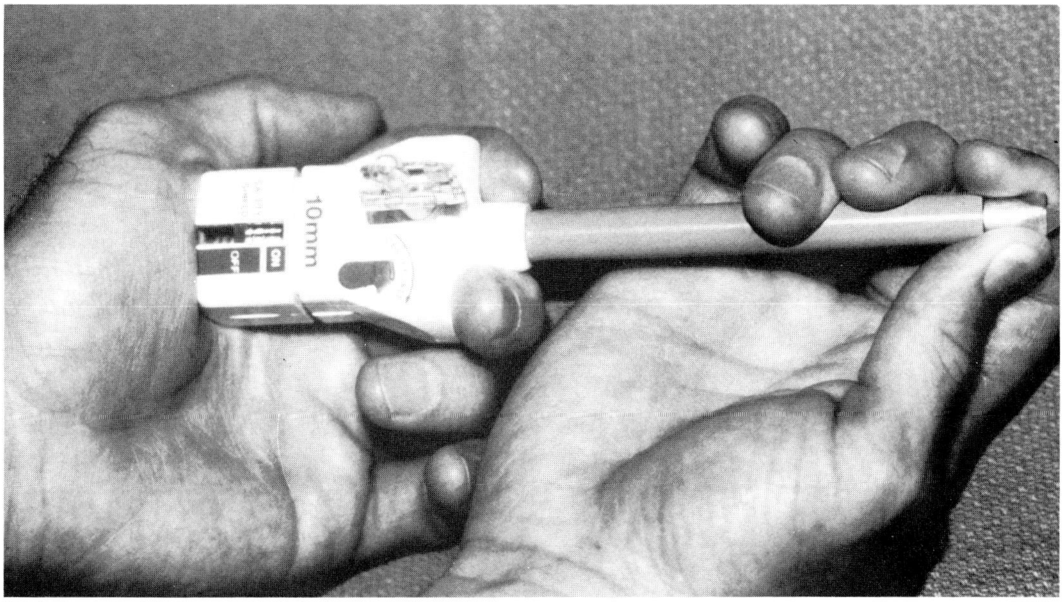

FIG 2–9.
The safety shield in the disposable Surgiport cannula/trocar unit is being pulled back to simulate passage through the abdominal fascia. Upon entry into the peritoneal cavity it immediately returns and is locked into the original position.

body wall and make a blind puncture hazardous. The major differences of the Hasson device from the standard cannula-trocar unit that has been described are a blunt obturator trocar, a cone-shaped sleeve, and a suture-holding component (Fig 2–10).

The blunt obturator serves as an atraumatic guide and pushes away intraperitoneal organs that contact the cannula. Because its insertion follows surgical incision of the abdominal wall, the risk of trauma is lessened. The cone-shaped sleeve is mounted on the cannula casing and adjusts for different thicknesses of the abdominal wall. The main function of the sleeve is to obliterate the fascial opening and thereby help maintain the pneumoperitoneum. Its final position on the cannula must be set prior to the attachment of the anchoring sutures.[16] Fascial sutures are wrapped around attachments on either side of the trocar sleeve under tension to hold the cannula firmly in position.

TABLE 2–2.
Endosurgical Energy Sources

Criteria	Laser	Electrocautery
Energy leaks	Rare	Frequent
Precision	+	Varies
Operative speed	Varies	Rapid
Learning curve	++	+
Reliability	−/+	+
"Appeal"	++	+
Cost	10*x*	*x*

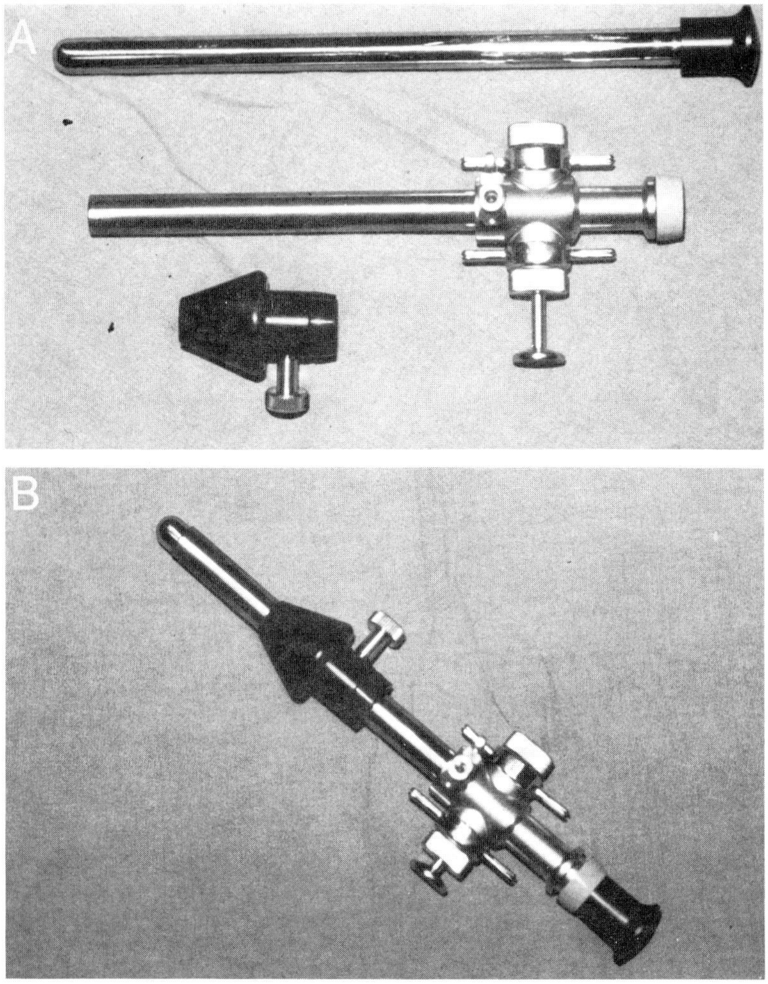

FIG 2–10.
A, Hasson cannula. Components of the instrument (from top to bottom) include a blunt obturator trocar, a sleeve with the suture-holding wings on either side of the trumpet-shaped valve, and a cone-shaped sleeve that obliterates the fascial opening. **B,** assembled cannula. The position of the cone-shaped sleeve can be adjusted for varying thicknesses of the abdominal wall.

Electrosurgery Units and Lasers

Electrosurgery units and/or lasers are an integral component of endoscopic surgical procedures. The surgeon wishing to employ either or both methods must be thoroughly acquainted with the principles, risks, and safety features.[9, 16, 17] Table 2–2 compares the two devices for endoscopic surgical applications.

Electrosurgery Units

The basic component is the electrosurgical generator. Historically, the early generators were "spark gap" units that were primarily hemostatic in nature and therefore referred to as "coagulators." Such units have been used for many years but have no place in modern endoscopic surgery.[18]

Two types of electrical methods are employed in modern electrosurgical units: unipolar and bipolar. In the unipolar system, current passes from the generator to the instrument, then through the patient to a return or dispersive electrode (ground plate), and then back to the generator to complete the circuit. In the bipolar system, current passes from the generator along one of the insulated jaws of the instrument, then through the grasped tissue to the other insulted jaw, and then back to the generator (Fig 2–11). No dispersive electrode is employed in bipolar devices. In both types of units, the heat generated by the passage of current through the tissues results in coagulation.

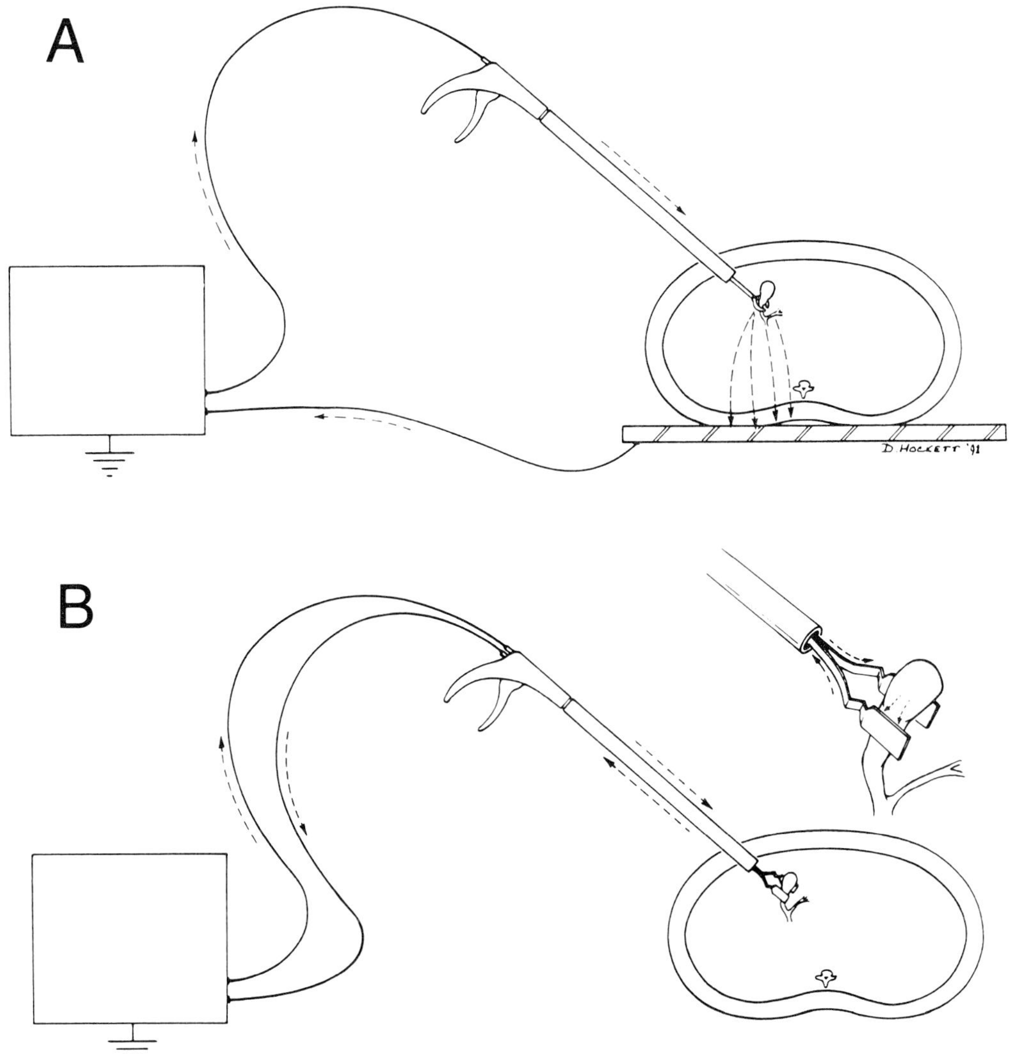

FIG 2–11.
Circuitry for the unipolar **(A)** and bipolar **(B)** modes of electrocautery. Under most circumstances the unipolar unit is satisfactory for endoabdominal surgery.

The majority of modern electrosurgical units can be employed in both unipolar and bipolar modes. Specialized single-purpose bipolar generators are available but are costly.[9] Contemporary electrosurgical generators are low-voltage, high-frequency solid-state units with insulated circuitry (Fig 2–12). Although some surgeons favor biopolar electrocautery, we have found the unipolar mode satisfactory for virtually all endoscopic surgical procedures.[11] When the unipolar technique is to be employed, the use of a ground plate is mandatory. Metal ground plates must be covered with the appropriate conductive jelly to obtain optimal contact with the patient. The manufacturers of most modern units offer disposable ground plates that must be fixed properly to the patient. In newer models, the ground plate has a sensor that recognizes the resistance of human tissue.[17] In the event of any change in the resistance, e.g., because of the malplacement or displacement of the ground plate, the generator stops automatically and emits a warning sound.

Cutting and coagulating current can be used separately. The intensity of the current is regulated for each mode. The intensity should be tested to ensure the desired tissue effect before using the device on vital structures. Energy delivery is triggered by depressing a foot pedal; one pedal activates the cutting and the other, the coagulating current. For safety, the current intensity should be adjusted properly before usage, and the foot pedal should be activated only by the surgeon. At all times the tip of the electrocautery instrument should be held within the field of view to prevent inadvertent injury.

Argon Beam Coagulator

Recently the argon beam coagulator (Birtcher Medical Systems, Irvine, Calif.) has been introduced for use during open surgical procedures (Fig 2–13). This technology is being evaluated for endosurgical applications and may be useful in the future for coagulation and cutting.

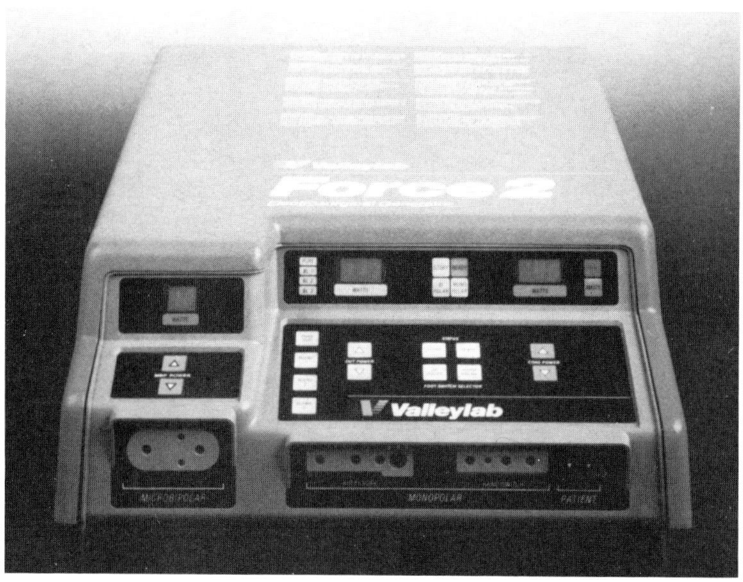

FIG 2–12.
Contemporary solid-state electrosurgical generator with both unipolar and bipolar capabilities.

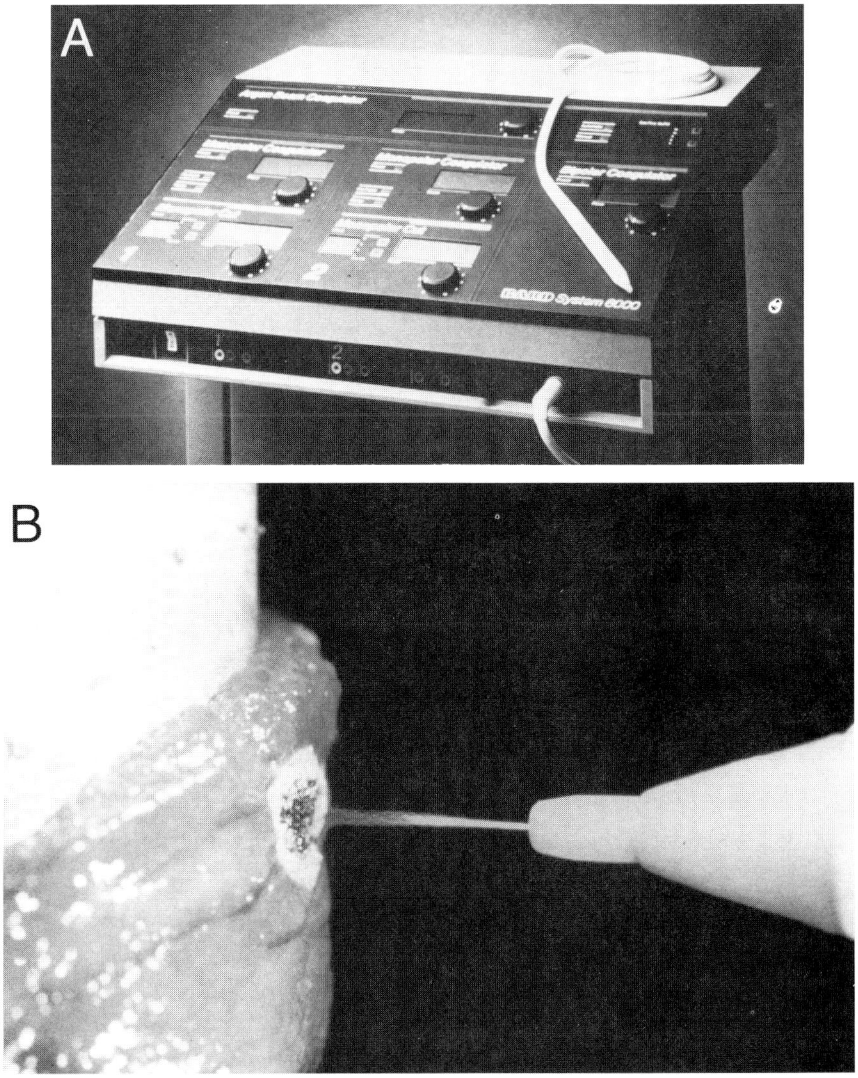

FIG 2–13.
A, the argon beam coagulator uses argon gas as a coagulation or cutting medium. This device has monopolar and bipolar modes. **B,** The gas beam is cauterizing a tissue surface.

Lasers

The word *laser* is an acronym for *l*ight *a*mplification by *s*timulated *e*mission of *r*adiation, a concept initially described by Einstein in 1917.[19] Currently, many of the early industrial prototypes (e.g., carbon dioxide, argon, and Nd:YAG) have been developed into commercially available units that are used in surgery.[20, 21] A more recently introduced unit, potassium titanyl phosphate (KTP) is becoming more widely applied in surgery because of favorable physical characteristics.[7, 21] Current costs of laser units range from $75,000 to $150,000. The biophysical principles and safety issues regarding lasers are addressed in Chapter 4.

To enable precise delivery of laser energy at some distance from the source such as the operating table, flexible delivery systems are desirable. For certain types of lasers (Nd:YAG, argon, KTP) this is easily accomplished with quartz fiber optics (Fig 2–14). For wavelengths that are absorbed by the quartz fiber or those that destroy fibers by high-peak energies such as carbon dioxide laser energy, current delivery is by articulated arms or hollow waveguides.

Laser fiber optics may be used to deliver the light energy at the target tissue in a noncontact fashion (free beam) or by directly touching the fiber to the tissue (contact). The Nd:YAG can be used as either a free-beam or contact instrument, whereas the frequency-double wavelength of the KTP laser is restricted to the free-beam mode. Free-beam applications require careful manipulation of the fiber to control the focal point. Obviously, important structures must not get into the path of the beam or serious damage can result that may become apparent in an immediate or delayed fashion.

Contact Nd:YAG laser devices deliver the laser energy to the tissue from the fiber-optic fiber through specialized tips made of sapphire, hardened quartz, or other heat-resistant optically transparent materials. The tips are expensive and tend to deteriorate. More recently, "hardened" fibers have become available, obviating the need for a special tip. When using a contact probe for endoscopic surgical procedures, a power of approximately 15 W is appropriate. Although there is no dependence on focal point control with a contact fiber, unintentional contact with neighboring structures can produce serious damage. In addition, there have been reports of the tips breaking off the fiber and air embolism produced by gas used to cool the laser fibers or for insufflation.[22]

Irrigation-Aspiration Systems

Combined irrigation and aspiration is commonly employed in flexible endoscopic diagnostic and therapeutic procedures. The potential constraints imposed by major surgery make it mandatory to have available a means to keep the operative field clean and dry as well as remove debris at the conclusion of the procedure. A variety of techniques are available to provide irrigation in sufficient volume over a short interval. Effective means include gravimetric urologic systems that use relatively large bore tubing to deliver the irrigant. The alternative is to use a pump to propel irrigant through conventional intravenous tubing.

More recently the hydroxylator has been adapted for endosurgical procedures.[6] The device is powered by a tank of pressurized carbon dioxide and is connected to 1-L containers of irrigating solution. The device has off/on controls and two pressure gauges; one measures the pressure directly from the carbon dioxide tank, and the other gauge is adjustable to regulate the irrigating pressure of fluid between 0 and 600 mm Hg. A pressure of 300 mm Hg generally is used to irrigate the abdomen.

Several endoscopic surgical instruments are designed to enable irrigation and aspiration simultaneously (Fig 2–15). Regardless of the device used, it is imperative that the surgeon ensure that irrigation and aspiration are available and that devices are functioning properly prior to commencing an operative procedure.

Specialized Endoscopic Surgical Instruments

The instruments used for endoscopic surgery are not only conventional and modified pelviscopy instruments but also specially designed devices for specific applications in areas with

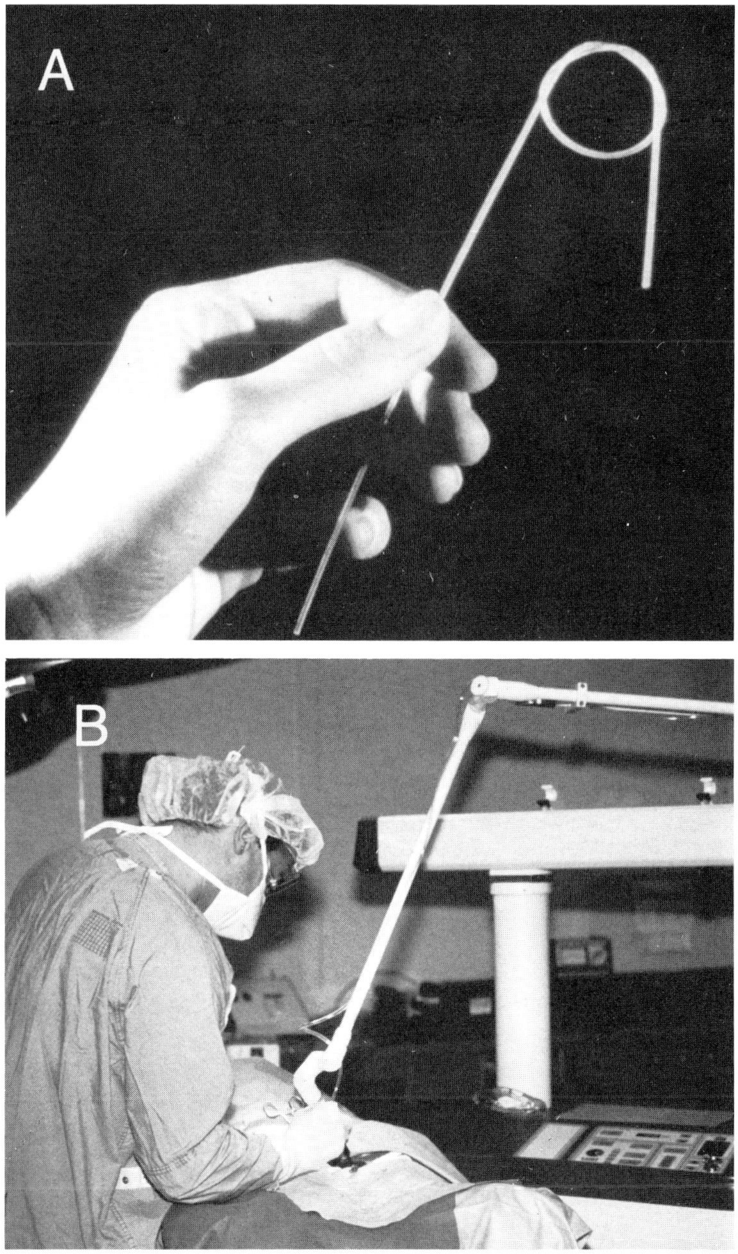

FIG 2–14.
Laser delivery systems. **A,** optic fiber used to transmit both Nd:YAG and KTP laser energy to the target site. **B,** articulating arm used to deliver carbon dioxide laser energy.

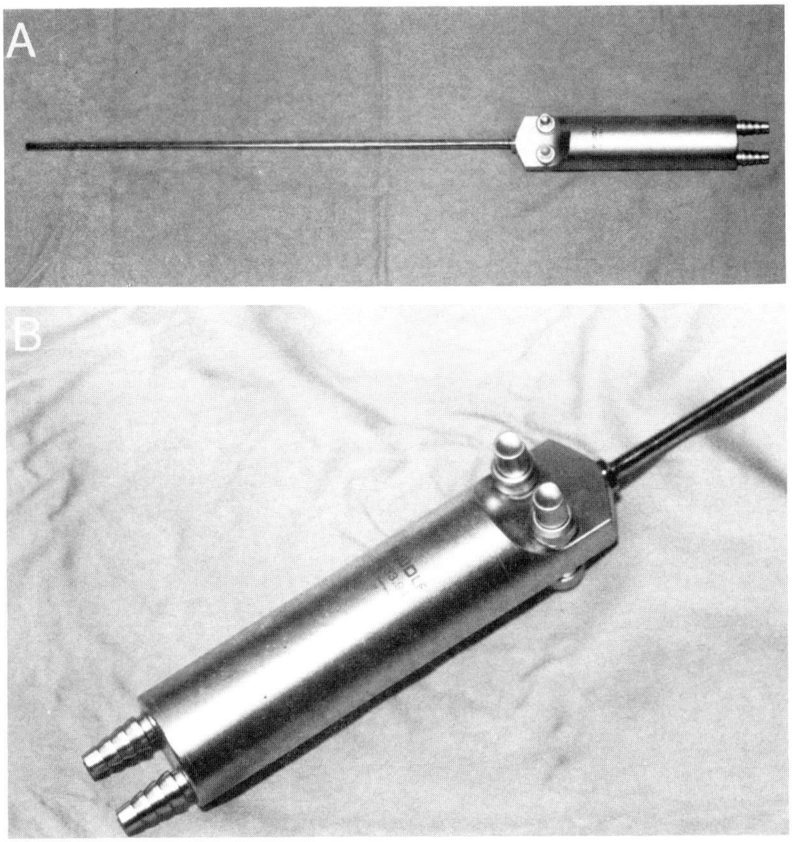

FIG 2–15.
A, Wolf irrigation-aspiration instrument. Introduced through a cannula, it connects irrigation to tubing via one port and aspirates by also connecting to standard operating room wall suction. **B,** demonstration of the valve mechanism for performing these maneuvers.

limited operative exposure.[6, 7, 9] Reusable metal instruments can be obtained with or without electrical insulation. When insulated, most instruments are adaptable for unipolar electrocoagulation and tend to have less light reflection. Several manufacturers produce a range of disposable instruments that are very popular.

It is impossible and unnecessary to catalog all of the available specialized instruments. Comments will also be restricted to the use of instruments through ancillary cannulas in contrast to introduction through the operating channel of a laparoscope because the later technique is not practical for most endoscopic surgical procedures. The ancillary instruments range in diameter from 3 to 10 mm depending on their function. Appropriately sized trocars and cannulas are available to accommodate these, although small-diameter instruments can be passed through larger-diameter cannulas fitted with appropriate reducing gaskets (see Fig 2–6).

Exploration Probes

Probes are essential for displacing the intraperitoneal structures in order to achieve complete visualization. They must be blunt to reduce the possibility of trauma during manipulation. The majority of these probes are marked with centimeter graduations so that structures can be measured. The magnification properties of many endoscopes make accurate estimation of size difficult by visual means alone. (Fig 2–16).

Grasping or Retracting Forceps

Grasping forceps are designed to hold structures firmly yet atraumatically (Fig 2–17). They are usually 5.0 mm in diameter and have a spring or ratchet mechanism handle that controls motion of the jaws. The ratchet handle expedites grasping and positioning of structures to gain surgical exposure by maintaining a constant grip on the tissue. Graspers are available with a variety of jaw configurations for different manipulations. For example, a 10-mm-diameter jaw grasper is particularly effective in attaining surgical exposure and retrieving debris and other objects (e.g., surgical clips, gallstones) from within the peritoneal cavity. Biopolar electrosurgical forceps are also available and have two prongs that are insulated individually. Claw forceps are designed for manipulating sturdy structures, but puncture of a hollow viscus is a hazard with this configuration.

Dissecting Instruments

A variety of devices are used to dissect structures from one another or from the surrounding tissue. Dissecting forceps usually have long round-edged jaws with small teeth or ridges to maintain a firm hold on tissue (Fig 2–18). When the jaws are opened, they are used to separate structures. The Maryland dissecting forceps have the jaws slightly bent to facilitate encircling tubular structures such as a blood vessel.[6] It serves the same purpose as a right-angle clamp during open surgery.

"Hook" and "spatula" dissectors are insulated for connection to electrocautery, and in some designs they can be combined with irrigation and aspiration equipment. The geometry of the hook or spatula metal tips are critical to effective dissection.[11] Both have to protrude several millimeters past the blunt end of the probe to avoid the probe acting as a coagulation device. The spatula can be used to push tissue in a fashion analogous to a Kittner dissector. When encircling a structure, the hook can be used much like a right-angle clamp for dissection.

Scissors

Scissors of various designs are available (Fig 2–19). Under all circumstances, both jaws of the scissors must be carefully visualized when they are utilized to avoid inadvertent injury. Scissors can be used to combine unipolar electrocoagulation capability with the mechanical cutting action. In general, scissors should have a smooth, rounded tip when closed even if one of the blades is somewhat curved or hooked. This feature permits tissue manipulation with the closed instrument without the risk of trauma. Hook scissors have sharp tips that overlap and are dangerous since they may inadvertently cause trauma if not carefully visualized. Special care must also be taken with microscissors to avoid damage to the delicate blades when introducing them into the endosurgical cannula.

Biopsy Forceps

Several types of biopsy forceps are available. Differences are primarily in the function and shape of the biopsy mechanisms. Some devices have one fixed and one movable jaw, whereas others have two movable jaws. The size and configuration of the jaws determine the size of the biopsy. Biopsy forceps with jaws that overlap and have sharp cutting edges are safer and

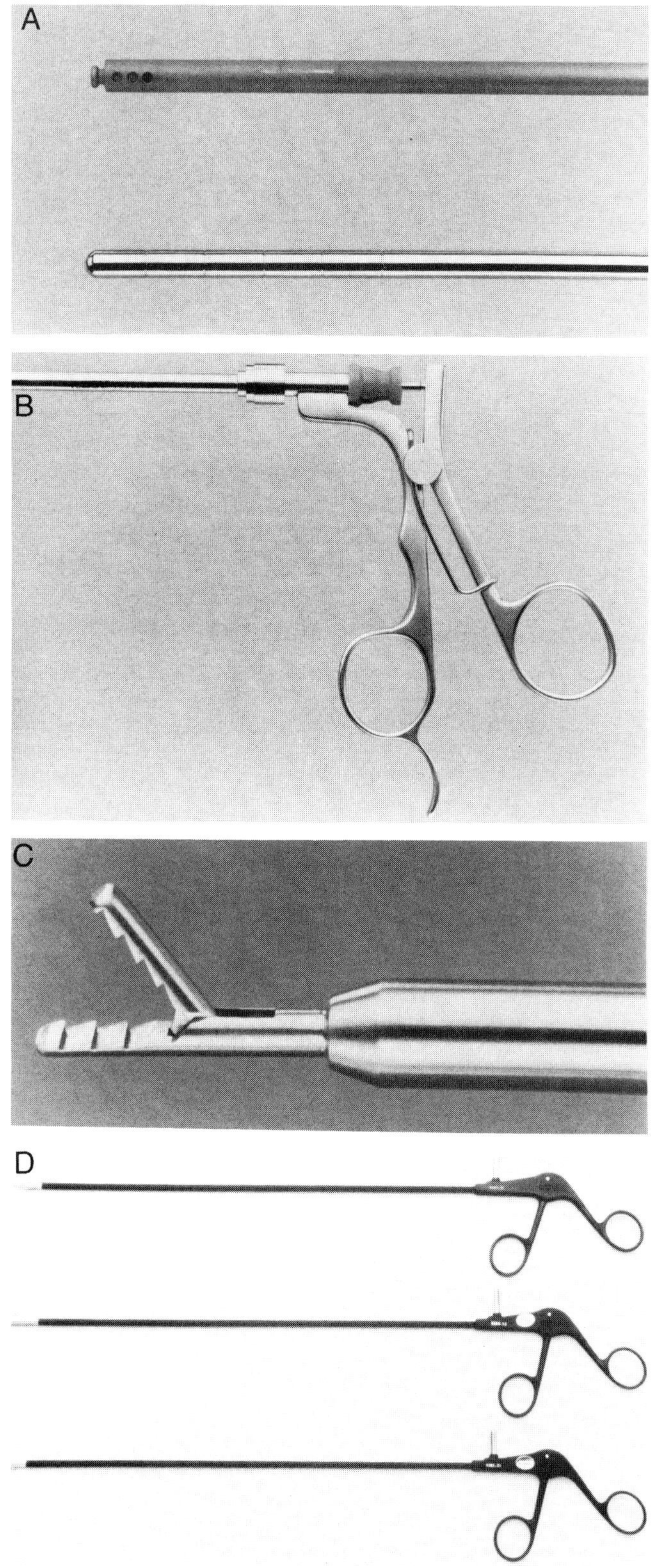

FIG 2–16.
A, exploration probes are calibrated in 1-cm increments. They are used to displace intraperitoneal structures and estimate dimensions. **B,** grasping or retracting forceps have a ratcheted handle and remote jaws **(C)** to manipulate structures. **D,** insulated instruments enable electrocoagulation and usually reduce light scatter.

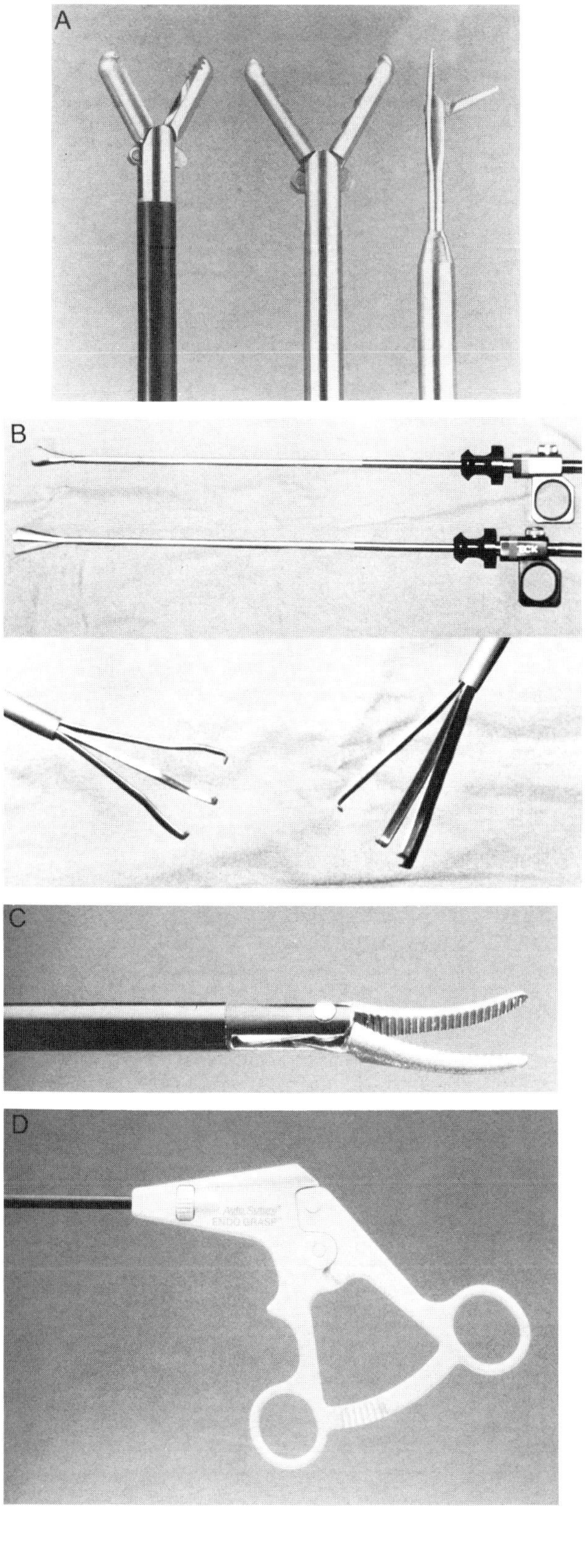

FIG 2–17.
Examples of grasping and retracting instruments with a "jaw" mechanism **(A)** and the "claw mechanism" **(B).** The instruments come in multiple diameters. The 5-mm and 10-mm devices are appropriate for most procedures. **C** and **D,** disposable versions of a grasping instrument.

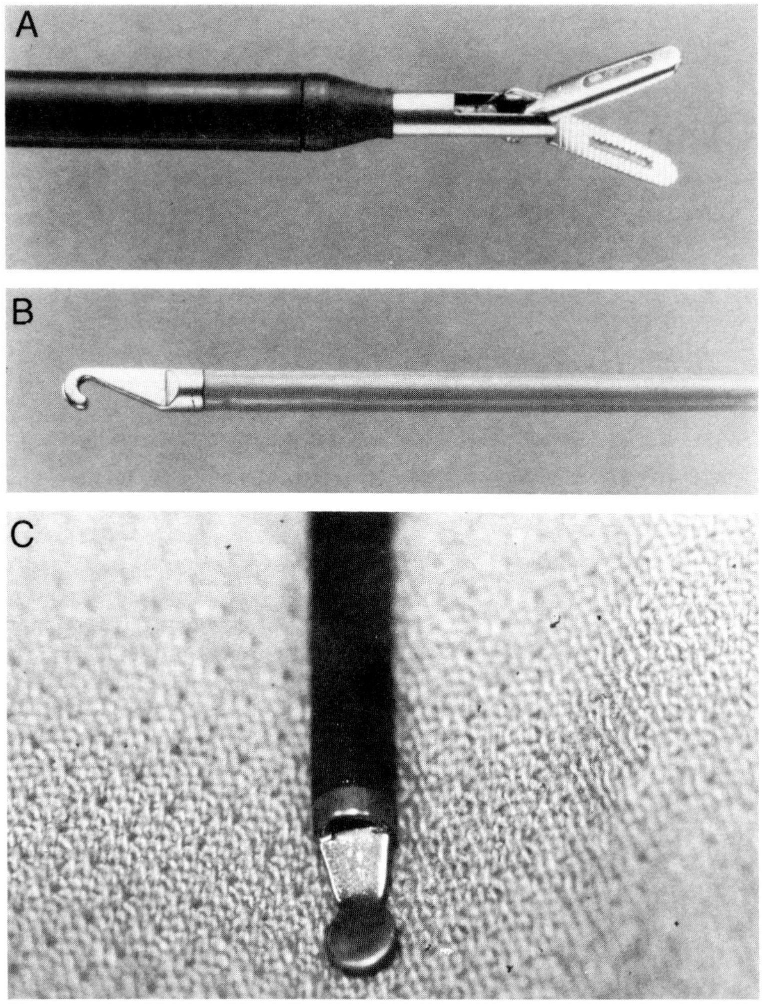

FIG 2–18.
Dissecting instruments have the same overall design as the grasping devices except that the jaws have different configurations. **A,** Elongated "alligator nose" jaws. **B,** "hook" and "spatula" **(C)** geometries are particularly effective for separating tissues and for conducting electrocautery.

provide better biopsy specimens without tissue tearing or bleeding. Almost all biopsy forceps are insulated so that the biopsy sites may be electrocoagulated. Punch biopsy forceps have a mobile, hollow upper jaw that, when closed, fits snugly within the sharp cutting edges of the fixed, hollow lower jaw. A biopsy sample is obtained readily by the scissor-like cutting action of the edges as they cross (Fig 2–20).

Surgical Clips, Stapling Instruments, and Ligating Loops

Clip appliers are introduced through the endosurgical cannula and place titanium U-shaped clips across a hollow structure for occlusion and hemostasis (Fig 2–21). During use, both prongs of the clip applier must be visible prior to clip placement to avoid inadvertent injury. Some reusable models permit placement of only one clip at a time. These devices are durable

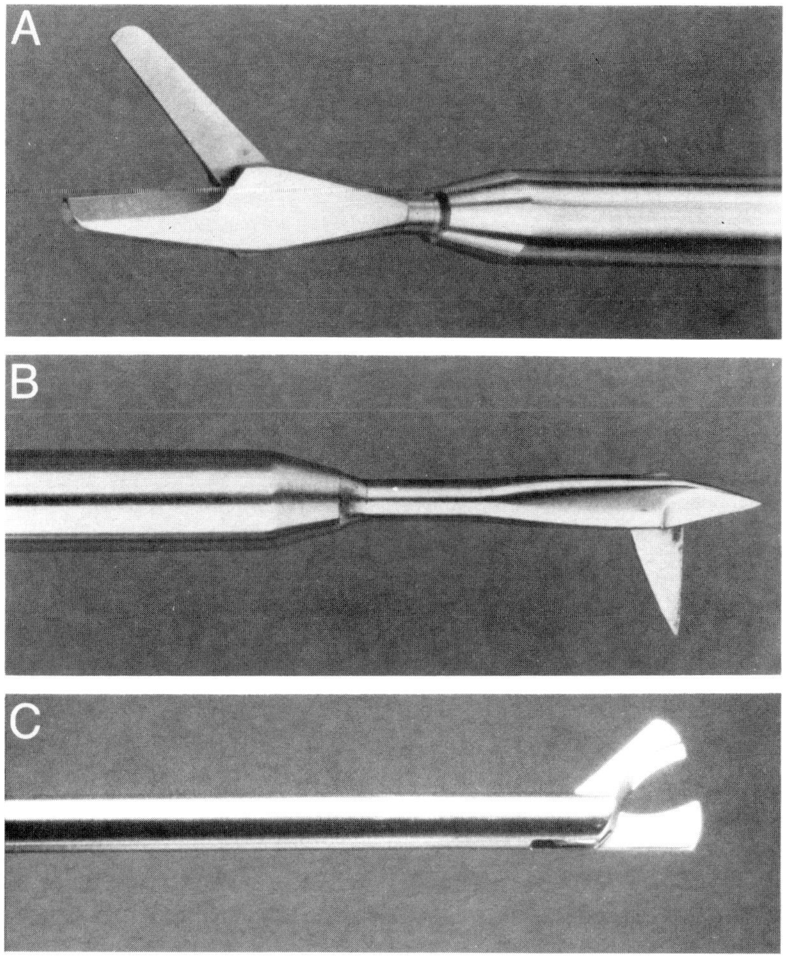

FIG 2–19.
Scissors are available in several designs. **A,** straight scissors with serrated jaws are effective for dissection and transection. **B,** microscissors. **C,** "hook" scissors.

and economical but require removal of the instrument and reloading after each clip is applied. In contrast, both reusable and disposable clip appliers (Endoclip, United States Surgical Corp, Norwalk, Conn) are available and contain twenty 9.0-mm titanium clips that are loaded sequentially without instrument removal. In addition, the disposable instrument shaft can be rotated without turning the handle, thus facilitating clip placement under direct laparoscopic vision. At the present time, both 6.0 and 9.0 mm disposable clip appliers are available, and other sizes are to be introduced in the near future. Future designs will also enable tissue approximation and sequential loading during endoscopic application.

Recently, the gastrointestinal stapling instrument (GIA, United States Surgical Corp) has been introduced in an endosurgical version (Fig 2–21). It places six rows of titanium B-shaped staples and cuts between the third and fourth row. The staple lines are 30 mm in length and are designed to have indications similar to the current available gastrointestinal stapling devices.

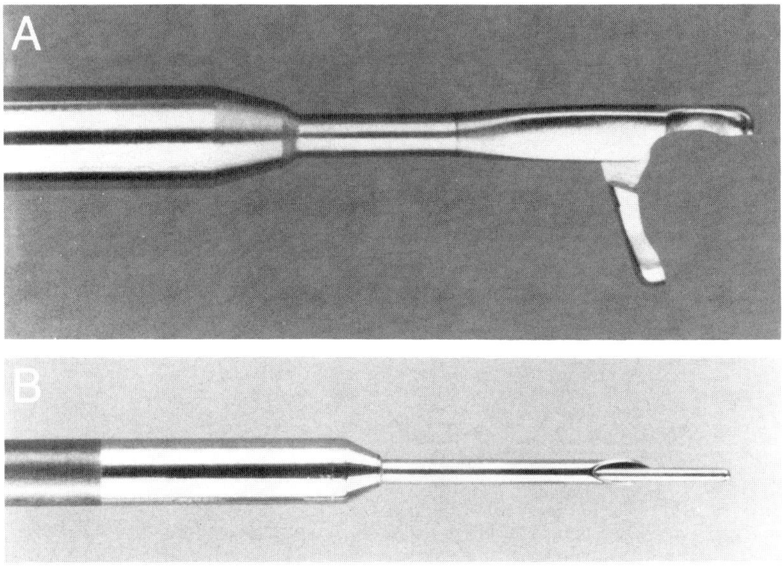

FIG 2–20.
Biopsy forceps **(A)** and aspiration needle **(B).**

Although any needle with a swaged-on suture may be passed down an appropriate-sized cannula and used in an endosurgical application, knot tying requires considerable dexterity. A pretied suture in the form of a loop (Endoloop, Ethicon, Inc, Sommervile, NJ, or Surgitie, US Surgical Corp, Norwalk, Conn.) can be passed down a 5-mm cannula and secured from outside a body cavity (Fig 2–22). Currently Endoloops are manufactured only with chromic suture and are effective for vessels as well as hollow viscera.

OPTICAL INSTRUMENTATION

The choice of optical systems is highly subjective, but there are several factors that should be considered. Only issues relating to the endoscope will be discussed here. Considerations regarding the imaging equipment, cameras, and light sources are found in Chapter 3.

The laparoscope is similar in construction to other endoscopes in common use. It consists of an optical system that conducts the light to illuminate the region to be explored and to return the image to be viewed or photographed. The illumination for the endoscope is generally conduced by way of fiber-optic bundles. These waveguides must provide sufficient illumination to the entire field of view. Inadequate illumination (less than 300 W) jeopardizes the safety of the procedure. The imaging portion and the mechanism by which the image is delivered to the observer determines the type of endoscope. If a bundle of aligned (coherent) optical fibers is utilized to convey the image back to the operator, the resulting fiberscope has some inherent flexibility (Fig 2–23). At present, flexible scopes are mainly used for thoracic or gastrointestinal visualization; these should be kept in mind as alternative instruments for laparoscopy. If the images are obtained by a system of relay lenses, the optical transmission requires that the endoscope be rigid (Fig 2–23). The number and size of the lenses inter-

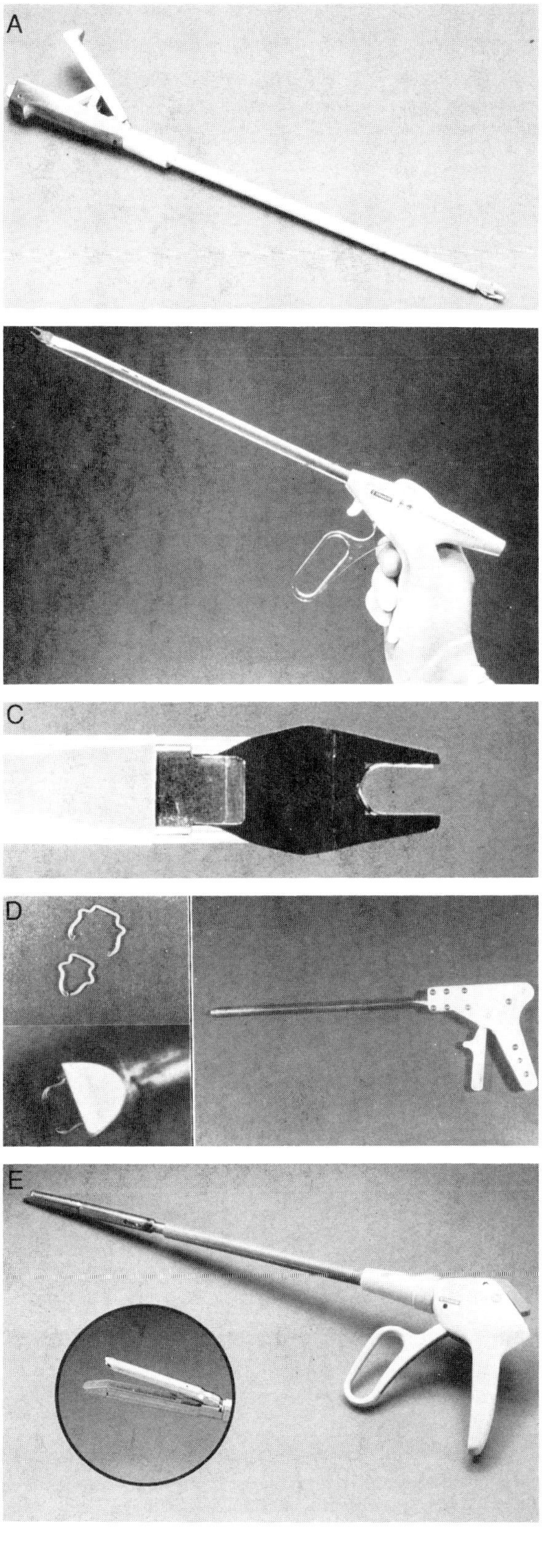

FIG 2–21.
The Endoclip is available in reusable **(A)** and disposable **(B)** versions. Each contains a cartridge with twenty, 6.0- or 9.0-mm staples. **C,** staples are in the "U" configuration. **D,** A experimental tissue joining stapler. This mechanical device functions in a manner analogous to a skin or fascia staple. **E,** The endosurgical version (Endo GIA) of the gastrointestinal (GIA) stapling device that joins and divides tissue to facilitate anastomoses.

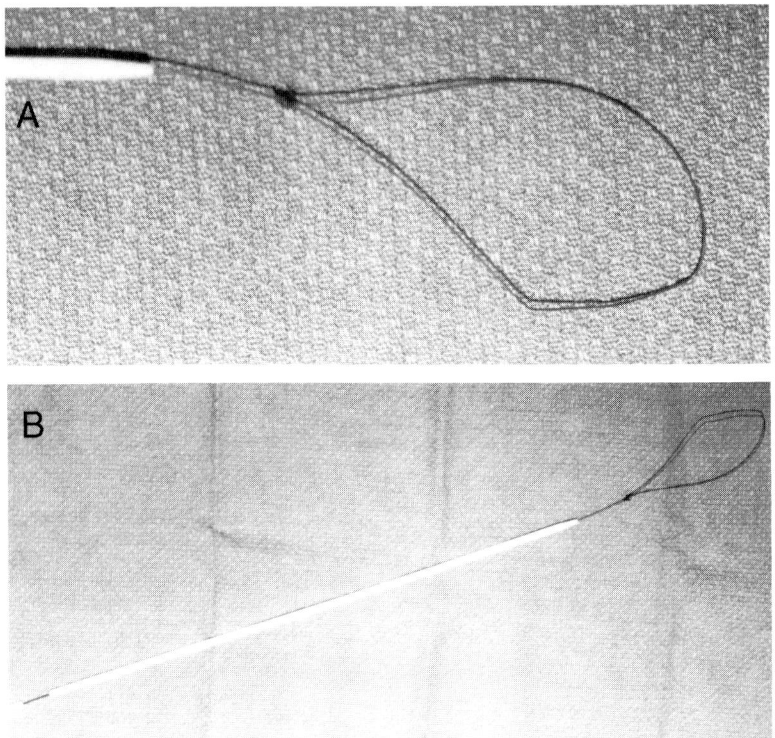

FIG 2–22.
A, a Surgitie ligature is a pretied chromic suture that is placed over the desired structure and tied by pulling up on the extracavitary part of the plastic stem **(B).**

posed between the objective lens and the eyepiece lens distinguish the different varieties of rigid endoscopes. As a standard practice, gynecologic and urologic diagnostic and operative procedures utilize rigid laparoscopes.

The quality of a laparoscopy is determined by the quality of the image it produces. Aspects to be considered when evaluating a scope include (1) the image quality including color, contrast, resolution, depth of focus, and magnification; (2) the scope diameter, ranging from 2.0 to 12 mm, (3) the angle of view by the objective lens, namely, straight, oblique, or foroblique (135 degrees); and (4) the service provided by the supplier or manufacturer.

Image Quality

Color

A true impression of the color of the tissues within the surgical field is an important consideration. The observed image is dependent on the spectrum and intensity of the illuminating light and the light loss in the imaging optics.

Contrast

The greater the difference between the intensity of the image and that of the background, the greater the object contrast obtained.

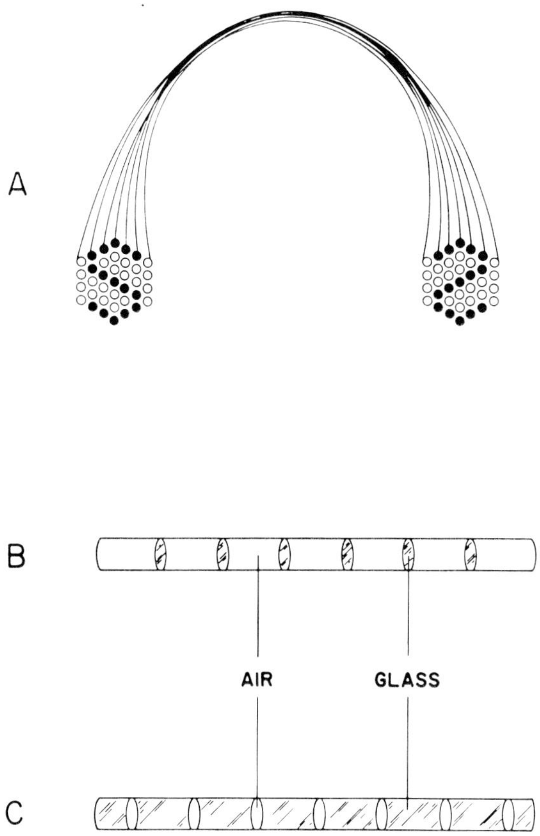

FIG 2–23.
Imaging optics. **A,** coherent fiber bundles within a flexible endoscope. **B** and **C,** the rod lens system within a rigid endoscope. In **B,** the pre-1960s arrangement, small lenses were interspersed with large air volumes. To improve the transmission of light (related to the refraction of the medium between the lenses) and image quality, Hopkins interchanged the air and glass spaces in the lens system **(C).**

Resolution

The ability of the optical system to separate two adjacent points in the resulting image is a measure of the resolution power of that particular lens system. The greater the resolution and contrast, the clearer the image obtained.

Depth of Focus

Just as with a photographic camera, some endoscopes have a variable-focus objective. Conventional laparoscopes have a fixed focus because variable-focus objectives are difficult to use and troublesome to sterilize. In order to obtain a panoramic view, it is necessary to compromise by sacrificing clarity at the periphery of the visual field. Newer optic systems provide a field of depth that ranges from 1 to 10 cm, but scopes that cannot focus close to the operative field should not be used.

Laparoscopic Diameter

Considerable progress in the design and manufacture of optical systems has made it feasible to produce smaller-diameter laparoscopes with little loss of image quality (Fig 2–24). "Non-operating" laparoscopes (endoscopes with no operating channel) generally range from 5 to 10 mm in diameter, although smaller, specialized endoscopes are also available. Use of a "non-operating" laparoscope mandates the use of ancillary puncture sites through which auxiliary

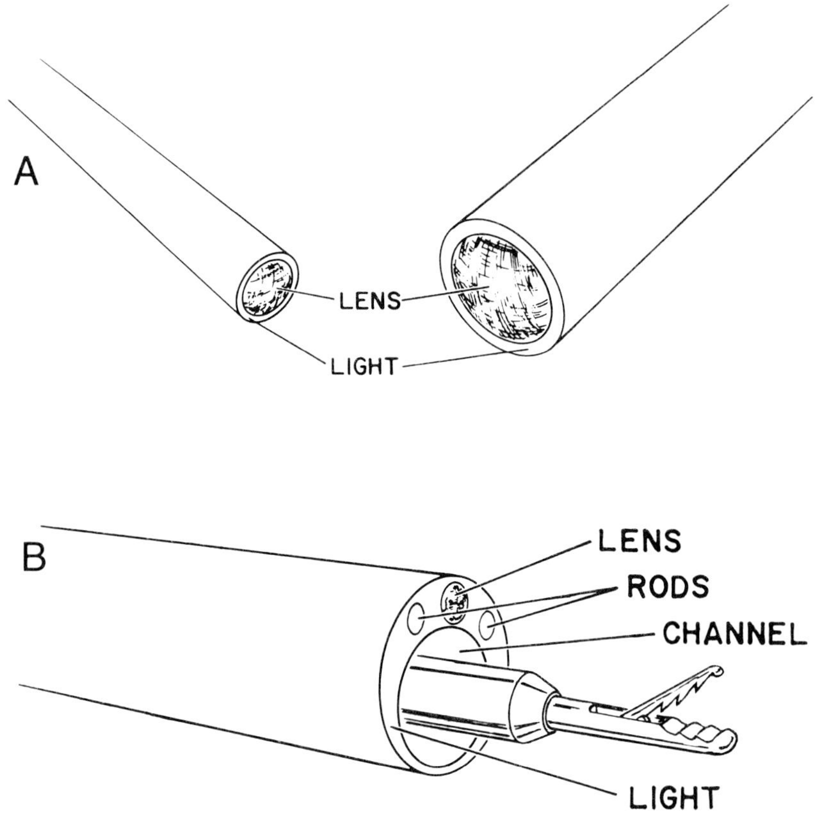

FIG 2–24.
Configuration of commonly used laparoscopes. Nonoperative **(A)** and operative **(B)** laparoscopes are distinguished by a channel for the passage of auxiliary surgical instruments.

surgical instruments are placed. Multiple cannulas provide the best security in terms of maximum visibility and control of procedures. This is the current procedure of choice (Fig 2–25).

Endoscopes are available with different angles of view. These include a straightforward, a 5-degree, and a 45-degree (foroblique) angle from the axis of the scope (Fig 2–26). The selection of the viewing angle is the surgeon's choice; it has been our experience that the novice laparoscopist does better to gain early experience with the straightforward view telescope. The angulated endoscopes have the advantage of permitting visualization of relatively inaccessible areas. In the future, angled views of the operative field will be enhanced by the use of flexible endoscopes.

Small-diameter endoscopes (approximately 5-mm in diameter) are more than adequate for diagnostic and operative laparoscopy. If, however, photographic documentation is desirable, large-diameter endoscopes (8 to 10 mm) are preferable since greater light transmission is possible.

Translaparoscopic surgery through a single endoscope (so-called single-puncture laparoscopy) is possible by the use of a large-diameter laparoscope with an operative instrument channel (see Fig 2–24,B). The single-puncture operative laparoscope has been developed as a result of improvements made in the optical systems. Miniaturization of the endoscopic com-

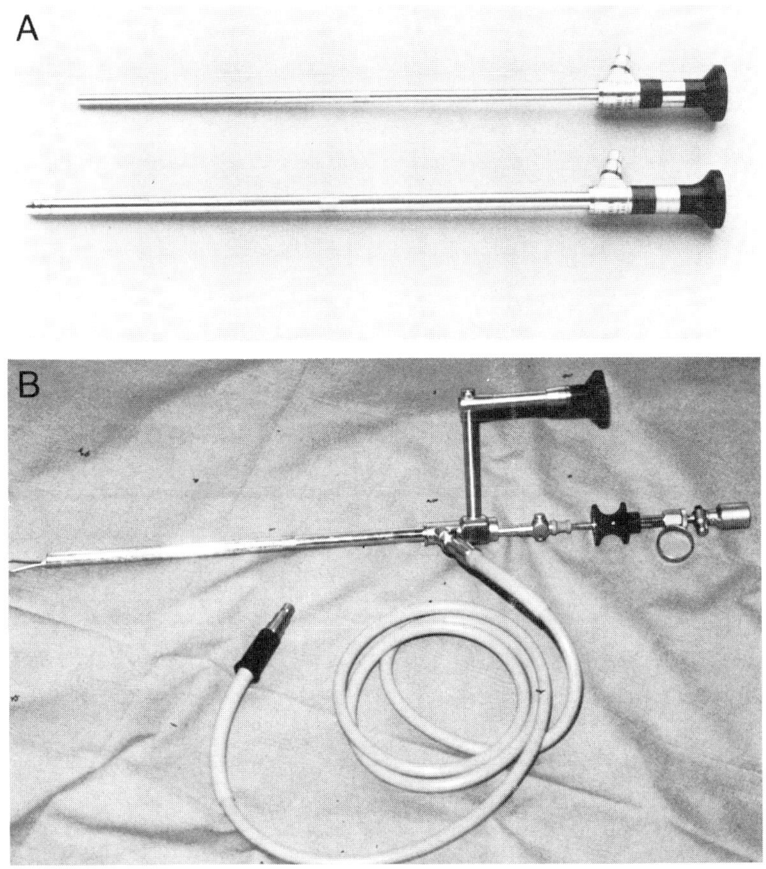

FIG 2–25.
Rigid laparoscopes with and without an accessory instrument channel. **A,** rigid laparoscope: 5- and 10-mm diameter. Both instruments have a 0-degree angle of observation (180 degrees or straight ahead from the observer). **B,** the Jacob-Palmer single-puncture operative laparoscope. A built-in instrument channel permits the insertion of auxiliary instruments.

ponents has enabled the addition of other component channels so that diagnostic and therapeutic instruments can be passed through auxillary channels in the device. Operative laparoscopes up to 12 mm in diameter with ancillary channels up to 7 mm accommodate various devices including metal clip or Silastic band applicators. The most commonly used instrument is 10 mm in outer diameter and contains a 5-mm visual lens system and a 5-mm operative channel (see Fig 2–24,B).

Advantages attributed to the single-puncture operative laparoscope range from cosmesis related to the single incision to the capability it offers for performing minor surgery such as lysis of omental or peritoneal adhesions. If using a single-puncture operative laparoscope is planned, a 10-mm cannula is advisable in most applications. This applies even when two or more cannulas may be required because it provides the operator with the flexibility to exchange a 10-mm laparoscope for a 10-mm operative scope.

Shortcomings of the operative laparoscope are mainly technical in nature and not easily resolved. They range from limitations of the operative field to inadequate mobility during the

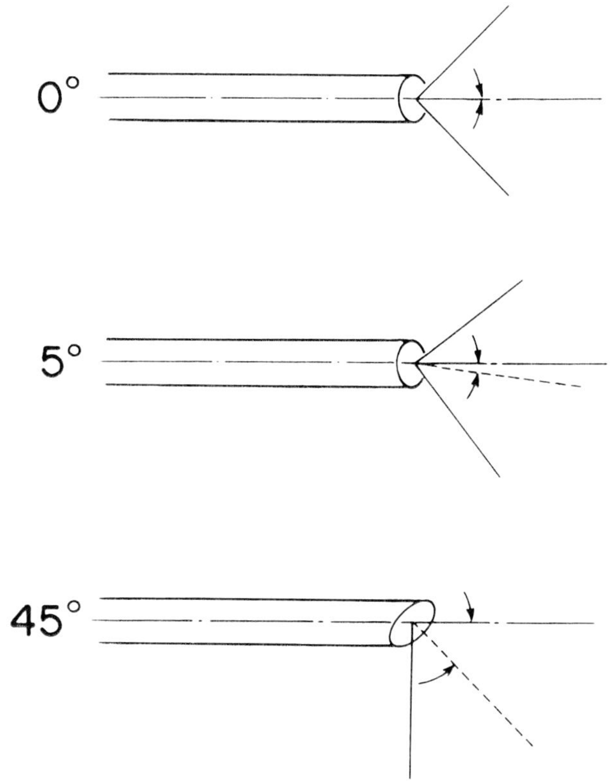

FIG 2–26.
Visual angles of the most frequently used laparoscopes: (from top down) 0-degree angle view (180 degrees or straight ahead from the observer), 5-degree view (175 degrees from the observer), and 45-degree view angle (135 degrees from the observer).

operation. Additional problems that restrict application of the operative laparoscope to endoscopic surgery include a limited unidirectional visual field deficit close to the tip of the endoscope and an inability to mobilize adjacent structures with devices introduced through ancillary ports. The initial enthusiasm for this concept has diminished recently as complications and technical limitations have become apparent. There is still controversy about whether electrosurgical procedures can be safely performed through an operative laparoscope.[9] The future of this concept is yet to be determined.

It is also undesirable to possibly have to remove an operative laparoscope during the course a procedure when the objective lens becomes fogged. All laparoscopes have a tendency to fog when first inserted into the abdominal cavity. This clouding of the lens can be overcome by touching the tip of the laparoscope to the fundus of the uterus, a loop of bowel, or the parietal peritoneum. This may cause a slight coating of the lens with serous peritoneal fluid and some loss of sharpness of the image when photography is being performed. Lens antifog detergent solution is also available. Although endoscope warming units have been produced by several manufacturers, their value is questionable.

CLEANING, STERILIZATION, MAINTENANCE, AND STORAGE OF INSTRUMENTS

The component instruments and equipment for endoscopic surgery must be cared for by knowledgeable personnel.[23] In order to maximize the useful life of the devices and minimize replacement and maintenance costs, each instrument has to be thoroughly cleaned and properly stored between operative procedures. It is a wise investment of time for the surgeon to explain appropriate care for instruments and equipment to the operating team.[23, 24] A well-maintained set of instruments properly stored and examined prior to every procedure is an essential safeguard to prevent frustrating intraoperative equipment delays.

Cleaning

All instruments used during an endoscopic surgical procedure should be soaked in warm water and washed with mild soap immediately upon the completion of the operation.[24, 25] With the exception of the laparoscope, camera, and the fiber-optic light cord, all other instruments have to be thoroughly cleaned and dismantled into their primary components. Each piece should be handled individually.[24] Special brushes are available for dealing with the in strument channels. The optical parts at the end of the laparoscopes or fiber-optic cables should be cleaned gently and dried with alcohol swabs.

Sterilization

Most fiber-optic illuminated endoscopes and their accessories can be gas sterilized or cold disinfected. Despite some manufacturers' recommendations that their equipment can be steam autoclaved, our experience has shown that autoclaving the lens and fiber optics shortens the life span of these instruments. When heat sterilization is used, one should remove all rubber sealing cups from reusable trocar sleeves to prevent melting.

The following are general rules for handling endoscopy equipment:

- Do not steam autoclave or boil any instrument containing fiber optics or a lens system.
- Do not use solvent solutions other than alcohol to clean the instruments.
- Do not use any corrosive agent such as a germicide.
- Do not leave instruments soaking in sterilizing solutions for prolonged periods of time (longer than 30 minutes).

Several methods can be followed in the process of sterilizing the instruments.[25] Since each instrument has different specifications, it is most important to conform with recommendations made by the manufacturer. There are three presently available sterilization techniques.

1. **Disinfection or Cold Sterilization.** This process is the most commonly used. It involves the use of an activated solution of glutaraldehyde (Cidex or Omnicide). This solution is germicidal and viricidal and adequately disinfects with 20-minute immersion of the instruments. The solution should be activated just before the procedure to ensure maximum efficacy. This method of disinfection is best for optical parts and rubber connections of the endoscopes to prevent damage or deterioration of the device. It is essential to not exceed the recommended immersion time, or the endoscope may be damaged.[24]
2. **Gas sterilization.** This technique uses a range of temperatures and pressures and requires aeration of devices following sterilization. So-called cold gas cycles limit the maximum temperature and are appropriate for certain devices.
3. **Steam Autoclave.** This process uses hot steam for sterilization. It is suitable for most nonoptical components. The process uses 210° F, 30 lb pressure for 10 minutes.

Maintenance and Storage

Even though the optical systems are the most delicate and frequently damaged components, proper maintenance of all equipment and instrumentation is essential. Routine inspection of instruments used for electrosurgery is required to identify disruptions in insulation that can cause a short circuit and electrocautery burns. In this regard, the integrity of the entire electrical circuit should be tested prior to each procedure to assure safety.

Trocars should be inspected periodically and sharpness of the tips maintained. A dull trocar markedly increases the force required to penetrate the abdominal wall during introduction. Added force depresses the abdominal wall and compresses underlying vessels and bowel. This markedly increases the risk of injury.

Metal trays with sponge or cloth partitions are desirable for storing delicate instruments. Fiber-optic cables should be stored in an extended position, if possible. Bending of fiber-optic devices produces fiber breakage and adversely affects light transmission and imaging.

REFERENCES

1. Epstein M: Developments in optical instrumentation. *Science* 1980; 210:280–285.
2. Ancona-Berk VA, Chalmers TC: An analysis of the costs of ambulatory and inpatient care. *Am J Public Health* 1986; 76:1102–1110.
3. Politser P: Ambulatory surgery: Some issues and considerations. *Bull Am Coll Surgeons* 1988; 73:26–28.
4. Haug JN, Politser P (eds): Average length of stay for selected operative procedures for patients discharged from short-stay hospitals 1987, in *American College of Surgeons Socioeconomic Factbook for Surgery 1989. Chicago, American College of Surgeons, 1989.*
5. Natof HE: Complications associated with ambulatory surgery. *JAMA* 1980; 244:1116–1120.
6. Gadacz TR, Talamini MA, Lillemoe KD, et al: Laparoscopic cholecystectomy. *Surg Clin North Am* 1990; 70:1249–1262.
7. Reddick EJ, Olsen DO: Laparoscopic laser cholecystectomy. *Surg Endosc* 1989; 3:131–133.
8. Gotz F, Pier A, Bacher C: Modified laparoscopic appendectomy in surgery: A report on 388 operations. *Surg Endosc* 1990; 4:6–9.
9. Hulka JF: Facilities and equipment, in *Textbook of Laparoscopy.* Orlando, Fla, Grune & Stratton, 1985.
10. Rioux JE, Yuzpe AA: Gynecologic endoscopic equipment. *Curr Probl Gynecol* 1981; 5:13–41.
11. Phillips E, Daykhousky L, Carroll B, et al: Laparoscopic cholecystectomy: Instrumentation and technique. *J Laparoendosc Surg* 1990; 1:3–15.
12. Sharp JR, Pierson WP, Brady CE: Comparison of CO_2 and N_2O-induced discomfort during peritoneoscopy under local anesthesia. *Gastroenterology* 1982; 82:453–456.
13. Neely MR, McWilliams R, Makhlouf HA: Laparoscopy: Routine pneumonperitoneum via the posterior fornix. *Obstet Gynecol* 1975; 45:459–460.
14. Veress J: Neues Instrument Zur Ausfuhrung von Brust-oder Bachpunktionen und Penumothoraxbehandlung. *Dtsche Med Wochenschr* 1938; 64:1480–1481.
15. Semm K: *Atlas of Gynecologic Laparoscopy and Hysteroscopy.* Philadelphia, WB Saunders Co, 1977.
16. Hasson HM: Open laparoscopy: A report of 150 cases. *J Reprod Med* 1974; 12:234–238.
17. LoCicero J, Quebbeman EJ, Nichols RL: Health hazards in the operating room. *Bull Am Coll Surgeons* 1987; 72:4–9.
18. Glover JL: The Bovie: A new look at an enduring technology. *Bull Am Coll Surgeons* 1986; 71:4–6.
19. Einstein A: Zur quantem Theorie der Strahlung. *Phys Zect* 1917; 18:121.

20. Keye WR: *Laser Surgery in Gynecology and Obstetrics.* Chicago, Year Book Medical Publishers Inc, 1985.
21. Dixon JA (ed): *Surgical Application of Lasers,* ed 2. Chicago, Year Book Medical Publishers Inc, 1987.
22. United States Department of Health and Human Services, Food and Drug Administration Bulletin, vol 20, No 2., October 1990.
23. Soderstrom RM: Safeguards in laparoscopy: Education, equipment care and electron control. *Contemp OB/GYN* 1978; 11:95–107.
24. Association of Operating Room Nurses Ad Hoc Committee on Infection Control in the Handling of Endoscopic Equipment. Guidelines for preparation of laparoscopic instrumentation. *AORN J* 1980; 32:65–66.
25. Hulka JF, Wisler MG, Bruch C: A discussion: Laparoscopic instrumentation sterilization. *Med Instr* 1977; 11:122–123.

Chapter 3

Image Production and Visualization Systems

Anthony Nobles, Ph.D.

SELECTING A VISUALIZATION SYSTEM

Choosing a visualization system for endoscopic procedures involves several important considerations. These include not only identifying the appropriate equipment but also assembling a system that can be easily used by physicians, nurses, and ancillary personnel to provide reproducible, high-quality images. This chapter discusses the technical aspect of the components of imaging systems and details methods to choose equipment appropriate for specialized applications.

Resolution

The resolution or sharpness and detail produced by a video system is a particularly important aspect for endoscopic visualization. All components of the system including the camera, monitors, fiber optics, and video cassette recorder (VCR) affect the quality of the image obtained. The video image is composed of lines of dots projected from left to right on the screen, called scan lines. The number of horizontal and vertical scan lines determines the quality of the image. Images are produced when phosphorescent dots, or photons, are stimulated by an electronic beam. The intensity of the beam determines the brightness of the image. Resolution is measured by the density of the individual dots that create an image. The greater the density, the better the resolution. Figure 3–1 illustrates this principle by displaying the same image at two different magnifications.

Vertical resolution is determined by the number of lines displayed vertically. Horizontal resolution is the number of visible lines as compared with those on a calibrated resolution chart. When evaluating imaging devices, the greater the number of vertical or horizontal lines available, the higher the resolution. The industrial standard for describing resolution is determined by the number of horizontal lines. As a point of reference, the maximal resolution that can be appreciated by the human eye is approximately 650 lines. Thus, horizontal image resolution greater than 650 lines is of no value in enhancing visualization.

Each electronic component of the video chain (i.e., the monitor, camera, etc.) has a spe-

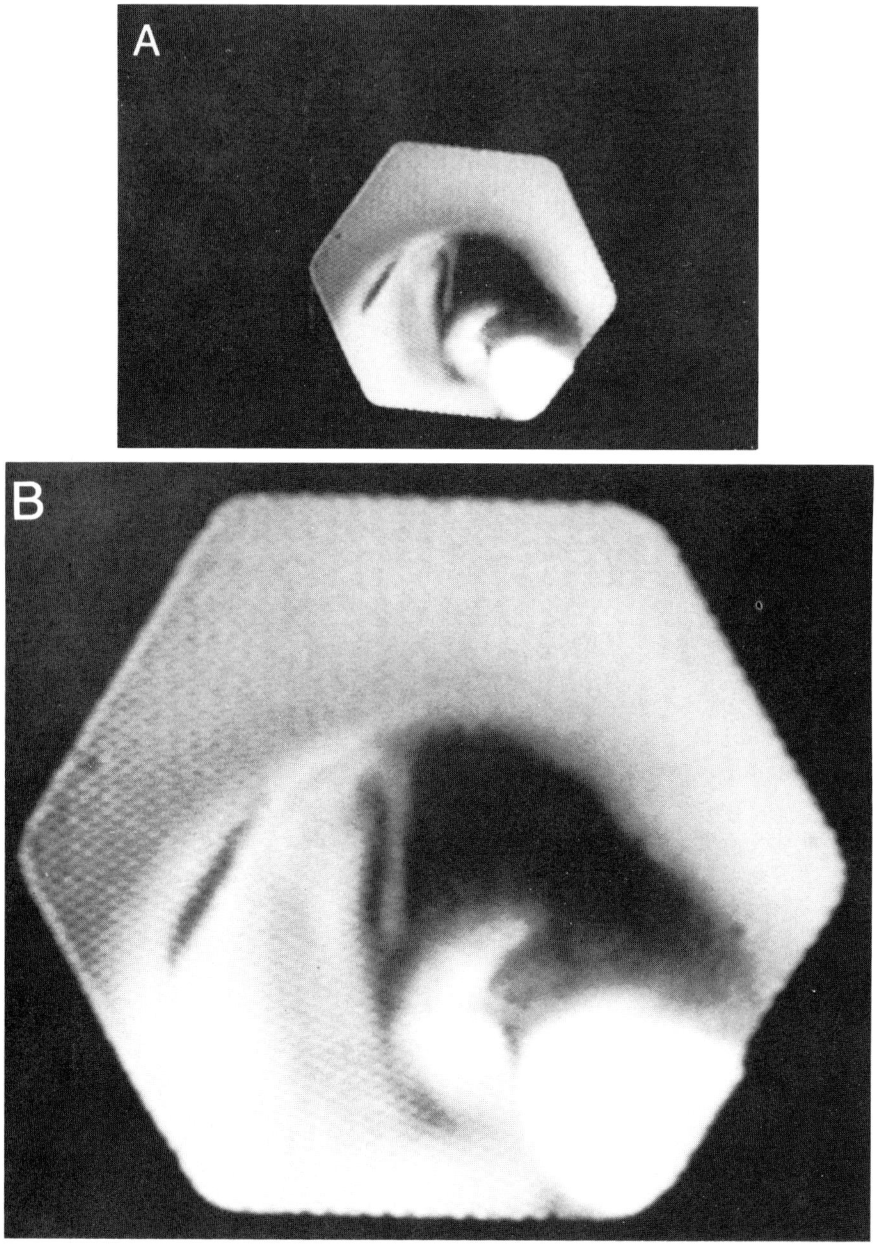

FIG 3–1.
Clear resolution **(A)** as compared with the poorer image **(B)** 4× magnification, i.e., one-fourth dot density per unit area.

cific horizontal resolution. Each nonelectronic component has a resolution that is equivalent to the amount of transferred light. In image coupling devices, the resolution is dependent upon the configuration and design of the lenses and is usually much greater than all other components of the system. It is therefore usually not necessary to consider the effect of the coupler on final image resolution.

In fiber-optic endoscopes, resolution is measured in pixels. The number of pixels are determined by the number of individual fibers that make up an image. Most fiber-optic endoscopes contain between 2,500 and 10,000 pixels. The number of pixels used in a particular endoscope is usually determined by the size and expense of the device. The smaller the size, the fewer the number of pixels. The greater the number of pixels, the greater the cost. For these reasons, most fiber-optic endoscopes have from 3,000 to 6,000 pixels. Very small devices (i.e., <2 mm in diameter) such as cornary artery angioscopes or percutaneous choledochoscopes may have less than 3,000 pixels for size limitations. A good-quality 1.0-mm or smaller scope should have approximately 2,000 to 3,000 pixels and incorporate high-quality light delivery fibers. In larger scopes with diameters of 1.0 to 3.0 mm, which include both light fibers and irrigation channels, quality images are produced by approximately 6,000 pixels. Figure 3–2 demonstrates the transmission of an image through a fiber-optic scope.

To obtain a quality video image when using fiber-optic endoscopes, one must choose a magnification on the video screen that gives the highest resolution without displaying the spaces between the pixels. When using a 6,000-pixel fiber magnified 30 times, the maximum resolution produced is 350 lines. Because most fiber-optic endoscopes available today for medical use are approximately 2,500 to 6,000 pixels, it is not possible to achieve an image magnified greater than approximately 5 in. without displaying the spaces between the pixels and degrading the visual resolution. At present, it is not possible to obtain greater resolution with fiber-optic scopes because of physical limitations.

Rigid- or single-fiber glass endoscopes are not limited by pixel resolution as are the fiber-optic endoscopes. These devices are essentially couplers between the lens and the video

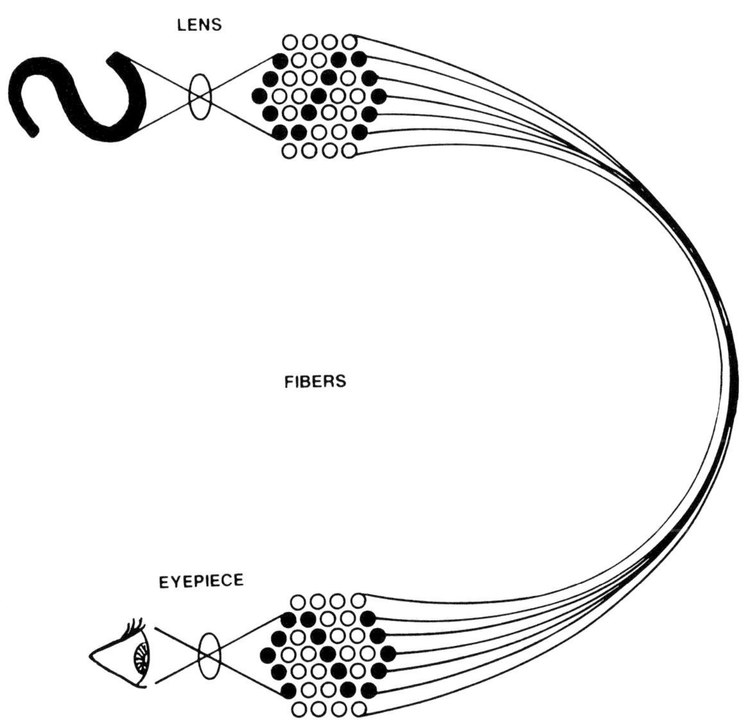

FIG 3–2.
Optical transmission via coherent fiber optics.

screen and do not affect the resolution of the system. For this reason, the images obtained from single-fiber scopes require less light and are better than those obtained when using fiber-optic endoscopes. The major disadvantages of most single-fiber devices are size and rigidity, which precludes manipulation into inaccessible areas. Most single-fiber scopes do not have accessory channels for irrigation or passage of instruments, and those that do are quite large. Most rigid-fiber scopes are also expensive to purchase and repair.

THE VIDEO CHAIN

The video chain is composed of all components involved in creating the video image (Fig 3–3). The components of the video chain are the monitor, camera, lenses and couplers, endoscopes, and VCR (optional). Light sources will be discussed later in the chapter.

When choosing the video components it is important to consider the resolution, light sensitivity, ease of use, overall quality of each component, and the compatibility of the individual parts. For example, having a camera with 600 lines of resolution and a monitor with 525 lines of resolution will produce a 525-line image.

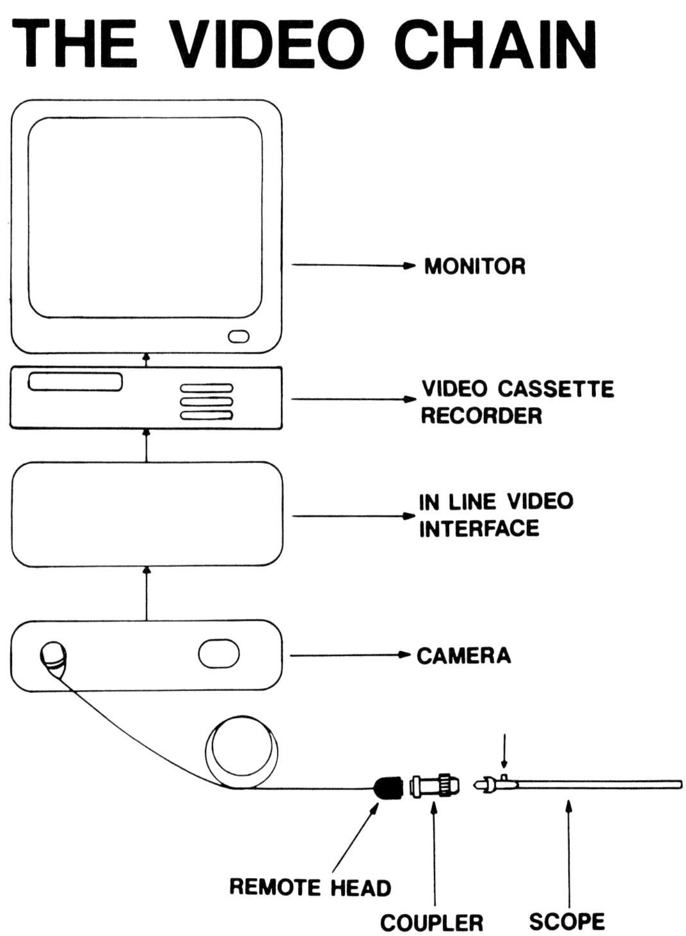

FIG 3–3.
Video chain. The VCR is optional.

When selecting video equipment, properly matching components is as important as maximizing the quality of each component. One must also consider the future upgradability of certain components. For example, purchase of a low-resolution camera to match a low-resolution monitor may not be desirable if a higher resolution camera can be acquired for a comparable cost. The monitors can be upgraded easily for less expense at a later time if the need arises. Developing an understanding of the most restricting factors in component development allows one to optimize a system based on these considerations and provides for future improvements in a cost-effective manner.

The Monitor

It is important to select a monitor that is professional quality. Using an inexpensive monitor or commercial television will not yield an acceptable image. One should select a monitor with the highest possible resolution that does not greatly exceed the resolution of the camera. Select a screen size that best fits your needs. Larger is not necessarily better, particularly when using fiber optics where image size is critical, i.e., using a larger monitor will provide a lower-quality image. A 13-in. monitor is best for most systems, although a 19- or 20-in. screen is desirable for multiple images. It is important to compare color and sharpness side by side to determine the best monitor. There are many monitors available, and those skilled in selecting professional video equipment can purchase a monitor from sources other than the company supplying the system. However, it may be more convenient and cost-effective when purchasing a system to acquire the monitor included with the system.

Line Loss

Line loss is the reduction of the vertical resolution when a picture is transmitted to a video monitor. As an example, in a 525-line monitor 41 lines are lost due to time lag during scanning of an image. Thus, approximately 484 lines of resolution are available in a quality medical system. In inferior-quality monitors, some picture elements are also lost because the scanning beam cannot pick up details in the image. The loss of this information is directly proportional to the angle of the scanning beam. The lower the angle, the greater the line loss. As a result, as few as 340 lines of vertical resolution may remain to construct the final image.

The Camera

The camera is the most important device in the video chain. Select a camera that has the highest resolution that is desirable for the proposed procedures. In general, a camera with at least 330 line of resolution is required for fiber-optic scopes and at least 360 for rigid scopes. Higher resolution of 480 or greater is desirable if possible. Miniaturized remote cameras are either part of the endoscope or can be passed separately onto the operative field to enable the surgeon to control the focus of images. One should select cameras that are easy to operate; most cameras for endoscopic procedures require only a white balance and gain adjustments. Other options are not necessary for routine procedures. Some remote heads can be sterilized in etheylene oxide gas or by immersion in antiseptic solutions. If possible, it is desirable to purchase a second remote head for use when the other requires sterilization or repair. Remote cameras can also be used nonsterilely if they are passed through a sterile sleeve (Fig 3–4).

When choosing a camera one should evaluate the quality of the image, color, sharpness, and depth of field. Because it is not very often possible to compare the image from different systems side by side, one must pay particular attention to detail. The camera should also be compatible with various manufacturers' couplers (lenses) and scopes. This is best accomplished by using a standard C-mount camera. Most but not all manufacturers provide a C-mount (Fig 3–5). Those who do not will require an additional purchase of a conversion coupler, which may be expensive and also degrades the image.

Couplers and Endoscopes

Couplers function like lenses and magnify and focus the image for the camera. It is usually advisable to purchase a coupler from the same manufacturer who supplies the endoscope you select. Most couplers are gas sterilizable; however, most cannot be prepared by using liquid antiseptics.

Endoscopes come in many different sizes and configurations. In many endoscopic procedures such as laparoscopy, arthroscopy, etc., rigid scopes made of glass that are not flexible or steerable are used. In locations where small flexible scopes are desirable such as gastrointestinal endoscopy, choledochoscopy, angioscopy, etc., smaller fiber-optic scopes are used. These do not provide the same-quality resolution as the rigid scopes and usually produce a much smaller image. Flexible endoscopes are easily made steerable and may be disposable. Selecting an appropriate endoscope is more dependent on the procedure than the selection of any other component of the video chain. When selecting an endoscope one must consider the size, diameter, and length of the device. These considerations include the overall working distance and the need for channels in the lumen of the endoscope for irrigation, guidewires, or interventional tools.

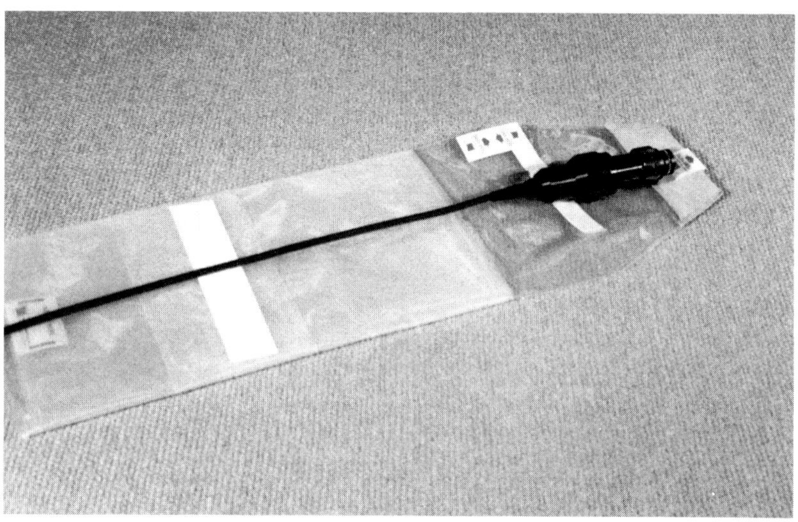

FIG 3–4.
Sterile plastic sleeve used to pass unsterile couplers and cables to the procedure site.

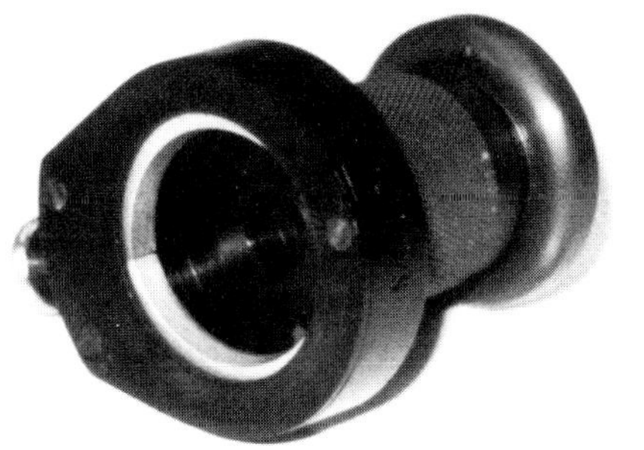

FIG 3–5.
C-mount camera adaptor.

The VCR

A VCR is not an essential component of the video system but is desirable to store images and maintain procedure records. The VCR is not required to provide imaging during the procedure and does not affect the image on the monitor. To acquire simultaneous recording of a procedure, one must be sure that the VCR is activated because the image visualized on the monitor does not indicate that the VCR is operational. One should select a professional-quality VCR with resolution as high as possible without greatly exceeding the resolution of the camera. This will ensure that the recorded images are the best available from the system. Most professional-quality, standard four-head VHS machines are adequate for this function. Selecting a VCR that is compatible in format to one's office and/or home VCR is frequently desirable. In general, commercial home entertainment VCRs offer features that are too complex for procedure recording. High-quality industrial units provide better images and are simpler to use.

ADDITIONAL VISUALIZATION SYSTEM COMPONENTS

Insufflation and Irrigation Systems

Gas insufflation systems are critical to perform adequate intraperitoneal examinations. The CO_2 gas insufflation devices for laparoscopic procedures are discussed in detail in Chapter 2. CO_2 gas is also being investigated as a method to enhance visualization in other applications such as angiography and angioscopy.

Visualization during other endoscope procedures including angioscopy, arthroscopy, and gastrointestinal endoscopy is frequently achieved by saline irrigation. Saline perfusion can be achieved by a pressurized bag of saline to provide a continuous rate of flow or by a syringe if a lower-volume and high-pressure infusion is desired. To overcome the limitations of these methods, infusion pumps have been developed to provide an easily controlled volume and rate of irrigation (Fig 3–6). For most applications it is desirable to have at least two infusion rates, particularly if more rapid flow is required to enable visualization such as during angioscopy. Some irrigation systems offer devices to detect air and bubbles in the infusate. In many endoscopic procedures infusion of air is not a problem, but it is a critical concern for visual-

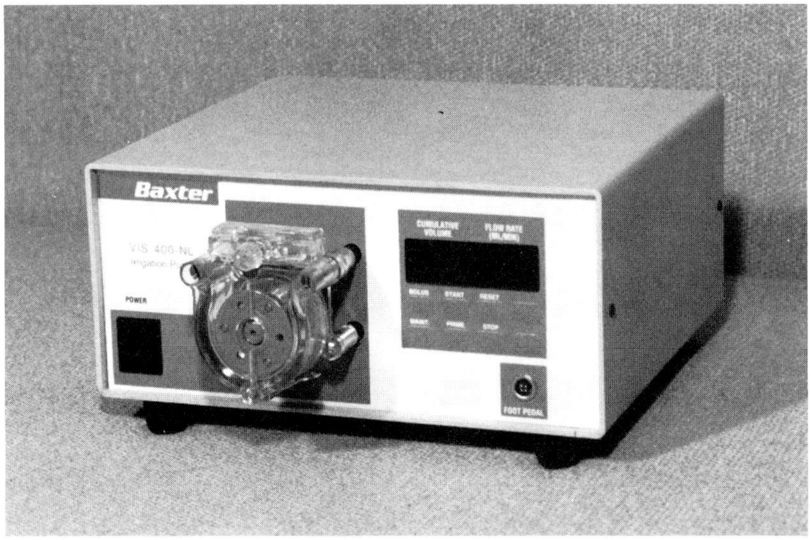

FIG 3–6.
Irrigation pump.

ization and patient safety during intravascular and some closed-space examinations. In these instances, it is mandatory that all air be evacuated from the infusate before connecting it to the irrigation system and that the infusion lines be monitored for air. It is desirable to select a pump that is easy to operate and has only the necessary controls to perform the procedure. It is also convenient to have a foot pedal control with "on/off" and rate of infusion adjustments (Fig 3–7).

The Light Delivery System

The light delivery systems consists of the light source, which generates the light; the light cable, which transmits the light to the endoscope; and the light delivery fiber, which transmits light to the imaging site.

Light sources are available in a range of powers, color temperatures, and gas compositions. A light source should be selected that accommodates the maximum required light and color temperature to perform a particular procedure. Most cameras are designed to accommodate a broad range of color temperatures but function best at a color temperature of 5,600 degrees, i.e., equivalent to daylight. In general, lower-cost light sources will have lower color temperatures. For example, a quartz light source provides a yellowish light that has an ambient color temperature of approximately 2,800 to 3,200 degrees. For this reason quartz light sources provide poorer color reproduction and image quality. Xenon light sources have an approximate color temperature of 5,600 degrees and provide the best light for most applications. The wattage of the light source is also a critical factor. Most light sources range from 150 to 300 W. One hundred fifty watts is adequate for many rigid laparoscopes, while 300 W or more may be needed for long, flexible fiber-optic devices. The only necessary control on a light source for most applications is brightness, with a continuous or volume-type adjustment being most desirable (Fig 3–8). Lamp life meters are usually inaccurate, and light filters are not nec-

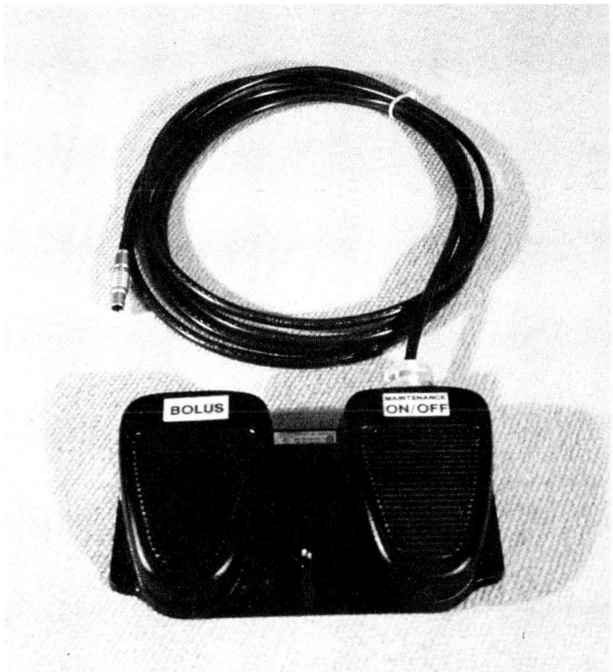

FIG 3–7.
Foot pedal for an irrigation system featuring on/off and bolus infusion control.

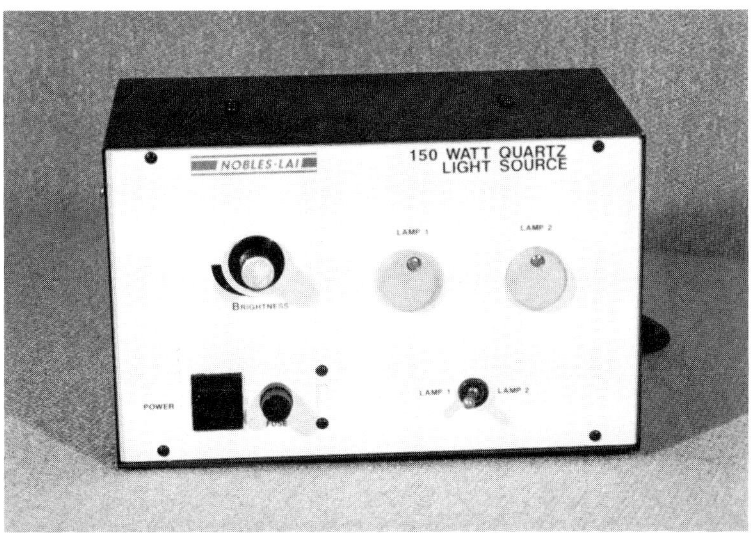

FIG 3–8.
Light source with variable brightness control.

essary for most applications. Power and brightness meters are not necessary because the image is the best brightness meter. Light cables that connect the light source to the endoscopes should be compatible with various systems, if possible. Conversion couplers are readily available and do not significantly degrade light transmission.

The light fibers in a rigid endoscope are usually glass and are quite effective in delivering a large percentage of the light provided by the light source. In fiber-optic endoscopes, the light delivery may be accomplished by either single larger fibers or multiple smaller fibers. In general, fiber-optic scopes have approximately 30% more light loss during transmission due to nontransparent spaces between fibers. For this reason, higher-intensity light sources are required with fiber-optic scopes to obtain adequate images.

It is important to note that approximately 50% to 75% of the light is lost during transmission through either fiber-optic or rigid systems. Light attenuation occurs at several interfaces including approximately 5% at air/glass transitions at either end of the scopes and an additional 20% at each connector, so the number of connections should be minimized.

Carts and Integrated Systems

Most companies that sell visualization equipment also offer carts that are specifically designed for their system, or they recommend an available cart that will accommodate all the components required. The cart should have adequate space for accessories, including video tapes, cables, etc. It is also advisable to have copies of instructional manuals for the devices in the cart. Some carts offer monitor stands that rotate or can be extended out and away from the cart. Placement of the component of the video chain in a logical and accessible manner is important. Some companies offer integrated systems that are usually built into or onto mobile carts. However, when cost is a factor, many types of available carts can be modified to accommodate ones need.

Integrated systems are designed to function as a unit (Fig 3–9). All of the individual components are preconnected. The video, audio, and power connections are hidden from the user. The systems usually only has one main power line and one power switch. This allows for greater flexibility with less error. Many integrated systems have their own intravenous fluid pole for irrigation systems as well as storage space for necessary accessories.

When purchasing an integrated system, be sure that the individual components can be easily removed without affecting the operation of the other elements. This will allow the integrated system to operate even though a particular component is missing. Many integrated systems also have useful accessories that may be purchased initially or added at a later time. These include video printers, video disc storage systems, and video character generators for labeling images. For many reasons including convenience and simplicity, integrated systems are often desirable.

Digital Techniques

Some companies offer devices that provide digital processing of the images generated by the visualization system. An example of this is digital angioscopy, which allows the user the flexibility of multiple images, freeze frame, and special storage and reproduction of procedure records.

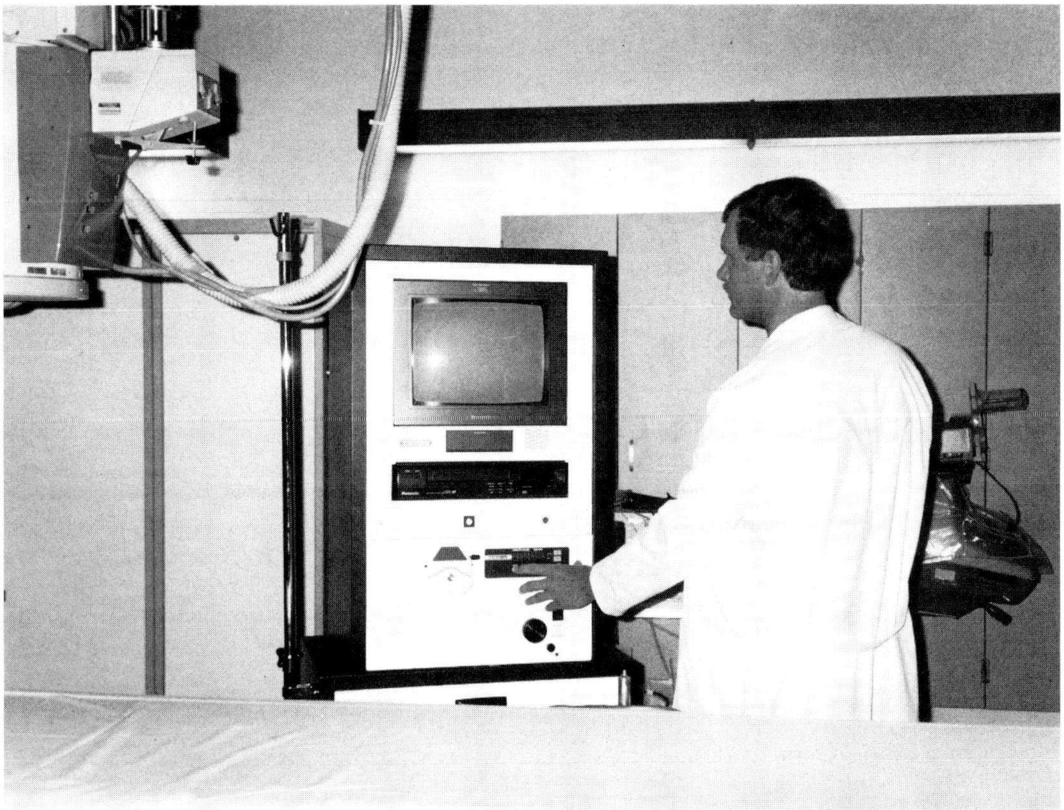

FIG 3–9.
Example of an integrated system containing all necessary components and accessories of the video chain.

Manufacturers

One of the most important considerations in selecting a visual system is choosing a manufacturer who will provide ongoing cost-effective repair and upgrade to the system. Accessibility to new technology, prompt service, and quality equipment are all critical to enhancing utility of the system.

Chapter 4

Hemostatic and Dissection Devices: Safety Considerations and Comparison of Various Modalities

George E. Kopchok, B.S.

Rodney A. White, M.D.

The continuing evolution of laparoscopic procedures offers an exciting, technology-dependent enhancement to conventional surgical practice. In this regard, it is essential that users become knowledgeable of potential hazards and methods to protect patients and personnel.

The instruments with the greatest potential for hazard are the dissection and/or coagulation devices. These include electrocautery, lasers, and ultrasonic scalpels. In these devices, electricity poses the greatest risk, with each modality having additional unique liabilities such as injury from high-intensity energy emission with lasers. This chapter reviews the considerations relevant to safe use of these devices and includes a discussion of the pertinent differences in utility, including the tissue effects, hemostasis, and the ease of use. Special considerations required for facility, personnel, and patient safety are presented.

ELECTROSURGICAL PRINCIPLES

Electrosurgical Principles

Electrosurgery has been extensively used since the early 1930s. Prior to this time the standard method for coagulation was thermal cautery. In 1928 Harvey Cushing described the advantage of using electrical current for control of hemorrhage during brain surgery.[1] The high-frequency current was generated for this procedure by a device designed by William T. Bovie. This radio frequency electrosurgical device, also known as the "bovie," was a major advance over thermal cautery. The bovie was quickly accepted throughout the medical field because it was faster and had more effective coagulation than thermal cautery did.

Although electrocautery equipment has evolved throughout the years and is now safer to use, the basic physical principle of diathermy are unchanged. Medical diathermy is based on the fact that high-frequency alternating current can be passed through the body with no effects other than the production of heat.[2] Low frequencies result in nervous system stimulation. The amount of heat produced by the alternating current is inversely proportional to the electrode area. With medical diathermy both electrodes are large ($>100\ cm^2$); therefore, the current is evenly dispersed with no current concentration or cell destruction. With electrosurgery, one electrode (ground, patient plate) is large, and the other is quite small ($\leq 1\ cm^2$). This small electrode, referred to as the "active" electrode, is used to control the current density. Current density is the measure of current concentration or current per unit area. The rate of heat production and resulting therapeutic effect is a direct function of the current density. Current density behaves much like laser power density in that the higher the current (or laser energy) per given area the greater the effect. The current density (just like laser power density) depends on (1) applied voltage (laser power), (2) resistance of tissue (absorption of photon energy), and (3) the area of active electrode in contact with the tissue (laser spot size).

As Professor William Bovie and Dr. Harvey Cushing continued their experiments at Peter Bent Brigham Hospital, they discovered that a continuous high-frequency current would produce a cutting effect while intermittment high-frequency current caused coagulation of vessels with little or no cutting effect. To use both effects in the operating room at that time required two entirely separate high-frequency oscillators installed in a single cabinet. Today, however, current waveforms for cutting, coagulation, or a combination of the two can be delivered from small solid-state electrosurgical units. If the waveform is continuous, uninterrupted high-frequency energy, it will cause cutting alone. Hemostasis alone is accomplished when the waveform is pulsed on and off, with on times being one fifth to one tenth as long as the off times. A modified or blended effect of cutting and coagulation is produced by longer on/off time ratios (Fig 4–1).

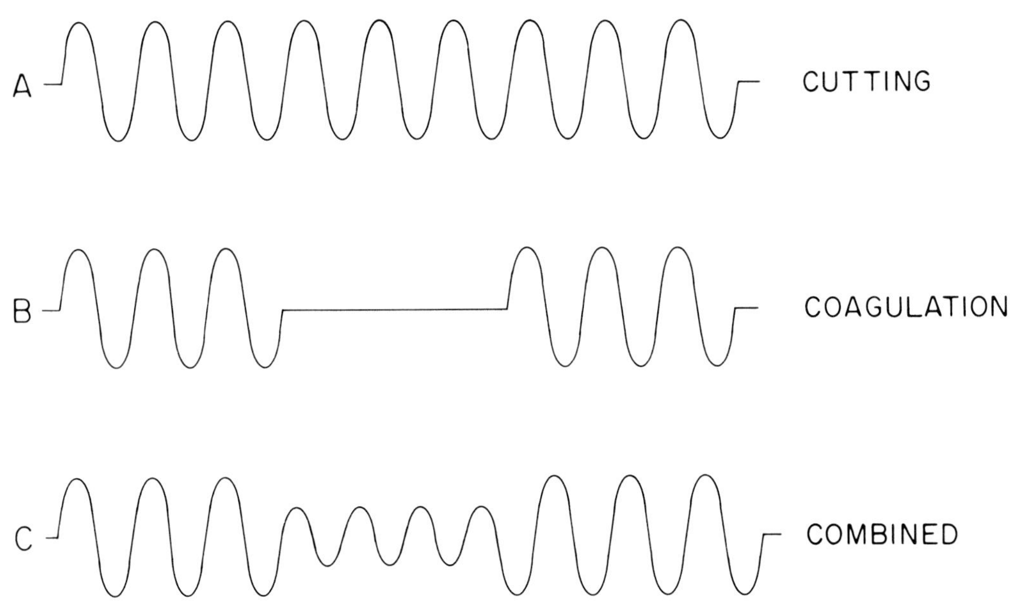

FIG 4–1.
Current waveforms for electrosurgical units. **A,** cutting; **B,** coagulation; **C,** combined.

Electrosurgical Safety

The arc is an important feature of electrosurgery that produces various tissue reactions. In prior years when explosive agents (ether and cyclopropane) were routinely used for surgical anesthesia, the electrosurgical arc was a hazard for gas ignition. Following several operating room fires in the 1930s, safety standards were developed to reduce the potential of gas ignition. Although explosive anesthetics are rarely used now, there still exists the potential for explosion due to arc formation in bowel gas. Bowel gas contain hydrogen, and in about one third of the adult population it also contains methane. Either of these two gases are combustible when mixed with the oxygen from swallowed air. In one study it was found that approximately 43% of unprepared bowels contain an explosive mixture.[3] As one might expect, the combination of the electrosurgical arc and flammable gas has caused incidents of fatal bowel gas explosions. In one case an electrosurgical snare was being used through a colonoscope to remove a polyp. When the electrical current was activated to begin the cutting process, the arc caused the combustible mixture to ignite.[4] To prevent these explosive incidents from occurring, the bowel must be carefully prepared in advance for any procedure involving electrosurgery.

Another source of electrosurgical hazard is the patient grounding plate. Although most dispersive electrodes marketed today are constructed with a significant safety factor, there have been several cases in which the electrodes were accidently tugged or dislodged while moving the patient. The decrease in grounding contact area increases the power density, and electrical burn results. Other grounding problems have occurred due to insufficient amount of conducting gel. Areas of severe skin damage between the grounding plate and the patient have been reported when a gel pad was 50% to 80% dry.[5]

The surgical current in monopolar electrocautery must travel from the active electrode to the patient ground. In most cases this is a low-resistance, highly conductive pathway. The large bowel, however, has a very high resistance (low conductivity) because the bulk of the fluid and electrolytes from intestinal contents are resorbed in this area. This may cause the electrical current to travel through the wall of the intestine at a power density high enough to cause a burn. There have been a number of complications, some fatal, due to bowel perforations following monopolar tubal ligation procedures.[6] The deaths reportedly resulted from thermal bowel injury following an electrical accident with a unipolar coagulating device. In these reports it was noted that the laparoscopic procedures were thought to have proceeded without complications. Most electrical injuries to the bowel are unrecognized at the time of occurrence. Intervals between the time of injury to the onset of symptoms (fever and abdominal pain) vary from 18 hours to 14 days.[7]

Most of these grounding plate and nonconductive tissue problems can be eliminated by using bipolar electrocautery. Bipolar means that both electrodes (active and ground) are placed at the tip of the forcep. In this mode, the current flows only between the two active electrodes. This virtually eliminates patient burns and reduces internal organ damage due to localized current flow. It is highly recommended, especially when working near the bowel as in laparoscopic tubal ligation, that bipolar electrocautery be used for coagulation.

Proper insulation of all endoscopic instruments is required to prevent burns to the skin or bowel. Instruments should be checked on a regular basis to verify that the insulation along the shaft is not cracked, chipped, or defective in any manner. When utilizing an electrosurgical unit, one must ensure that the electrode is in contact only with the appropriate tissue. If the electrode comes in contact with the endoscopic or other noninsulated metal instruments, a conductive path is created. This short circuit may lead to skin burns at the trocar insertion site or burns to the skin and eyes of the operator. Nonconductive fiberglass and Teflon sheaths are available and should be used when electrocoagulation is to be performed.

An improvement in the current electrosurgery units, which may be beneficial for endoscopic surgery, is the argon beam coagulator (ABC; Bard, Bellerica, Mass). The ABC uses a stream of argon gas to conduct the current to the target tissue. The inactive gas serves the dual purpose of delivering a uniform arc and blowing the blood or fluids away from the tissue. The reticulum formed by the uniform arc is more regular and homogenous than conventional electrocautery. Ward et al. reported that the ABC reduced blood loss by up to 50% when compared with convention electrosurgical units.[8] Although this device is not approved for endoscopic surgery, research is being conducted to determine whether the ABC is safe and more effective than conventional electrosurgery.

LASERS

Laser Physics

Laser is an acronym for *l*ight *a*mplication by *s*timulated *e*mission of *r*adiation. The theoretical principles of the lasing process were first described by Albert Einstein in 1917.[9] In that paper entitled "Quantum Theory of Radiation," he described the process of stimulated emission. This theory combined with other works was the basis for Einstein's being granted the Nobel Prize in physics in 1921.

Before one can understand the concept of stimulated emission, an understanding of spontaneous emission is required. Under normal conditions, atoms interact with protons and absorb their energy by elevating an electron from a lower energy orbit to a higher energy orbit. This process will only occur when an atom interacts with a photon that has enough energy to elevate an electron one orbit. An atom with an electron in an elevated energy state (excited atom) quickly releases the energy in the form of a second photon as the electron returns to its normal orbit. The wavelength and energy of the emitted photon corresponds to the differences between the higher and lower energy orbits. This process, because it occurs naturally in all matter, is called spontaneous emission (Fig 4–2).

Lasers work by a process known as stimulated emission (Fig 4–3). The lasing process occurs when an atom is excited with photons from an external source. When a second photon having identical wavelength and energy to the first photon that excited the atom interacts with the excited atom, it stimulates emission of a photon. The second stimulating photon is not absorbed by the excited atom, but only causes the atom to emit a photon that has characteristics identical to the stimulating photon. In a laser, when the majority of the atoms have been charged by photons from the external source (population inversion), a poorly understood phenomenon called stimulated emission occurs. All of the stimulated photons are released simultaneously in a coordinated wave. Since the atoms being stimulated are identical, only a limited number of orbital changes are possible. Thus, by using pure elements as the laser medium, the particular wavelength of the released energy is specific for the limited possible energy changes between orbits.

Laser light has three unique characteristics: the light is monochromatic, directional, and coherent. Monochromicity means that the laser light consists of a particular wavelength or a very narrow range of wavelengths. If the wavelength of the energy is in the visible range, it is

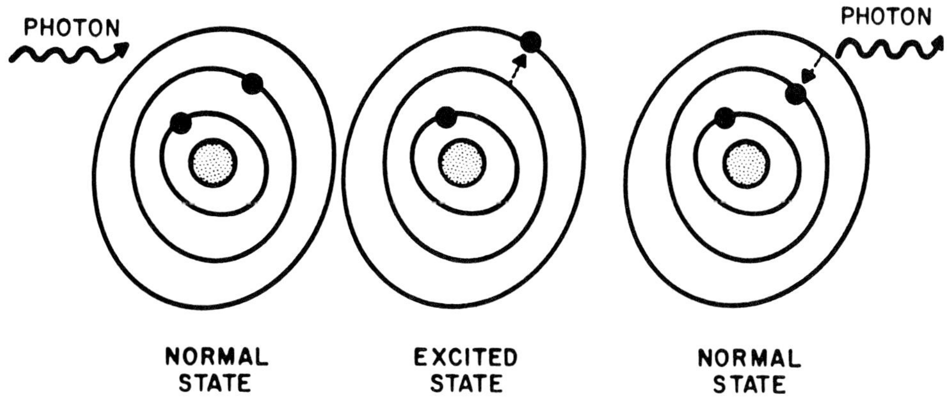

FIG 4–2.
Spontaneous emission. An atom absorbs the energy of a photon by elevating an electron to a higher orbit and then spontaneously releases the energy as a second photon. (From White RA: Basic physics of laser energy in arterial surgery, in Bergan J, Yao JST (eds): *New Diagnostic and Operative Techniques.* New York, Grune & Stratton, 1988, pp 33–45. Used by permission.)

correctly called laser light and will have a color corresponding to its particular wavelength. Normal white light from a source such as a lamp contains the entire spectrum of wavelengths of visible light. When the light is passed through a prism, the individual wavelengths are separated to produce the characteristic colors in the pattern of a rainbow. When laser energy is passed through a prism, because of the select wavelength distribution, only one wavelength or color is visible (Fig 4–4).

Laser light is also described as directional. Directionality or collimation means that the laser energy is released in a highly concentrated, parallel beam with minimal amounts of light spread. As an example, light emitted from a light bulb is not directional and spreads so that it lights up the whole room. In contrast, laser light emitted in a dark room only illuminates a very small spot the same size as that of the laser light source. Spread of laser energy is so minimal that a point source aimed at the moon only spreads to the extent that it would illuminate a circle approximately one-half mile in diameter on the moon's surface.[10] The direc-

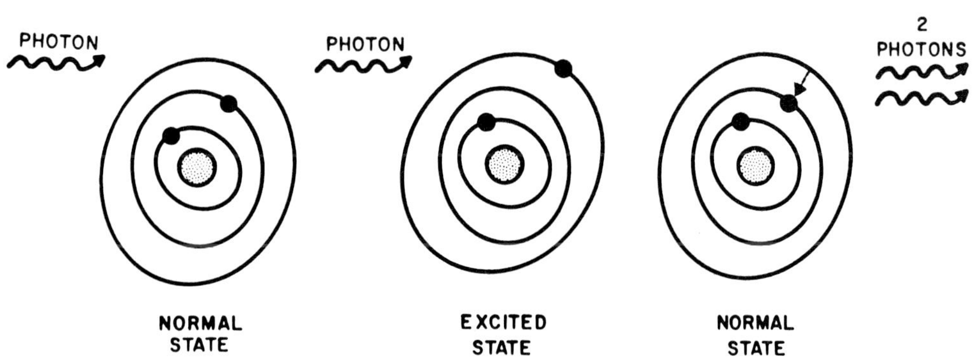

FIG 4–3.
Stimulated emission. (From White RA: Basic physics of laser energy in arterial surgery, in Bergan J, Yao JST (eds): *New Diagnostic and Operative Techniques.* New York, Grune & Stratton, 1988, pp 33–45. Used by permission.)

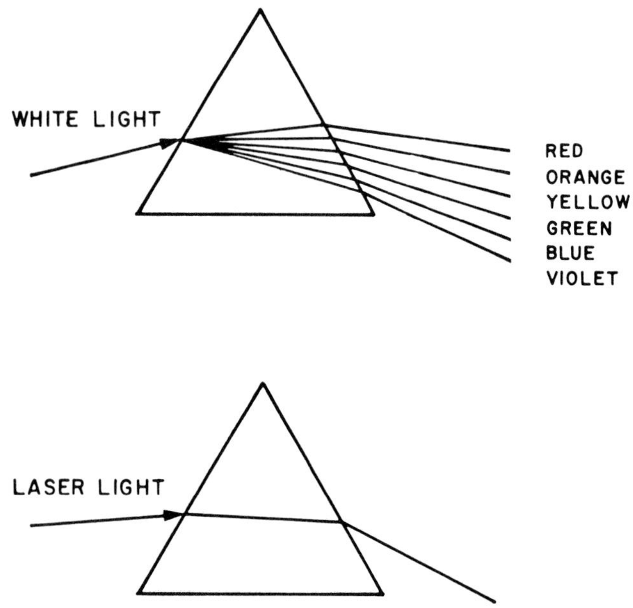

FIG 4–4.
Monochromacity of laser energy. White light passed through a prism is separated into its component wavelengths to produce the colors of the rainbow. Laser light has a select wavelength spectrum. (From White RA: Basic physics of laser energy in arterial surgery, in Bergan J, Yao JST (eds): *New Diagnostic and Operative Techniques.* New York, Grune & Stratton, 1988, pp 33–45. Used by permission.)

tional characteristics of laser energy are important factors in the ability to precisely control its use. The amount of divergence of laser light is quantitated in millirads. One millirad is 1,000th of a radian (a radian is the length of circumference of a circle that is equal to the length of the radius of the circle). The amount of divergence of the laser energy in millirads is an important descriptive specification for a particular laser because any amount of divergence of the energy from the laser results in an exponential decrease in the amount of energy delivered to the tissue.

The third unique property of laser energy is that it is coherent. According to the wave theory of electromagnetic radiation, the waveform of laser energy can be characterized according to wavelength, amplitude, and frequency. Amplitude is the ventricle height of the wave, wavelength (λ) is the distance between two successive wave peaks, and frequency *(f)* is the inverse of the wavelength with the velocity of light *(c)* being 186,000 miles per second ($c = \lambda f$). The light waves emitted from a normal lamp are incoherent in that the waveforms have different amplitudes and different frequencies and are not aligned spatially as to peaks and valleys of the waveform. Laser energy is coherent in that all of the waveform amplitudes, frequency, and temporal distribution of the peaks and valleys of the curves are the same (Fig 4–5).

The most important parameter that is used to describe the overall laser-tissue interaction and enables quantitation of the amount of energy distributed so that a particular interaction is reproducible is the power density, or energy fluence. These two terms are used interchangeably in the literature and may be referred to as fluence. The energy fluence is described in joules per centimeter squared and is equal to laser power output (watts) times the exposure

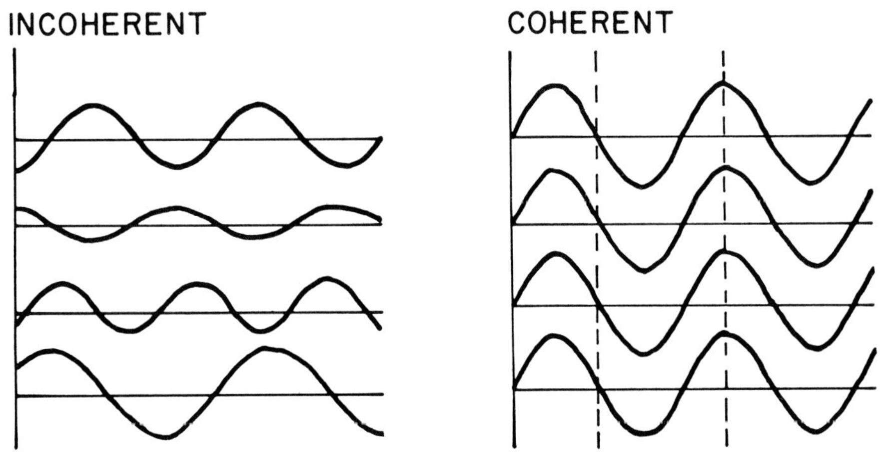

FIG 4–5.
Incoherent vs. coherent waveforms. (From White RA: Basic physics of laser energy in arterial surgery, in Bergan J, Yao JST (eds): *New Diagnostic and Operative Techniques.* New York, Grune & Stratton, 1988, pp 33–45. Used by permission.)

time (second) divided by the laser cross-sectional area (cm^2) where it interacts with the tissue.

$$\text{Energy fluence} = \frac{\text{Laser power output (W)} \times \text{exposure time (s)}}{\text{Laser beam cross-sectional area } (cm^2)}$$

To enable precise delivery of laser energy at some distance from the source, such as into the abdomen during laparoscopy, various types of delivery systems are available. For certain types of lasers (Nd:YAG, potassium titanyl phosphate [KTP], and argon) this is easily accomplished by using quartz fiber optics. CO_2 laser energy is absorbed by the quartz fibers and therefore must be transmitted by other methods. CO_2 laser energy is currently delivered to the operating field by articulating arms (series of reflective mirrors) or through hollow waveguides.

In most cases the fiber-optic delivery systems absorb approximately 10% to 20% of the laser energy. The amount of energy transmitted also varies with wavelength of the light, the diameter and quality of the fiber, and the shape of the fiber tip. Upon transmission through the fiber, the collimated laser light bounces from side to side as it travels through the fiber. This change of direction causes the laser light to diverge 10 to 15 degrees as it exits the fiber tip (Fig 4–6). The divergence property can be used to vary the power density (watts/area) and resultant tissue effects (cutting or coagulating) by changing the distance between the fiber tip and the tissue.

When laser energy interacts with the tissue, it may be absorbed, transmitted, scattered, and/or reflected. Laser-tissue interactions are dependent upon how the laser energy is dissipated and the absorption characteristics of the tissue for the particular wavelength. When tissue absorption occurs, the laser energy produces variable effects depending on the type of interaction. These include laser photochemical effects (chemical bond disruption), laser fluorescence (re-emission of photons), or photothermal changes (heat-producing vibration and collision of atoms).

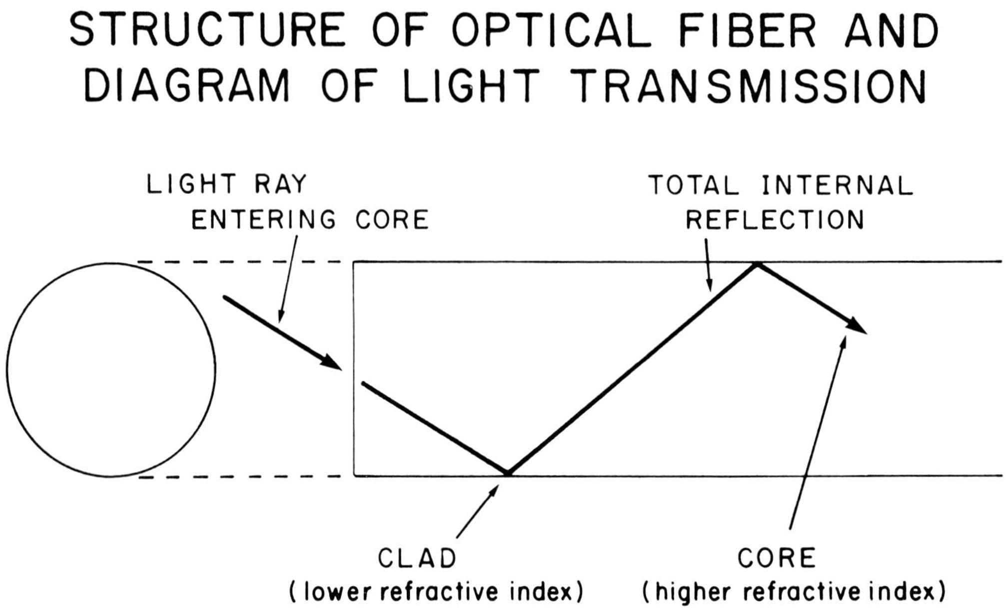

FIG 4–6.
Transmission through the optic fiber causes the laser light to bounce from side to side, thus losing its coherent property. For this reason, laser light diverges at an angle of 10 to 15 degrees following emission from the fiber tip.

Currently the lasers most commonly used for endoscopic surgery are argon (480 to 540 nm), Nd:YAG (1,060 nm), and the combined Nd:YAG and frequency-doubled Nd:YAG (532 nm). Argon energy and the 532-nm component of the KTP laser (Laserscope, Inc, San Jose, Calif) have similar hemostatic effects and depth of penetration (400 to 800 μm). Both are primarily absorbed by chromagens such as hemoglobin or melanin, and this enhances their superficial coagulative effects. The Nd:YAG laser is not particularly well absorbed by any tissue elements; thus it penetrates deeply (1 to 4 mm) and is used for tissue coagulation and necrosis.

Another commonly used laser in endoscopic procedures is the CO_2 laser. CO_2 laser energy is primarily absorbed by water. For this reason it is good for cutting applications because it rapidly vaporizes the water and tissue at the surface. CO_2 lasers have been used extensively in laparoscopic gynecology procedures. The CO_2 energy is delivered by articulating arms and hollow waveguides.

When using a laser with a laparoscope or video camera system, it is advisable to install a filter in front of the lens or camera adapter that absorbs the particular laser wavelength being used. The filters protect the photosensitive elements within the camera and enhance visualization by eliminating the glare of light from visible wavelengths.

Laser Safety

Establishment of a laser safety protocol, facility specifications, approvals, in-service training sessions, and continuing education for personnel are essential to maintain a safe environment.

Personnel training regarding operating procedures and precautions to prevent personal injury and property damage must be given to all laser users. Only certified personnel should be permitted to set up, use, and discontinue use of laser equipment. Although laser radiation can cause eye damage, skin burns, and combustion of flammable materials, these hazards can easily be averted by a carefully planned program.

The physician and all key operating room personnel should be fully versed with an understanding of laser physics, appropriate nomenclature regarding laser energy, and laser-tissue interactions.[11, 12] The physician user is ultimately responsible for selecting the wattage and appropriate lens or fiber for each procedure. However, a laser safety officer or his designee should be present at all cases (American National Standard for the Safe Use of Lasers in Health Care Facilities, American National Standards Institute [ANSI] Z136.3, 1988).

Laser procedure and operating rooms must have all windows covered with nontransparent barriers to prevent the inadvertent passage of laser light. All doors must be closed, and access to the room should be restricted while the laser is activated. Clearly visible warning signs with flashing lights to signify that the system is activated are mandatory. The laser should remain in the off position or with the safety shutter closed until ready for use. Control of laser emission by a foot pedal and direction of the beam by hand control greatly enhance the safety. As with the electrocautery or any active device used in laparoscopy, laser energy should be directed and activated only when the tip of the fiber is in the field of view and or in contact with the specific target. Control of fiber-optic laser delivery is similar to the use of electrocautery in that the system is activated only when it is in contact with the tissue being treated. Reflective surgical instruments should be avoided and reflective surfaces in the laser procedure room minimized. Moist sponges in the open operating fields can prevent combustion of dry or paper materials.

Laser energy can affect different parts of the eye depending upon which structure absorbs that particular wavelength. The three areas of most concern are the cornea, lens, and retina. Laser energy outside the visible range ($<$350 nm and $>$1,400 nm) is absorbed by the cornea and lens. Exposure to this energy can produce cataracts and corneal scarring. Laser energy in the visible wavelength is focused by the cornea and lens onto the retina and causes up to 100,000$\times$ amplification of radiant exposure.[13] Careless misdirection of the laser light even at low powers can result in instantaneous burning of the retina and consequent blindness in the visual field corresponding to the burn spot. Everyone in the operating room, including the patient, must have appropriate eye wear during the procedures. For the CO_2 laser, clear plastic or glass lenses are adequate, and wet gauze can be used to protect an anesthetized patients' eyes. Green lenses (nontransparent to 1,060 nm) are recommended for the Nd:YAG laser and amber lenses (nontransparent to 488 to 515 nm) are necessary to absorb the green or blue light of the argon laser. Other lasers with different wavelengths require specific lenses for eye protection as recommended by the manufacturer of the instrumentation.

Lasers are classified according to their potential to cause biologic injury. The parameters used for laser classification are laser power, wavelength, exposure duration, and beam spot size at the area of interest. Lasers are stratified into four classes. Class I, or exempt lasers, produce no hazard under normal operating conditions. The total amount of energy produced is less than the maximum permissible exposure level established by ANSI, and therefore no special facility or safety precautions are needed. Class II lasers are low-power lasers that do not present a visual hazard due to a normal aversion response. The eye normally closes in approximately 0.25 seconds when exposed to a noxious stimulus. This response avoids eye damage from a class II laser. Class IIIa lasers operate with maximum power output ($\leq$5 mW) and power density ($\leq$2.5 mW/cm^2). These lasers present a hazard if viewed through collecting optics but present no hazard if viewed momentarily with the unaided eye. Class IIIb lasers can damage the eyes if viewed directly but present no hazard to the skin. Class IV denotes high-power laser systems that are hazardous to the eyes, skin, and flammable material from a direct and/or diffusely reflected beam. Facility requirements vary with the class of laser being used. Generally, class IV lasers are used in surgical applications, and therefore operating facilities must be set up in accordance with requirements for this classification.[12, 13]

The most frequent cause of laser injury in industrial environments is electrical accidents. Activation of the laser systems frequently requires high current; thus the electrical outlets should be carefully positioned when the room is designed. Adequate warning signs and in-service training are essential to prevent inadvertent accidents. Maintenance is to be performed by trained technicians only. Laser use and maintenance records must be kept from the date of installation. The laser system should be stored so that components and the ignition key are secured when the laser is not being used. Table 4–1 summarizes the pertinent guideline and procedures that should be included in a laser standards of practice.

Although the risk of airborne contaminants with laparoscopic laser applications is minimal, users should be aware that precautions must be implemented to prevent exposure and inhalation of laser plume. There is still a controversy whether laser plume contains viable cancer and/or mutagenic cells or whether laser exposure destroys these organisms. A closed-system smoke evacuator should be used if exposure to laser plume is likely to occur. Dangerous by-products may also be released from inorganic materials. Plastic bottles, drapes, instruments, polytetrafluoroethylene (PTFE) prosthetic materials, and tubing may emit poisonous gases if exposed to laser energy.

TABLE 4–1.

Laser Standards of Practice: Operational Guidelines

A. Prior to beginning any laser procedure, the laser safety officer and the user must be sure that
   1. There are no flammable chemicals in the room.
   2. Opaque barriers are intact to prevent propagation outside the controlled access area.
   3. There is adequate ventilation to eliminate laser plume and hazardous concentration of by-products if plastics or combustibles are used in the procedure.
   4. Warning signs on the entrance door and laser and English labels on laser controls are intact.
   5. The entrance door to the controlled area is secured.

B. During procedures
   1. Appropriate protective eyewear must be worn by all personnel and by the patient.
   2. The user must be sure that the laser beam path is free of specularly reflective surfaces and combustible materials and that the beam is terminated in a noncombustible, nonreflective barrier.
   3. Lasers are to be activated, when possible, by foot pedal control and directed to the operative site by handpieces to maximize accuracy and safety.

C. Following laser operative procedures
   1. The laser is to be turned off before the controlled access entrance is opened.
   2. The key to the laser control is to be removed when the laser is not in use to prevent unauthorized operation.
   3. The laser operating entrance is to be locked at all times when the facility is not in use, or the instrumentation must be secured in some way to prevent unauthorized use.

ULTRASONIC SCALPELS

In 1880, Jacques and Pierre Curie discovered the piezoelectric effect of various crystals.[14] They found that mechanical stress applied to a crystal resulted in a electrical potential whose magnitude was proportional to the applied stress. Shortly after the initial discovery, the Curies verified the converse piezoelectric effect in which application of a voltage across these crystals created a mechanical stress. This reverse piezoelectric phenomenon and associated motor generator properties, when used at frequencies too high for human perception (above 20 kHz), create ultrasonic waves. The applications of ultrasound to medicine and biology have been to receive and analyze signals or to generate and transmit ultrasound waves.

High-power ultrasonic scalpels are other devices that may have application in the laparoscopic armamentarium. At the present time these devices consist of pencil grip surgical handpieces containing a transducer that oscillates a titanium tip longitudinally at 23 kHz. Figure 4–7 displays a modern ultrasonic surgical unit. The vibration is imperceptible (approximately 100 μm), but sufficient heat is generated to burn through the surgical glove on contact. Cooling is provided by saline irrigation over the tip of the device. Hodgson et al. have used the ultrasonic scalpel in general surgery for liver resection.[15] This device selectively fragments the target tissue and skeletonizes hepatic vessels so they can be secured before division. Other applications of ultrasound ablation devices that are being evaluated include percutane-

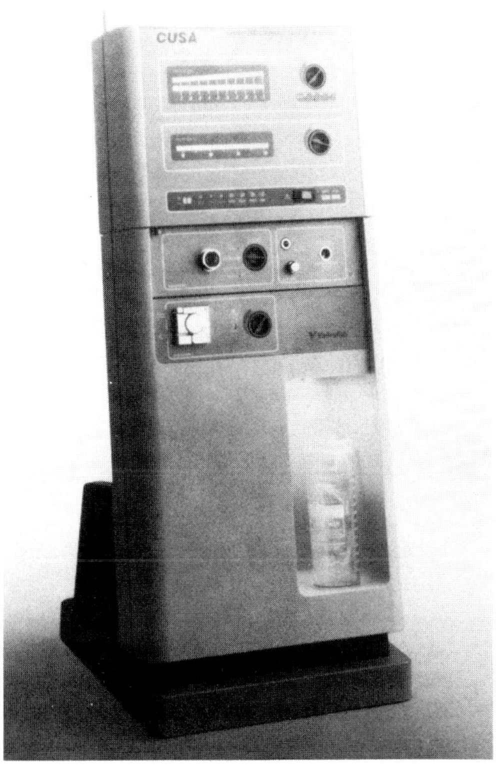

FIG 4–7.
Ultrasonic surgical unit.

ous dissolution of genitourinary stones,[16] excision of intracranial tumors,[17] decalcification of cardiac valves,[18] and recanalization of atherosclerotic arteries.[19]

UTILITY OF VARIOUS DEVICES

Lasers are expensive equipment that have unique space and facility requirements. Unless they fulfill a need or offer superior results that are not available by current, less expensive technologies, the use of lasers is not appropriate. As outlined below, there may be several potential advantages that lasers offer the endoscopic surgeon.

In an experimental study comparing endoscopic coagulative effects of monopolar electrocoagulation (MP), bipolar electrocoagulation (BP), argon laser photocoagulation (AR), and Nd:YAG photocoagulation (YAG), Johnson et al. found that each method was effective at stopping bleeding in the canine ulcer model.[20] They reported that the order of increasing tissue injury (or decreased margin of safety) was AR, BP, YAG, and MP.[20] Both lasers were found to be much easier to manipulate and control than electrocoagulation. The order of decreasing ease of application was YAG, AR, MP, BP. With electrocoagulation, visualizing, touching, and coagulating the bleeding point was often difficult endoscopically. Contact and tissue adherence during BP and MP treatment sometimes temporarily increased bleeding.

In another study Hunter et al. evaluated the colonic effect of MP, AR, and YAG.[21] This study on normal canine colonic mucosa found that at mucosal ablation energy levels, minimal energy was required to cause necrosis of mucosa and that AR and YAG caused significantly less necrosis of surrounding tissues than MP when applied at energies above the ablation threshold. Although the YAG injuries were deeper than with AR, this was not significant at low energy densities. The thermal tissue damage noted histologically with all three thermal devices was greatest 6 days after application. The conclusions drawn from this study were that transmural tissue necrosis occurred with AR, YAG, and MP at six, two, and one times the mucosal ablation energy respectively. This suggests that AR and YAG may be safer then MP.

In a subsequent report of 222 endoscopic gastrointestinal laser procedures, Hunter et al. noted that both the AR and YAG lasers were equally useful with separate therapeutic applications determined by the characteristics of wavelength.[22] The AR laser (penetration depth, approximately 1 mm) was most effectively used for the treatment of mucosal lesions in the small bowel and colon where wall thickness is less than 3 mm. The Nd:YAG laser (penetration depth of 3 to 4 mm) was more effective for gastrointestinal bleeding because of the deeper penetration and the ability to deliver up to six times greater energy. They also found that for large bulky lesions such as tumors, the YAG more rapidly vaporized the lesions than did the AR laser.

Corson et al. reported on the clinical and experimental animal results of laparoscopic treatment of endometriosis with the Nd:YAG laser.[23] The advantage reported for the Nd:YAG laser when compared with electrosurgical techniques was the ability to accurately deliver energy to a precise location with minimal damage to adjacent normal tissue. The investigators used the Nd:YAG laser because of precision provided by the fiber-optic delivery as compared with CO_2 lasers for this study, which require rigid delivery systems.

REFERENCES

1. Cushing H, Bovie WT: Electrosurgery as an aid to the removal of intracranial tumors. *Surg Gynecol Obstet* 1928; 47:751.
2. Dobbie AK: The electrical aspects of surgical diathermy. *Biomed Engin* 1969; 4:206.
3. Ragins H, Shinya H, Wolff WI: The explosive potential of caloric gas during colonoscope electrosurgical polypectomy. *Surg Gynecol Obstet* 1974; 138:554.
4. Bigard MA, Gaucher P, Lassalle C: Fatal colonic explosion during colonoscopic polypectomy. *Gastroenterology* 1979; 77:1307–1310.
5. Pearce JA: Electrosurgical arc burns at dispersive electrode sites. Presented at the Association for the Advancement of Medical Instrumentation, 19th Annual Meeting, 1984, p 65.
6. Peterson HB, Ory HW: Deaths associated with laparoscopic sterilization by unipolar electrocoagulating devices. *Am J Obstet Gynecol* 1981; 139:141–143.
7. Hoffer FD, Pent D: Indications, contraindications and complications of laparoscopy. *Obstet Gynecol Surg* 1975; 30:407.
8. Ward PH, Castro DJ, Ward S: A significant new contribution to radical head and neck surgery. *Arch Otolaryngol Head Neck Surg* 1989; 115:921–923.
9. Einstein A: Zur quantem Theorie dr. Strahlung. *Phys Zeit* 1917; 18:121.
10. Hallmark C: *Lasers, the Light Fantastic.* Blueridge Summit, Pa, TAB Books, 1979.
11. Arndt KA, Noe JM, Northam BC: Laser therapy-basic concepts and nomenclature. *J Am Acad Dermatol* 1981; 5:649–654.
12. American National Standard for the Safe Use of Lasers. New York, American National Standards Institute, 1980, ANSI Z 130.1.
13. A Guide For the Control of Laser Hazards. Cincinnati, American Conference of Governmental Industrial Hygienists, 1981.
14. Curie PJ, Curie PJ: Crystal physics: Development by pressure of polar electricity in hejhedral crystal with inclined faces. *Comptes rendus hebdom adaires des seances de L'Academis de Science.* 1880; 91:294.
15. Hodgson WJ, Delguercio LR: Preliminary experience in liver surgery using the ultrasonic scalpel. *Surgery* 1984; 95:230–234.
16. Segura JW, LeRoy AJ: Percutaneous ultrasound lithotripsy. *Urology* 1984; 23:7–10.
17. Chan KK, Watmoush DJ, Hope DT, et al: A new motor-driven surgical probe and its in-vitro comparison with cavitron ultrasonic surgical aspirator. *Ultrasound Med Biol* 1986; 12:279–283.
18. Brown AH, Davies PG: Ultrasonic decalcification of calcified cardiac valves and annuli. *Br Med J* 1972; 3:274–277.
19. Siegel RJ, Don Michael TA, Fishbein MC, et al: In vivo ultrasound arterial recanalization of atherosclerotic total occlusions. *J Am Coll Cardiol* 1990; 15:345–351.
20. Johnson JH, Jensen DM, Mautner W: Comparison of endoscopic electrocoagulation and laser photocoagulation of bleeding canine ulcers. *Gastroenterology* 1982; 82:904–910.
21. Hunter JG, Burt RW, Becker JM, et al: Colonic mucosal lesions: Evaluation of monopolar electrocautery, argon laser and neodymium:YAG laser. *Curr Surg* 1984; 41:373–375.
22. Hunter JG, Bowers JH, Burt RW, et al: Lasers in endoscopic gastrointestinal surgery. *Am J Surg* 1984; 148:736–741.
23. Corson SL, Unger M, Kwa D, et al: Laparoscopic laser treatment of endometriosis with the Nd:YAG sapphire probe. *Am J Obstet Gynecol* 1989; 160:718–723.

Chapter 5

Laparoscopic Principles and Techniques

Stanley R. Klein, M.D.

It is only by meticulous attention to detail, complete familiarity with the instruments, a thorough knowledge of abdominal anatomy, and increasing experience with laparoscopy that endoscopic surgery can be performed safely, accurately, and for the maximum benefit of the patient. It is the purpose of this chapter to outline for the reader those aspects of the techniques of diagnostic and therapeutic laparoscopy that form the basis of the author's practices. The details pertaining to availability and proper use of the described instrumentation or equipment are found in Chapter 2.

HISTORICAL PERSPECTIVE

It is a tribute to the usefulness of laparoscopy as a basic diagnostic examination and as a basis for operative procedures that there have been many modifications and innovations added since it was first popularized.[1–3] At the turn of the century, European internists invaded the abdominal cavity with specula and optics to visualize and diagnose diseases of the liver and gallbladder. "Peritoneoscopy" was practiced by internists as an office procedure using local anesthesia with the patient lying on an examining table. Gynecologists attempting visualization through the vaginal route encountered the small intestines when the optical scopes were introduced through the cul-de-sac. However, it was not until 1944, when Decker in the United States used the knee-chest position to create a pneumoperitoneum through the cul de-sac, that gynecologic endoscopy became clinically useful through culdoscopy. In the same year, Palmer of France used the transabdominal approach, Trendelenburg position, and general anesthesia to establish laparoscopy as a productive diagnostic endeavor.

In the mid-20th century, endoscopes were lenses illuminated with small, hot bulbs; when placed inside body cavities, there was a great risk of bowel burn, and photography was impossible. Rapid technological developments in the field of fiber-optic light cables that allowed powerful but cool light into the abdomen and the development of imaging optics led European innovators to explore the potential of laparoscopy more fully.[4] The recent trend toward "less invasive surgery" with more procedures performed through the laparoscope by using direct visual assistance as well as x-ray and ultrasound guidance is accelerating.[5] It is essential that the contemporary surgeon be appropriately familiar not only with the latest status of laparoscopic surgical procedures but their foundations and risks as well.[6]

ANATOMIC CONSIDERATIONS

A thorough knowledge of abdominal wall as well as internal anatomy is essential before undertaking a laparoscopic procedure. A review of the anatomy of the anterior abdominal wall and its variations is valuable even for surgeons who regularly perform major abdominal

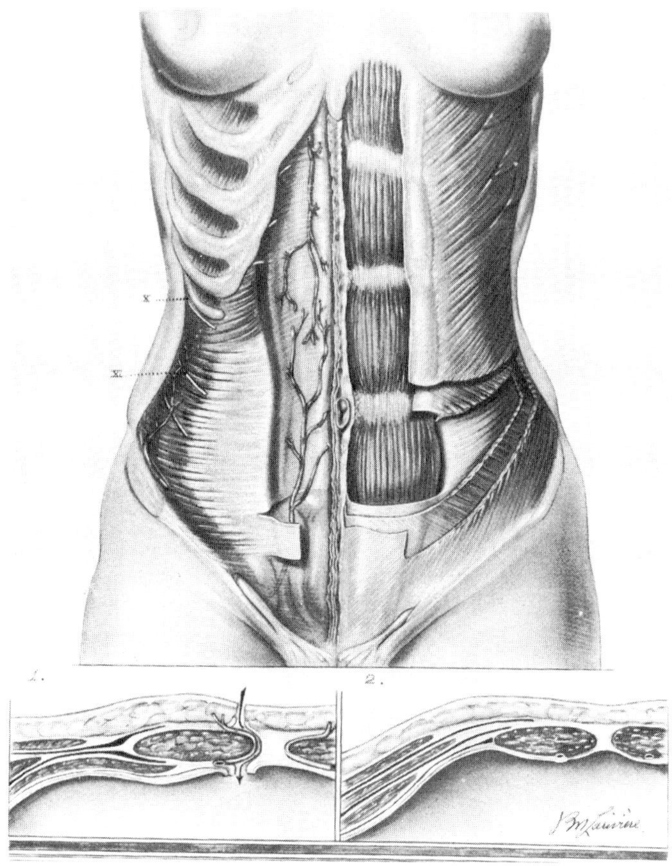

FIG 5–1.
Abdominal wall anatomy in the anteroposterior and cross-sectional projections depicting muscles, fasciae, nerves, and blood supply. *Top,* internal and external oblique muscles on the reader's left have been removed, leaving the transversus abdominis muscle. *Bottom,* (1) transverse section of the abdominal wall above the umbilicus and (2) transverse section of the anterior abdominal wall below the semilunar line of Douglas. Note the difference in the fascial origins of the rectus sheath (From Maingot R: *Abdominal Operations,* ed 5. New York, Appleton-Century-Crofts, 1969. Used by permission.)

operations. The umbilicus and its relationship to auxiliary puncture sites should be familiar to the laparoscopist not only for preventing iatrogenic morbidity but also to gain optimal surgical exposure as well as identify and correct an abnormal condition when it is encountered.

Muscles and Fasciae

The anterolateral abdominal muscles and their corresponding aponeuroses are illustrated in Figure 5–1. For all practical purposes, the linea alba is considered a single layer. The planes of the abdominal wall gain increased importance when ancillary trocar insertion sites are to be made lateral to the linea alba. Two layers of fascia as well as the peritoneum will be traversed when puncturing above the semilunar line of Douglas, whereas only a single fascial layer is encountered when entering below that line (Fig 5–1).

Vessels

The superficial epigastric artery arises from the femoral artery about 1 cm below the inguinal ligament. It ascends in the subcutaneous tissue of the anterior abdominal wall, lateral to the rectus muscle, until it reaches the level of the umbilicus.

The inferior epigastric artery arises from the external iliac artery just above the inguinal ligament. After crossing the line of Douglas, it ascends posterior to the rectus muscle but ventral to the posterior rectus fascial layer. It divides into several branches that anastomose with the terminal branches of the superior epigastric artery, a division of the internal thoracic artery. These arteries are accompanied by their corresponding veins. The terminal branches of the intercostal arteries, veins, and nerves run circumferentially around the trunk between the inner two layers of muscle, eventually penetrating the rectus sheath and joining the epigastric vascular arcade. Under conditions of portal hypertension the accompanying abdominal wall subcutaneous veins may significantly enlarge and are subject to potential injury.

The lower margin of the umbilicus provides the optimum location for inserting the Veress needle and primary laparoscopic cannula. At the level of the umbilicus, the skin of the anterior abdominal wall is attached to the fascial layer and parietal peritoneum with little intervening subcutaneous fat or muscular tissue. The fibrous tissue found at the lower pole represents the remnants of the obliterated umbilical vessels and the upper end of the urachus (Fig 5–2).

If the linea alba is penetrated for an ancillary cannula to gain access into the peritoneal cavity, few other organs or vascular structures should be encountered within the abdominal wall that are susceptible to injury. Infraumbilically, the major exception is a patent urachus or urachal cyst. By contrast, when one chooses a lateral lower quadrant site to enter the abdominal cavity, the location of the superficial and deep inferior epigastric vessels should be remembered.

Previous abdominal surgery or inflammatory conditions may distort normal textbook anatomy. The presence of an abdominal scar should make the endoscopic surgeon wary of a blind peritoneal cavity entry. Unusual intraperitoneal anatomic variants are encountered, and their recognition is described in subsequent sections of this text.

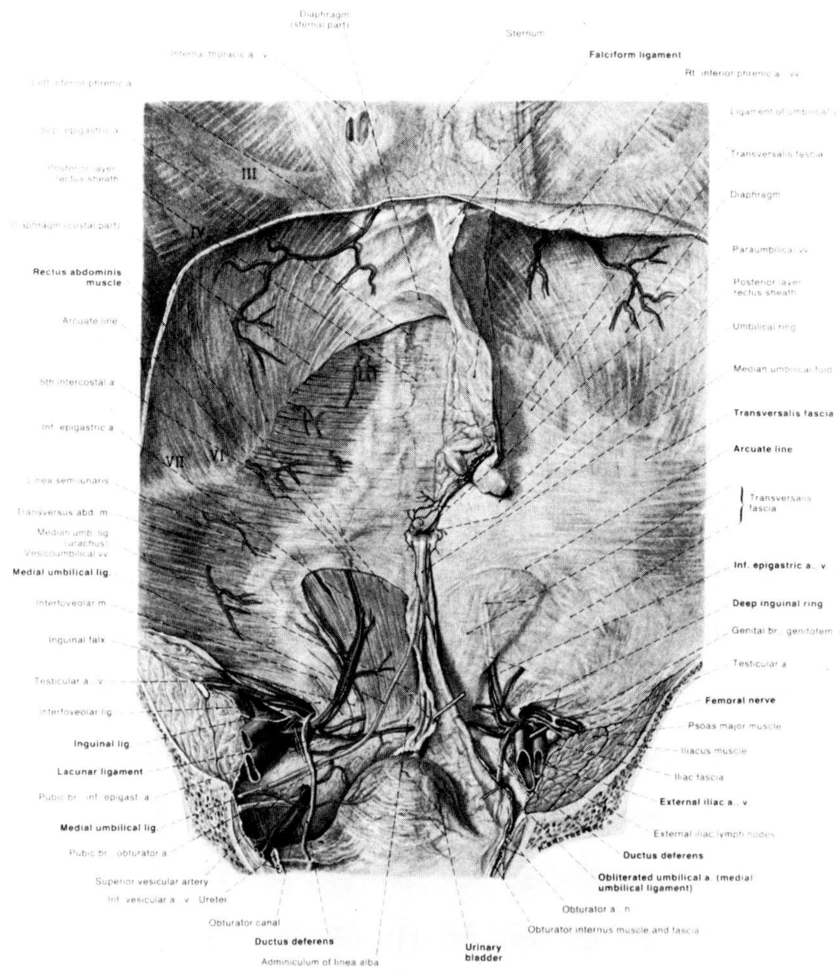

FIG 5–2.
A posterior view of the anterior abdominal wall demonstrates important laparoscopic anatomic landmarks. These include the umbilicus, urachus, obliterated umbilical vein, and falciform ligament. (From Clemente CD: *Anatomy: A Regional Atlas of the Human Body,* ed 3. Baltimore, Urban & Schwarzenberg, 1987. Used by permission.)

PREOPERATIVE PREPARATION

In order for the surgeon to be in control of the procedure, it is imperative that disciplined preparation of the patient, instruments, and equipment occur in a prescribed manner.[7]

THE PATIENT

Prior to performing an endoscopic surgical procedure, a complete history and physical examination should be performed. The patient's fitness to undergo general anesthesia (if appropriate) must be determined and appropriate consultation obtained. In general, evaluation should be no less rigorous than in the case of an open version of the same procedure because any endoscopic endeavor may require conventional surgical exposure during the operation. Particular attention should be directed to the patient's laboratory coagulation profile. A prothrombin time of 3 to 4 seconds above the control and a minimum platelet count of 70,000/mm^3 should constitute the tolerable upper and lower limits of safe feasibility for the procedure. In our opinion, known portal hypertension and pregnancy are contraindications for endoscopic surgery at this time.

Informed consent must be obtained in a manner that clearly demonstrates that the patient understands the nature of the procedure (laparoscopy and endosurgery) to be performed, its objectives, and its potential hazards. It is stressed that the patient should be counseled and the informed consent reflect that they have been apprised of the other available therapeutic options. Information in the form of a written pamphlet that details the procedure might be offered to the patient. If ambulatory surgery is contemplated, the patient should be given a separate information sheet (or video cassette) describing the specific preparatory steps for that procedure and laparoscopy in general. Pertinent preoperative instructions to the patient include the following:

1. No intake on the day of surgery (special counseling for the diabetic requiring insulin).
2. Avoidance of self-administered enemas.
3. The patient should empty his bladder immediately prior to premedication administration.
4. Information regarding what to expect after the procedure.

Laparoscopic Instruments and Equipment

Before the patient enters the operating room, it is the responsibility of the surgeon to ensure that all equipment is present and in working order. Appropriate ancillary surgical instrumentation should be sterilized and assembled to avoid intraoperative delays. The light source should be tested and the fiber-optic cable connected. The author would suggest that, if possible, backup equipment be available. Given the proliferation of endoscopic surgery in multiple surgical disciplines, integration of intrahospital system components is feasible.

Particular attention must be directed to the electrosurgical system, especially if the unipolar mode is to be employed. There should be no evidence of frayed wires or defects in insulated instruments, the ground plate should be well lubricated, and all electrosurgical laparoscopic instruments must be compatible with the electrosurgical generator.

ANESTHESIA AND PATIENT POSITIONING

Although diagnostic laparoscopy can be performed under local anesthesia, we find it necessary to use general anesthesia when operative procedures are planned. General anesthesia offers greater comfort to the patient and less stress for the operating team. While the nature of the general anesthetic agents used are in the province of the anesthesiologist, certain basic principles should be stressed. Because of the risk of hypercarbia, patients should be intubated and receive assisted ventilation. Standard monitoring including oximetry and capnography is helpful. For selective diagnostic indications, regional anesthesia will provide adequate pain relief to accomplish limited objectives.

If the patient is awake at the beginning of the procedure, local anesthetic should be administered prior to attempts at insufflation needle, trocar, or cannula insertions. Local anesthesia can best be accomplished with a 10-mL mixture of 0.5% lidocaine plus 0.25% bupivacaine mixture instilled into the abdominal wall along a tract in the same direction as planned for trocar and cannula insertion (Fig 5–3).[8] It is advisable to elevate the lower abdomen during injection of local anesthesia in the same way that the abdominal wall will be elevated to insert the trocar and sleeve so that the same tissue planes are anesthetized. Very obese patients require great effort to elevate the abdominal wall for the needle or trocar insertion, and hence general anesthesia is recommended.

Organization and positioning of the equipment around the operating table has been reviewed in Chapter 2. For the first few cases, instruments for a laparotomy should be available on the operating field. Subsequently, having them in the operating room will prove satisfactory.

If the surgeon is to stand on the patient's left side, any intravenous lines should enter through the patient's right arm. The presence of an intravenous system in an extended arm can interfere with optimal positioning of the surgeon or his assistant. If the arm is placed by

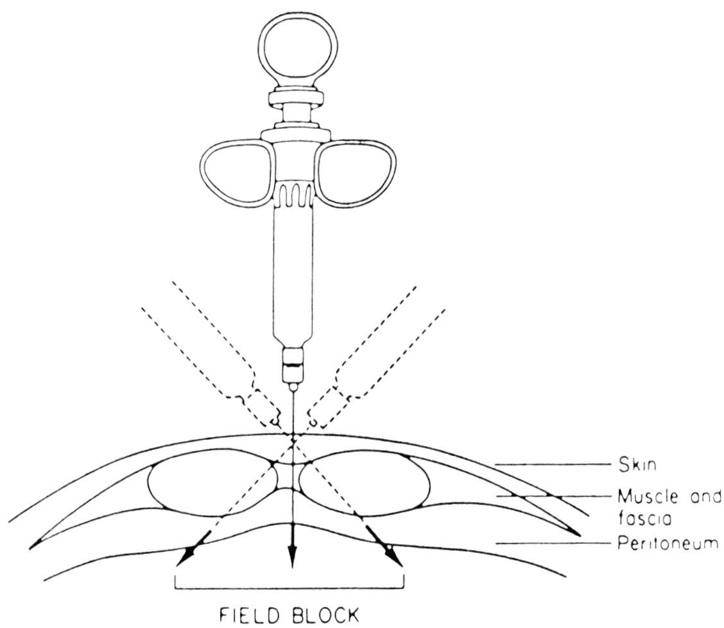

FIG 5–3.
Regional anesthesia for endoscopic diagnosis and/or minor surgery can be achieved by anesthetizing the anterior abdominal wall and cannula tract. The needle attached to a syringe containing the anesthetic agent is inserted to the peritoneum. A 5-cc aliquot of agent is injected. When the needle is withdrawn, 3 to 4 mL of anesthetic is instilled into that tract. The needle is turned 45 degrees to one side, the peritoneum is again reached, and another 3 to 4 mL is instilled while withdrawing the needle. This technique creates satisfactory local anesthesia by a small field block. (From Hulka JF: Gynecologic laparoscopy, in Droegemueller W, Sciarra JJ (eds): *Obstetrics and Gynecology,* vol 1. Philadelphia, Harper & Row Publishers, 1985, p 9. Used by permission.)

the patient's side rather than on an extended arm support, this inconvenience is avoided. Care must be taken that the arm be protected when the table is moved to facilitate laparoscopic manipulations. Appropriate provision for intraoperative x-ray procedures must be made preoperatively.

PNEUMOPERITONEUM

The establishment of an adequate intraperitoneal gas compartment or pneumoperitoneum is fundamental for the visualization of the intraperitoneal organs and for performance of the operative procedure. The risks of misadventure or injury increase dramatically when visualization and exposure are inadequate.[6]

Induction of the Pneumoperitoneum

The Veress needle is usually introduced at the lower border of the umbilicus. Alternatively, it may also be introduced in the area located midway between the pubic symphysis and the umbilicus, immediately supraumbilically in the midline, the lateral border of the rectus at either the left or right of McBurney's point, or the lateral border of the rectus two fingerbreadths below the left costal margin (Fig 5–4).

In patients with abdominal surgical scars, introduction of the Veress needle at the umbilical

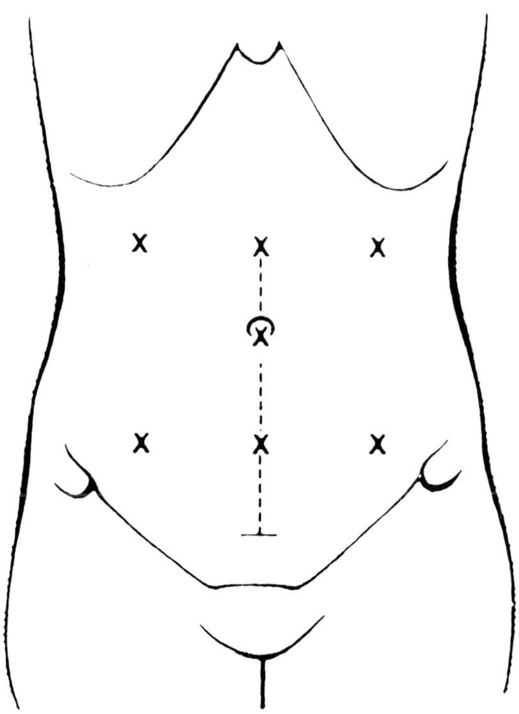

FIG 5–4.
Sites for insertion of the Veress needle to induce pneumoperitoneum.

site may risk injury to intra-abdominal tissues if they are adherent to the abdominal wall. In a small group of patients without prior surgery, tumors or enlarged organs may also be at risk. It is under these circumstances that alternate sites on the abdomen wall or alternate approach techniques (see below) may be selected for pneumoperitoneum induction.

On occasion, the stomach may be inadvertently inflated during induction of anesthesia. In this case, it is at risk of perforation. This can be averted if the upper portion of the abdomen is percussed and any areas of hyperresonance noted. If the stomach is inflated, a nasogastric tube should be introduced and the gas aspirated prior to introducing laparoscopic instruments. Routine placement of a nasogastric tube and Foley drainage catheter has been advocated by several authors, especially prior to upper abdominal endosurgery.

The most common approach to pneumoperitoneum induction involves the Veress needle being inserted through a small incision at the lower border of the umbilicus (Fig 5–5). The size of the incision is dictated by the diameter of the cannula to be placed. A reusable Veress needle must be sharp and the spring stylet checked for free movement. The blunt-ended inner spring-action stylet should protrude beyond the sharply bevelled outer sleeve. This permits one to verify the penetration of the abdominal wall tissue planes by upward displacement of this component of the device as each tissue plane is traversed.

The Veress needle is inserted by grasping it between the finger and thumb at a distance from the end of the needle equal to the thickness of the abdominal wall. If the shaft of the needle is grasped ... this point, a sudden advance beyond the posterior abdominal wall structures will be prevented by the grasping fingers.

To insert the Veress needle, the ulnar border of the hand is rested on the patient's abdomen and the tip of the needle inserted at a 45-degree angle to the abdominal wall through the skin incision (Fig 5–6). The other hand grasps the hypogastrium and elevates the parietes. This maneuver increases the distance between the anterior abdominal wall and retroperitoneal structures but *not* between the ventral body wall and small bowel until the intraperitoneal vacuum is disrupted. As the Veress needle penetrates the peritoneum, the spring-loaded central stylet will advance, thereby indicating that penetration of the peritoneum has occurred. With experience, the surgeon recognizes each layer of the abdomen as it is traversed and identifies peritoneal penetration by the sudden "pop" and decrease in resistence as the tip of the needle enters the peritoneal cavity.

Following peritoneal penetration, the abdomen wall is released, and proper placement of the neeuie tip is confirmed. Proper positioning of the insufflating needle is the most important step ensuring gas insufflation without complications. No gas should be insufflated prior to verification of the proper location of the insufflation needle, and the needle should be held stationary to avert intraperitoneal injury.

Several tests can be employed to document the correct intraperitoneal position of the Verres needle (Fig 5–6).[9] These include percussion of abdominal tympany over the liver, injection and attempted aspiration of 5 cc of saline, and the saline drip test. It must be emphasized that none of these tests is foolproof.

The saline injection test is performed by connecting a 10-cc syringe containing 5 cc of normal saline to the needle. Gentle withdrawal of the plunger should not produce any gas bubbles or blood. With the second maneuver, 5 mL of saline is injected into the peritoneal cavity and aspirated. If the needle is correctly positioned, no saline will be recovered. If the needle has inadvertently entered the bowel, clouded saline may be returned. Intravascular placement is signified by blood in the return. If the needle has not yet entered the peritoneal cavity and

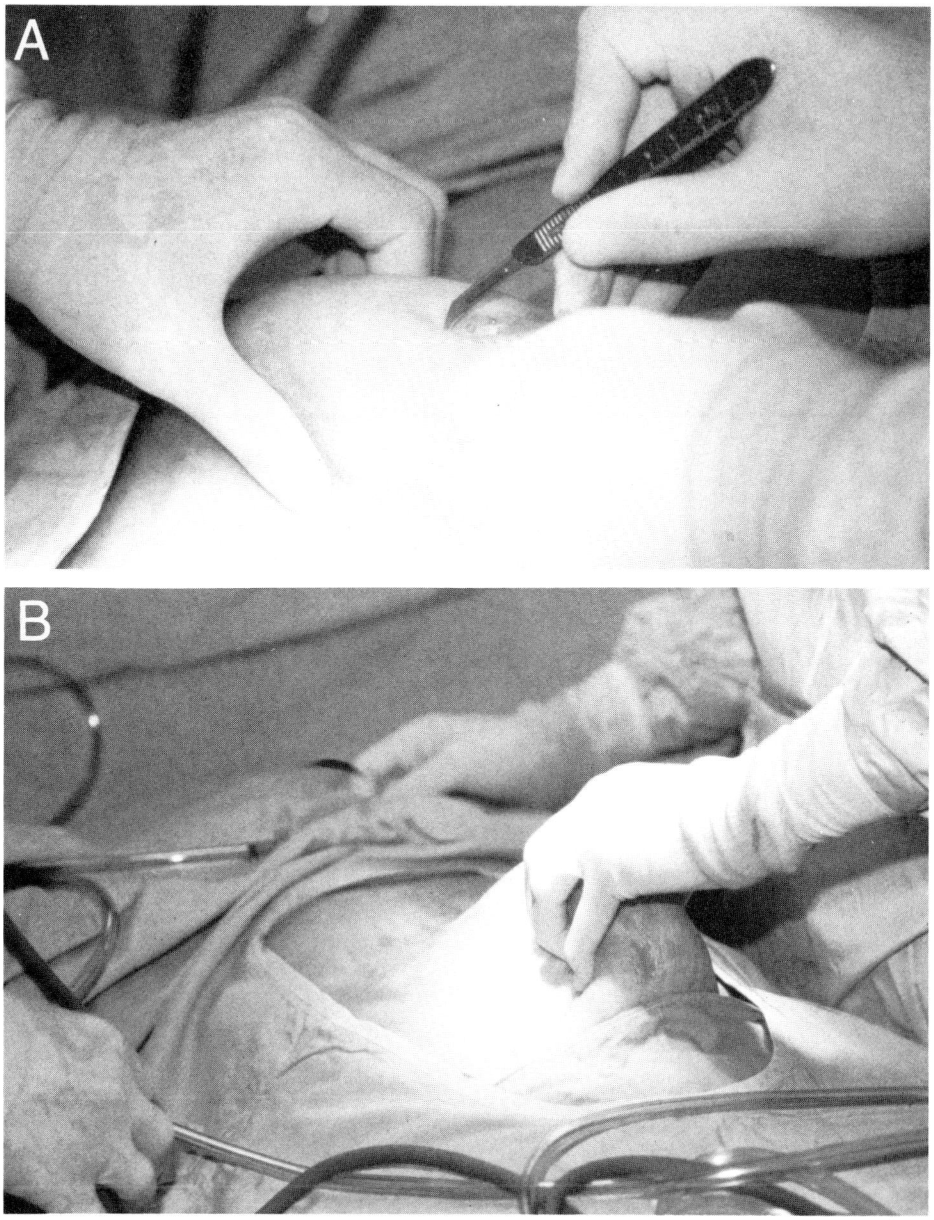

FIG 5–5.
Induction of pneumoperitoneum is most often begun by placing a curved incision at the lower border of the umbilicus **(A).** This is facilitated by using a no. 12 sickle-shaped surgical knife blade. At the time the Veress needle is placed into the peritoneal cavity the anterior body wall should be elevated **(B).** This maneuver does not eliminate risks associated with Veress needle placement.

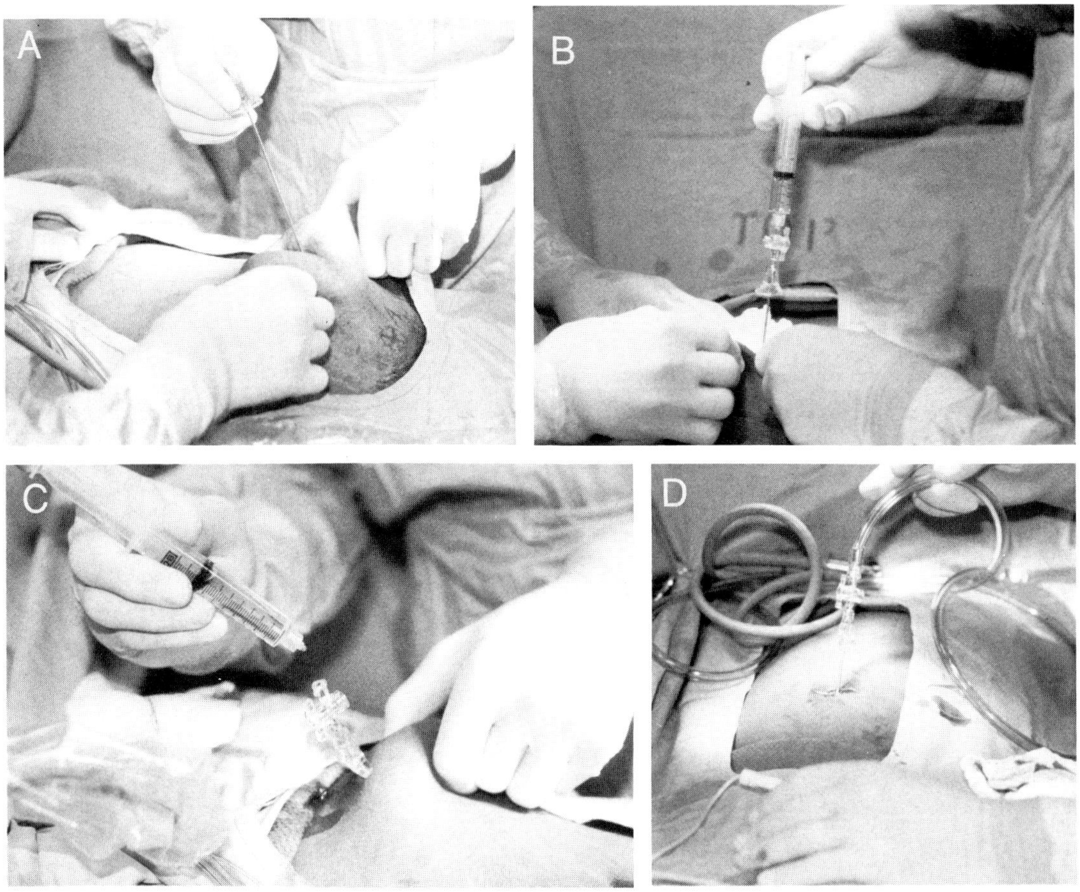

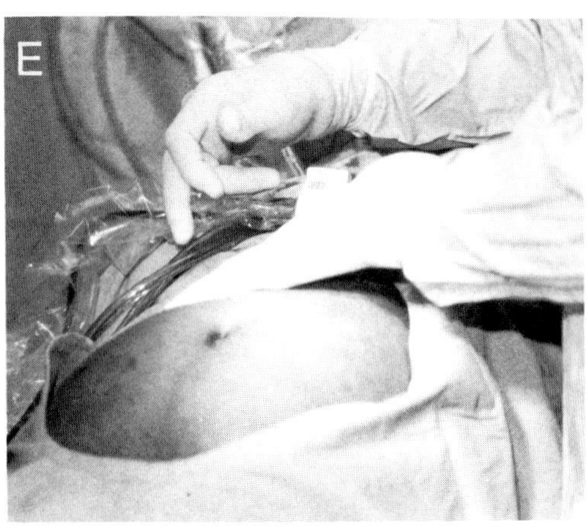

FIG 5–6.
Correct Veress needle insertion and tip placement verification are essential for the successful establishment of a pneumoperitoneum. The needle is usually introduced through a small incision at the lower border of the umbilicus in either a cranial or caudal direction. **A,** the shaft of the needle is grasped at a length equal to the thickness of the abdominal wall to prevent excessive entry. Intraperitoneal placement of the needle is verified by instillation and attempting aspiration of 5 cc of saline **(B)** or the drip test, which is described in the text **(C).** Following verification of Veress needle placement in the peritoneal cavity, the CO_2 insufflation tubing is attached to the hub of the Veress needle and gas instillation begun at a flow rate of 1 L/min **(D).** After 1 L of insufflation, percussion over the liver reveals tympany **(E).**

remains in the preperitoneal space, clear saline may be obtained. Identification of visceral or vascular perforation mandates laparotomy. The surgeon should leave the needle in place while opening the abdomen to facilitate localizing the injury.

The saline "drop test" is a third maneuver and verifies correct needle placement by instilling a single drop of saline on the Luerlock hub of the Veress needle and lifting the anterior abdominal wall. Correct placement is signified by prompt passage of the saline into the peritoneal cavity.

Insufflation

Failure to achieve and maintain a suitable pneumoperitoneum is the most common source of operative procedural failure and is a frequency cause of complications. Once the position of the Veress needle is confirmed within the peritoneal cavity, the CO_2 gas line is connected to the needle and flow begun at 1 L/min. In a well-anesthetized patient, the pressure differential during gas infusion should not be greater than 5 mm Hg. If higher pressures are recorded, the surgeon should suspect that the needle is either in the preperitoneal space, has entered an intra-abdominal viscus, or is tangled in omentum. If insufflation pressures are high, the lower abdominal wall should be grasped with both hands and gently agitated. This manuever will frequently dislodge the omentum from the tip of the needle. If this fails to relieve the increased pressures, the angle of the needle from the plane of the abdominal wall should be increased because, on occasion, the tip may be against the abdominal wall. If neither maneuver relieves the increased pressure, the Veress needle should be removed and replaced. If gas infusion pneumoperitoneum produces preperitoneal emphysema, the gas line should be disconnected from the Veress needle, the preperitoneal space emptied as much as possible, and an alternate site for pneumoperitoneum induction selected.

If gas pressures are normal with flow at 1 L/min, within 45 to 60 seconds percussion over the right costal margin should demonstrate a loss of liver dullness. This occurs without an incremental increase in pressure and is the most convincing demonstration that the Veress needle is within the peritoneal cavity. If, however, after passage of 1 L of gas liver dullness does not disappear, it is almost certain that the tip of the Veress needle is in the preperitoneal space or in a viscus. Under these circumstances, the needle should be withdrawn and repositioned. Continued infusion of gas into a needle in the preperitoneal space may also cause liver dullness to disappear.

Once the surgeon is satisfied that the gas is flowing into the peritoneal cavity, flow rates can be increased to 6 to 8 L/min until between 2 and 4 L has been insufflated. The volume required will depend on the depth of anesthesia, the size of the patient, and the diameter of the trocar and cannula to be inserted. The optimal amount of gas for an individual patient is assessed more by the amount of distension of the abdomen than by the volume of gas infused.

While the gas is flowing, the pressure recorded by the insufflator does not reflect the *true intraperitoneal pressure* unless a special insufflation needle with a separate gas inflow and pressure-monitoring channel is used to provide this information simultaneously. In order to accurately measure intraperitoneal pressure during insufflation, the gas flow is turned off at the insufflator, and the tap on the Veress needle is opened.

Following establishment of the pneumoperitoneum, automatic monitoring modes on the insufflator can be used to maintain the level of pneumoperitoneum, although it is mandatory for the surgeon to continuously monitor intra-abdominal pressures to avert mishaps.

INSERTION OF THE PRIMARY CANNULA AND TROCAR

Once an adequate pneumoperitoneum has been established, the next step is to introduce the principal cannula through which the laparoscopic endoscope will be passed. Depending on several factors relating to the ultimate safety of the procedure, it can be performed closed ("blind") or open. Both techniques will be discussed, and the instrumentation pertinent to both techniques is discussed in Chapter 2.

The risks associated with the closed introduction of the primary cannula and trocar are dependent upon the surgeon's experience, the patient's history of abdominal surgery or intra-abdominal inflammatory conditions, the dimensions of the cannula, and the location of cannula insertion on the abdominal wall.

Cannulas are inserted through a skin incision made at a length to provide a snug approximation of tissue to the device to avert subsequent gas leak. The cannula and trocar are introduced subcutaneously (trocar inside the cannula) for a distance of about 2 cm. The device is inserted at a 45-degree angle to the plane of the abdomen if directed toward the upper abdomen or at 60 degrees if directed toward the pelvis. The ulnar border of the hand not inserting the cannulas is placed on the abdominal wall and encircles the cannula to act as a stop to prevent sudden inadvertent advancement through the abdominal wall (Fig 5–7). The degree of force required to penetrate the different planes of the anterior abdominal wall is proportional to the size of the trocar/cannula unit and inversely related to the sharpness of the trocar. Some resistance to trocar penetration is produced by the distended abdomen, and this necessitates elevation of the subumbilical abdominal wall to avoid indenting the abdominal wall to a point that endangers the retroperitoneal structures. During insertion, gentle rotation of the cannula and trocar may facilitate gradual entry into the peritoneal cavity. Another method of cannula and trocar insertion that minimizes potential injury is for the operator to grasp the cannula with the index finger placed on the device at a level corresponding to the point of maximal planned penetration (Fig 5–8).

Most trocars are hollow, and a hole at the tip permits gas to escape through a proximal opening once the peritoneal cavity has been entered. This indicates to the surgeons that the peritoneal cavity has been entered. At this point, the trocar is retracted inside the cannula sheath, and the cannula is advanced an additional 1 or 2 cm to ensure that it is adequately placed within the peritoneal cavity. The retraction of the reusable trocar into the cannula or automatic safety shield deployment on the disposable version of the trocar is designed to prevent trauma to the intraperitoneal organs during further advancement of the cannula.

Following positioning of the cannula, the trocar is removed, and excess gas is allowed to escape so as to leave in the peritoneal cavity the optimal amount of gas required for the procedure. The endoscope, which previously has been connected to the light source and "white balanced" (see Chapter 3), is introduced. Viewing commences as the endoscope traverses the cannula. If any organ has been impaled by the cannula, it will be visualized by passage of the endoscope. If direct visualization confirms accurate cannula placement, the gas line is attached to the Luerlock on the side of the cannula (lock closed during the initial introduction of the trocar and cannula) and the insufflator changed to the automatic mode.

The major risks associated with the introduction of the primary cannulas and trocars are related to the force that must be exerted and the control that can be applied to the devices. Two factors influence the degree of force required: the tightness of the abdominal skin and the diameter of the cannula.

If insertion of the primary trocar and cannula cannot be accomplished in the umbilical

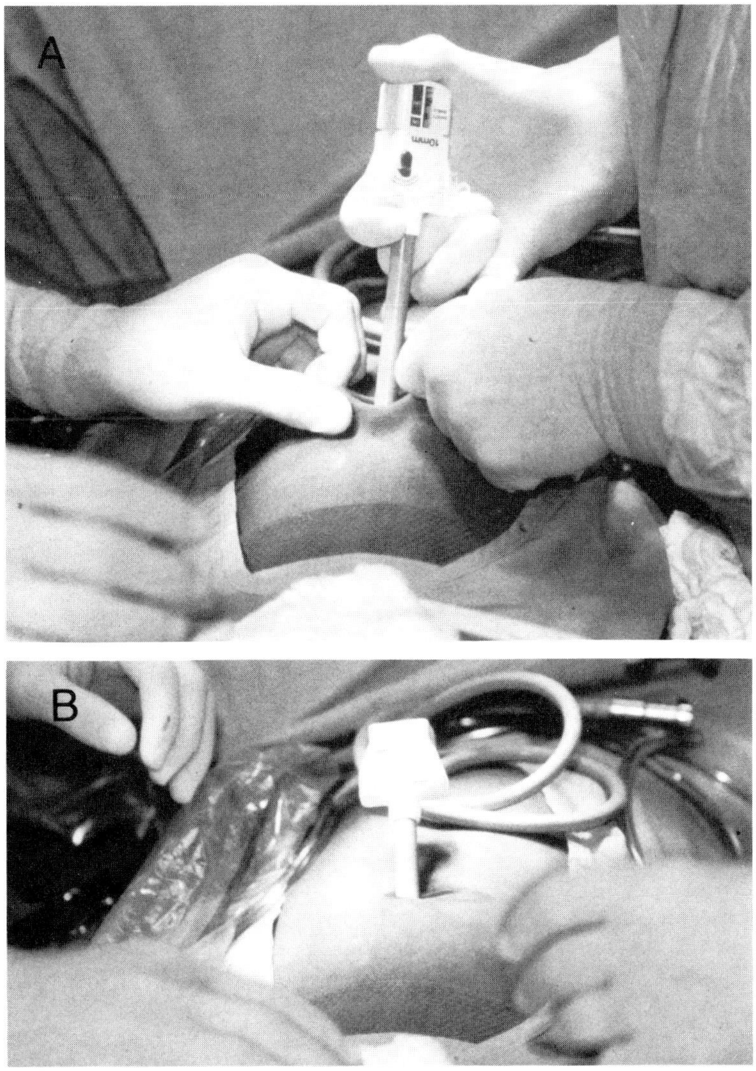

FIG 5–7.
Introduction **(A)** and advancement **(B)** of the primary cannula/trocar unit into the gas-filled abdomen through the periumbilical incision. Note the elevation of the anterior abdominal wall and the angle of trocar insertion.

area, it may be possible to gain abdominal access at another site. In this situation, ancillary cannulas and trocars can be placed initially. A 5-mm telescope is then inserted through the remote ancillary port to directly visualize the placement of the umbilical cannula. The initial 5-mm telescope is then withdrawn, and the cannula is used for subsequent instrument insertion (Fig 5–9).

Once the endoscope has been inserted into the primary cannula and the surgeon is satisfied that no intraperitoneal damage has been rendered by either placement of the Veress needle or primary trocar and cannula, a systematic diagnostic evaluation should be performed. Endoscopic videotaping and photography are part of the procedure.[10] At this point, with the table in the horizontal position, it is appropriate to inspect the upper portion of the abdomen first

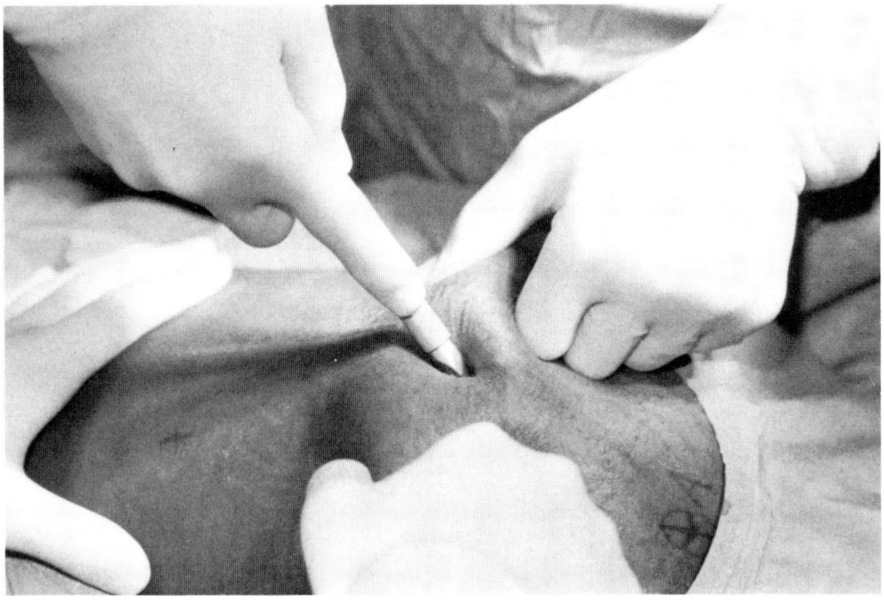

FIG 5–8.
Alternative method of primary cannula and trocar insertion in which the extended index finger marks the point of maximal planned penetration of the laparoscopic trocar.

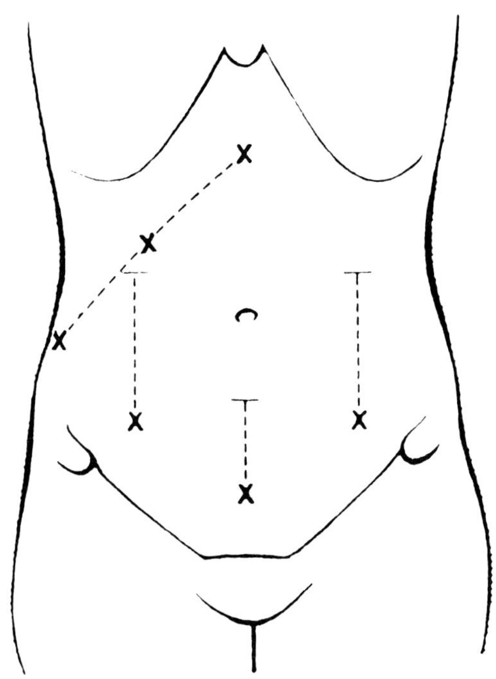

FIG 5–9.
Strategy for ancillary cannula placement is a function of the type of procedure and patient habitus. The midline and lateral rectus sheath borders are particularly safe. These placements usually follow the primary umbilical cannula and are done under direct visualization. Occasionally, one of these sites serves as the initial locus of peritoneal cavity entry.

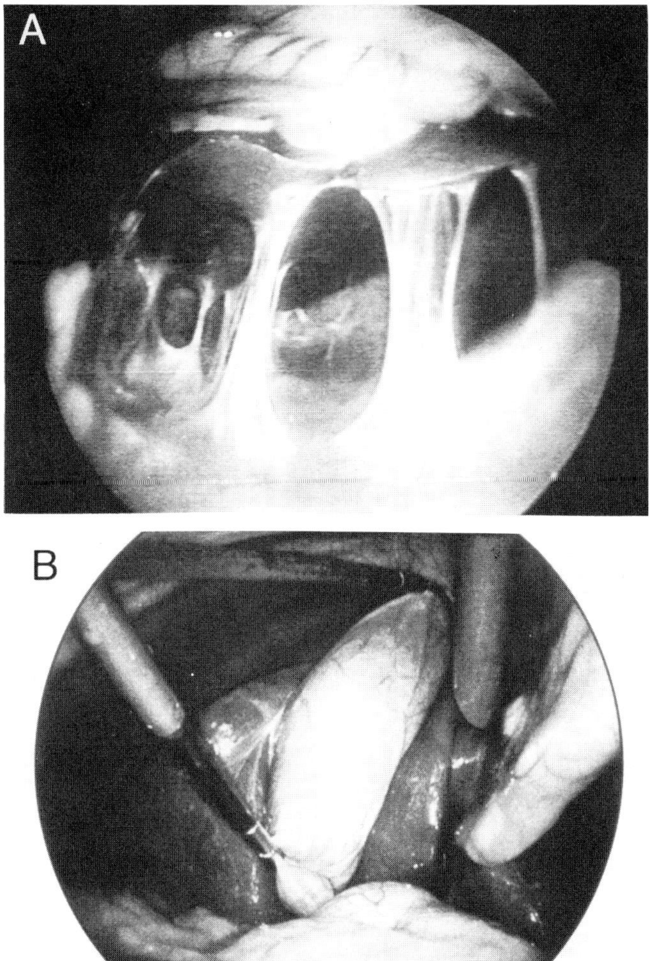

FIG 5–10.
Inspection of the upper abdomen demonstrates perihepatic adhesions **(A)** and the gallbladder **(B).** The appendical area is shown in **(C).** Color plates of the upper abdominal anatomy are presented in Chapter 6 and lower abdominal anatomy in Chapter 7.

(Fig 5–10). If a clear view cannot be obtained with the table in the horizontal position, the Fowler position will facilitate visualization. A normal spleen is usually not visible unless, in addition to a steep Fowler position, a right lateral decubitus rotation is added. The Trendelenburg position and manipulation of the bowel facilitate visualization of the appendix, terminal ileal loops, and possibly Meckel's diverticulum (Fig 5–10). Proper visualization of the pelvic organs also requires the patient to be in the Trendelenburg position. An inspection of female pelvic anatomy is enhanced if a uterine cannula is in place,[11] and this also enhances diagnostic procedures.[12, 13]

Obesity may pose special problems, and positioning of the obese patient is important. Any degree of flexion of the thighs will result in the abdominal panniculus doubling its thickness and folding in such a way as to make the procedure almost impossible. A longer Veress needle may be helpful in gaining peritoneal access. The infraumbilical approach is preferred and is facilitated by a deeper periumbilical incision.

Extremely thin patients are also at risk for complications because the distance between the anterior abdominal wall and the abdominal aorta is often quite limited. The force required to introduce the Veress needle may be less than anticipated in thin patients because the fascia is thin. To avoid this risk, the Veress needle should be grasped close to the tip, the abdominal wall should be elevated, and the angle of the needle directed toward the pelvis or head should be modified so that the Veress needle is more parallel to the plane of the abdominal wall.

Pediatric laparoscopy also requires unique instrumentation. The risks are similar to those for the asthenic patient because the fascia tends to be poorly developed. For these reasons, the Veress needle must be grasped close to its tip, the abdominal wall is aggressively elevated, and the angle of the needle pointed toward the pelvis is modified. Pneumoperitoneum is established quickly in the pediatric patient due to the small overall volume of the peritoneal cavity. In addition, small increments of gas cause dramatic changes in intraperitoneal pressure that necessitate close monitoring.

OPEN LAPAROSCOPY (ALTERNATIVE METHOD FOR PRIMARY CANNULA PLACEMENT)

Complications resulting from the conventional technique of insufflating the distending gas for the creation of pneumoperitoneum (closed technique) have created the need for alternative ways of entering the abdominal cavity. One of the methods that has gained recognized acceptance is open laparoscopy as described by Hasson in 1974.[14–16] The main advantage attributed to this method is that the peritoneal cavity is entered while using continuous visual surveillance.[17]

Open laparoscopy is based on the principle that direct opening of the abdominal cavity carries less risk than the blind introduction of sharp instruments does. The technique is usually performed by using a small, subumbilical incision through the outer parietes, and the peritoneum is identified and incised under direct vision. The technique is similar to that described for open peritoneal lavage in abdominal trauma. The open laparoscopy trocar and cannula are the key to this procedure (see Chapter 2). After the exposed fascia is separated from any adherent bowel or omentum, the trocar and cannula are introduced through a small peritoneal incision. Four hooks on the cannula for securing the device to the peritoneal edges with sutures and a funnel-shaped adapter that is inserted into the abdominal wound maintain an air-tight interface. With the trocar and cannula in place, the gas line is connected and the pneumoperitoneum established. The blunt obturator is removed and the endoscope inserted. Open laparoscopy then proceeds in the same manner as the conventional closed method.

While this technique should theoretically carry less risk than traditional laparoscopy, bowel damage has been reported to occur at the time of peritoneal entry. In addition, open laparoscopy takes longer to perform.

INTRODUCTION OF ANCILLARY CANNULAS AND TROCARS FOR INSTRUMENTATION

Virtually all endosurgical operative procedures require the insertion of ancillary cannula(s). In isolated diagnostic procedures, a separate puncture site for use of additional instruments allows better manipulation of the intra-abdominal organs so that they will be under direct vision at all times. Moreover, the approach does not limit the observer to a single visual plane. This contrasts with the constraints inherent in the single-puncture operative laparoscope (see Chapter 2). In operative procedures the secondary ports are used to introduce essential ancillary surgical instrumentation.

Selection strategy of entry site(s) and attention to proper technique are as important for inserting the secondary trocar(s) as for the primary laparoscopic trocar. The strategy for determining the location of the ancillary cannulas is a function of the type of operative procedure and the patient's habitus. Particularly useful loci include the midline and lateral border of the rectus sheath (Fig 5–9). It is important in selecting secondary puncture sites to maximize the internal distance between cannulas to avoid the instruments interfering (scissoring) with each other within the peritoneal cavity. In order to minimize trauma to the abdominal structures, the site of secondary puncture should be indented with the index finger and observed with the laparoscope in the abdomen (Fig 5–11). The site of indentation is inspected to ensure that it provides the necessary access. When the site has been chosen, the operating room lights may be temporarily turned off and the tip of the laparoscope pressed against this site, thus transilluminating the anterior abdominal wall to determine the absence of parietal blood vessels. Secondary incisions are made at selected points of sufficient size to accommodate the trocar and cannula. The trocar-cannula unit is inserted through the skin and fascia. Further advance of the trocar and cannula is controlled by direct laparoscopic observation to avoid peritoneal blood vessels, bladder, and abdominal organs (see Fig 5–10).

PROCEDURE TERMINATION AND ABDOMINAL WALL CLOSURE

At the conclusion of any laparoscopic procedure, a final survey is made to confirm that there is no unsuspected trauma or bleeding. Ancillary instruments and the cannulas are removed. The sites of secondary puncture are inspected with the laparoscope to ensure that there is no bleeding, and the endoscope is removed. With the patient in the Trendelenburg position, the valve of the principal cannula is opened and the gas expelled from the peritoneal cavity.[18] The abdominal wall is compressed with one hand, while the umbilical cannula is removed with the valve in the open position. Pressure from the hand will prevent the introduction of room air into the peritoneal cavity. Maintaining the valve open prevents a subatmo-

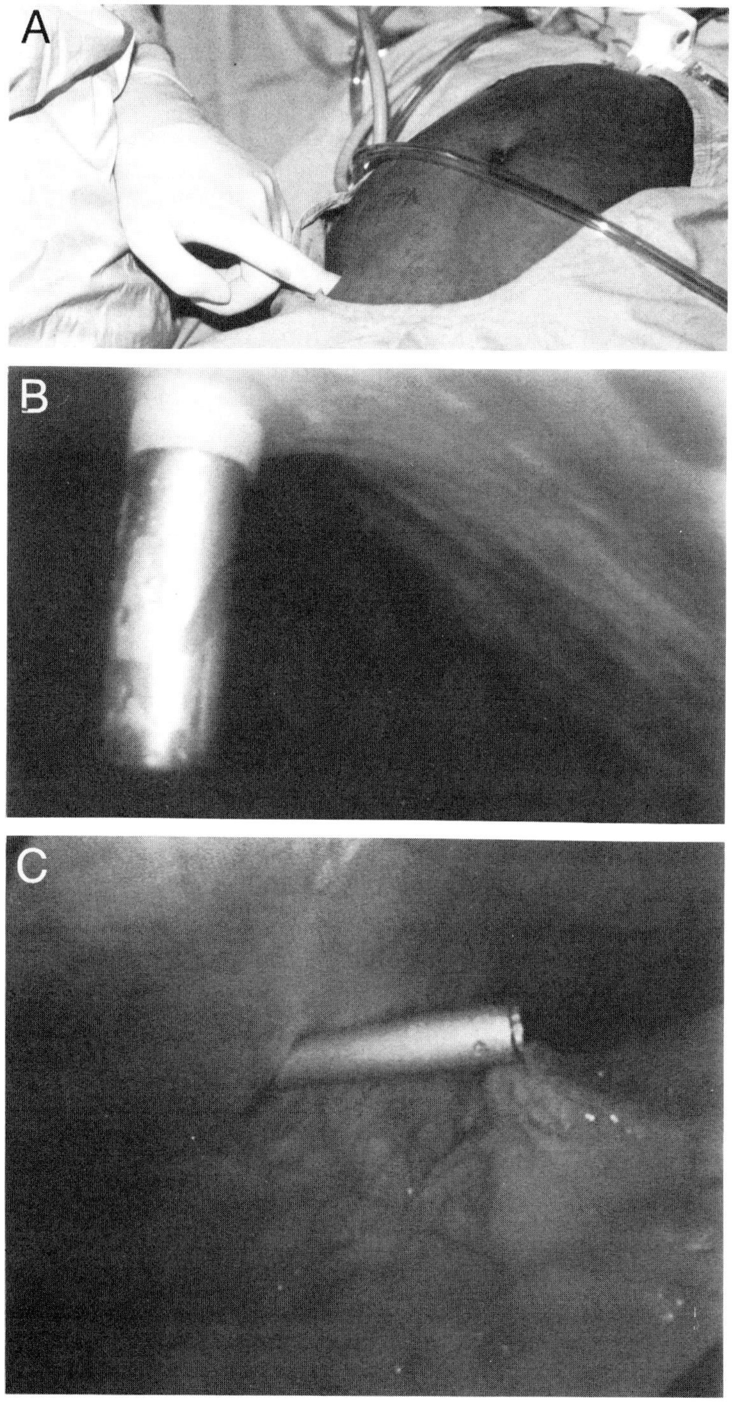

FIG 5–11.
Insertion of ancillary cannulas and trocars. The technique of insertion is similar to that used for the insertion of the primary access cannula except that it is done with direct intraperitoneal visualization. **A,** depression of the abdominal wall; **B,** the sheathed disposable trocar-cannula unit entering the peritoneal cavity; and **C,** the cannula in place with the trocar removed.

spheric pressure from sucking bowel or omentum into the puncture wound. When the instruments are removed, the incisions are closed. The author places an absorbable fascial stitch at the umbilical site and any ancillary cannula site of 10 mm or more to prevent potential visceral entrapment or hernia formation. Otherwise cutaneous sutures or steristrips are used.

Following the procedure and termination of anesthesia, the patient recovers in the standard fashion.[20] It should be recognized that hypercarbia can develop following extubation. If no problems are encountered, the patient is ready for subsequent triage.[21]

REFERENCES

1. Ruddock JC: Peritoneoscopy. *West J Surg Obstet Gynecol* 1934; 42:392–405.
2. Gomel V: Laparoscopy. *Can Med Assoc J* 1984; 111:167–169.
3. Berci G, Jensen D: Laparoscopy for the hepatologist and the general surgeon. *Acta Endoscopica* 1982; 12:3–12.
4. Levinson J: The role of laparoscopy in intra-abdominal diagnosis. *Del Med J* 1978; 50:259–270.
5. Frank L, Bliesze H, Beck K, et al: Laparoscopic sonography. A new dimension in the diagnostic approach to internal organs. *Dtsch Med Wochenschr* 1983; 10:902–904.
6. Wheeless CR: Gastrointestinal injuries associated with laparoscopy, in Phillips JM (ed): *Endoscopy in Gynecology.* Downey, Calif, American Association of Gynecologic Laparoscopists, 1978, pp 317–324.
7. Corson SL: Operating room preparation and basic technique, in Phillips JM (ed): *Laparoscopy.* Baltimore, Williams & Wilkins, 1977, p 88.
8. Hegarty JH, Brennan TG: Laparoscopy under local anaesthesia: Our experience in 400 non-gynecological patients. *Ir J Med Sci* 1983; 152:276–278.
9. Lacey CG: Laparoscopy: A clinical sign for intraperitoneal needle placement. *Obstet Gynecol* 1976; 47:625–627.
10. Marlow J: Endoscopic photography. *Clin Obstet Gynecol* 1983; 26:359–365.
11. Atanov YuP, Papin YuP: Combined manipulator for laparoscopy. *Khirurgiia (Mosk)* 1982; 8:103–105.
12. Gullini S, Cantarini D, Boccia S, et al: Cytological brushing. *Minerva Med* 1983; 18:215–218.
13. Jensen D, Berci G: Laparoscopy: Advances in biopsy and recording techniques. *Gastrointest Endosc* 1981; 27:150–155.
14. Hasson HM: Open laparoscopy: A report of 150 cases. *J Reprod Med* 1974; 12:234–238.
15. Hasson HM: Open laparoscopy vs. close laparoscopy: A comparison of complication rates. *Adv Planned Par* 1976; 8:41–50.
16. Hasson HM: Open laparoscopy, in Phillips JM (ed): *Laparoscopy.* Baltimore, Williams & Wilkins, 1977, p 145.
17. Hinojosa Mata MA, Morales Perez A, Garcia Luna AM, et al: Open laparoscopy. Analysis of 60 cases. *Gynecol Obstet Mex* 1982; 50:201–204.
18. Minoli G, Terruzzi V, Spinzi GC, et al: The influence of carbon dioxide and nitrous oxide on pain during laparoscopy: A double blind, controlled trial. *Gastrointest Endosc* 1982; 28:173–175.
19. Driscoll GL, Tyler JP, Simpson P: Closure of laparoscopy incisions. *Clin Reprod Fertil* 1982; 1:241–242.
20. Hovorka J, Lehtinen AM, Kalli I: Recovery after general anesthesia for laparoscopy. *Acta Anaesthesiol Scand* 1983; 27:396–399.
21. Krief JC, Levy B, Moret G, et al: Towards an outpatient surgical department. I. Test comparison of reawakening after three anesthetic protocols. *Agressologie* 1982; 23:109–113.

PART III

Clinical Applications of Endoscopic Surgery—Multispecialty Perspective

Chapter 6

Laparoscopic Biliary Surgery

Miguel Velez, M.D.

Stanley R. Klein, M.D.

Cholelithiasis is common and is the consequence of multiple etiologies. Approximately 10% (25 million) of the U.S. population has gallstones. Cholecystectomy is the most common abdominal operation performed by the general surgeon in the Western world, with approximately 550,000 cholecystectomies performed annually in the United States alone.[1] Following cholecystectomy patients are hospitalized for several days and disabled for 4 to 6 weeks.[2] In an attempt to reduce morbidity and disability, alternative methods to treat gallstones have been introduced.[3] Recent endeavors include chemical dissolution,[4–9] and percutaneous extraction and ultrasonic lithotripsy.[10–18] Although many of the newer methods are minimally invasive, most individuals require subsequent therapy for recurrent symptoms when the diseased gallbladder has not been removed. Because of the frequency of recurrent calculi after stone removal alone, cholecystectomy remains the gold standard for therapy.[1–3]

LAPAROSCOPIC CHOLECYSTECTOMY FOR CHOLELITHIASIS

Techniques of laparoscopic surgery have evolved rapidly over the last 20 years.[19–29] Initial development emphasized treatment of gynecologic diseases. The first laparoscopic cholecystectomy was performed by Mouret in Lyon, France, in 1987, followed by Dubois and colleagues in Paris in 1988.[19] Saye and McKernan performed the first laparoscopic cholecystectomy in the United States in 1989 and used a laser to remove the gallbladder.[21] Reddick et al. published their initial series of cases in 1989 and emphasized the principles of upper abdominal laparoscopic surgical technique, new instrumentation facilitating surgery, and training methods for laparoscopic general surgery.[20, 21] Several subsequent series have substantiated the initial reports of decreased patient morbidity and disability.[20, 23–25]

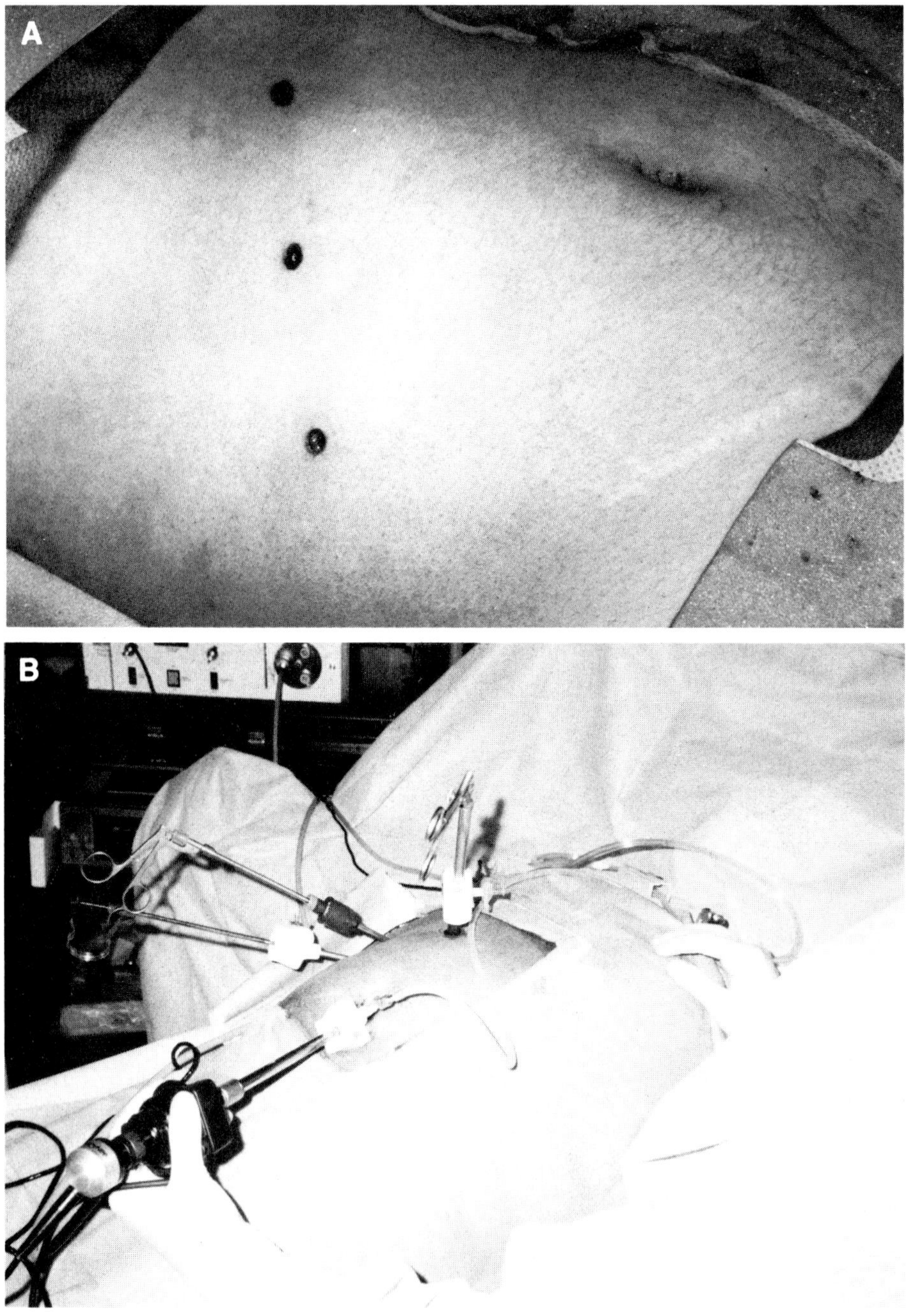

FIG 6–1.
A, incisions. **B,** cannula insertion sites. The patient's head is at the right of **B.**

Indications

The current indications for laparoscopic cholecystectomy are nearly identical to those for conventional cholecystectomy. This may include management of asymptomatic stones.[26, 27] Notable exceptions include the presence of portal hypertension and pregnancy.[21, 22, 24, 25] Choledocholithiasis, extreme obesity, previous upper abdominal surgery with extensive adhesions, and a bleeding diathesis are relative contraindications.[21, 23, 25, 28, 29] Considerations for conversion from the laparoscopic procedure to conventional open cholecystectomy may include gangrene of the gallbladder, impacted common bile duct stones, excessive adhesions, unsuspected remote pathology, excessive bleeding, and an inability of the surgeon to safely identify the regional ductal and vascular anatomy.[21–25, 29]

Preoperative Evaluation and Patient Preparation

Preoperative evaluation for laparoscopic cholecystectomy is similar to that for the traditional operative procedure.[24, 25, 29] Documentation of gallbladder calculi is based upon ultrasound or oral cholecystography.[30–32] B-mode ultrasound may yield additional information regarding the liver parenchyma as well as distension of the intrahepatic and extrahepatic biliary tree.[30, 31] A complete blood count, hepatic enzymes, and amylase level are usually docu-

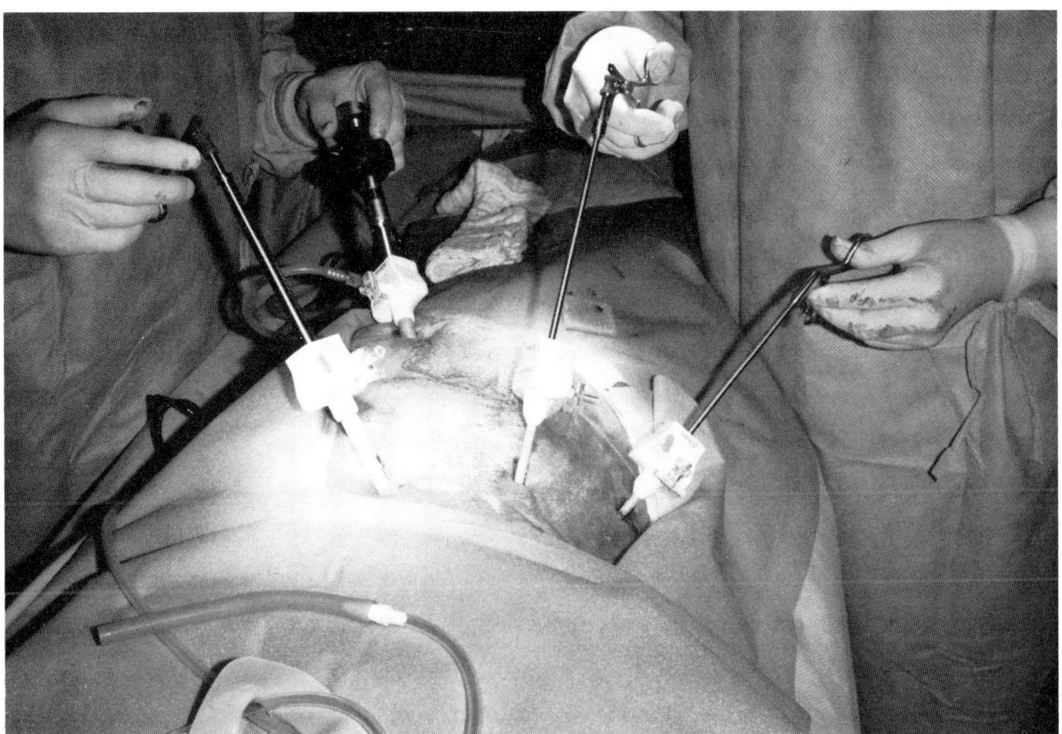

FIG 6–2.
Positioning of surgeon *(right)* and assistant *(left)*. The patient's head is at the bottom of the figure.

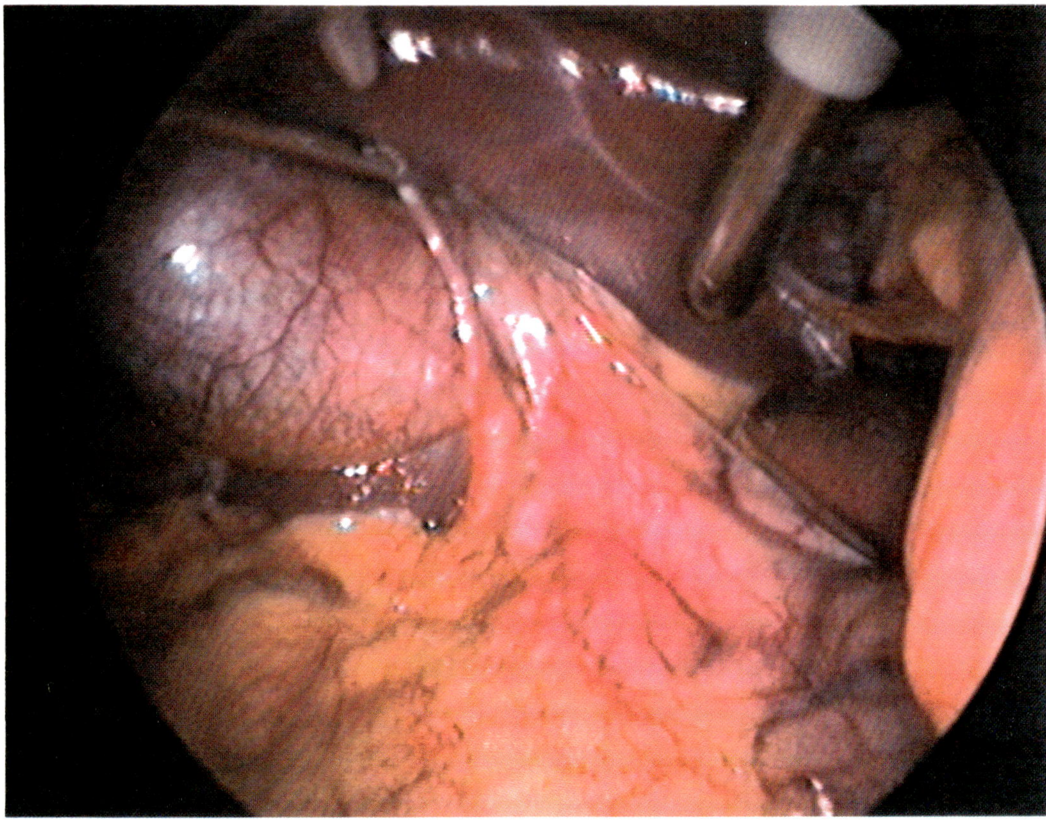

FIG 6–3.
Lateral and superior retraction of the gallbladder to expose the gallbladder fossae.

mented.[24, 25, 29] Preoperative anesthestic considerations include cardiopulmonary depression associated with general anesthesia as well as the potential pulmonary compromise produced by a pneumoperitoneum.[33, 34] Currently, fewer than 4% of laparoscopic cholecystectomies are converted to an open procedure.[20, 23–25, 29] Thus, operative consent must always be obtained for both endoscopic and open procedures. Surgical instruments in the operating room should include those for both the endoscopic procedure and laparotomy. Endoscopic surgical instruments, light sources, insufflation gas tanks, electrocautery devices, and lasers should be checked prior to each procedure.

Operative Technique

General anesthesia is administered via endotracheal intubation. A single dose of an effective preoperative antibiotic may be given.[35, 36] Insertion of a nasogastric tube and Foley catheter is optional. Both are recommended for anticipated lengthy procedures.[24, 25, 29] The surgical field is prepared and draped similar to that for a cholecystectomy. The operation is performed through endosurgical ports requiring four small incisions to enable passage of the instruments into the abdomen. (Fig 6–1). Appropriate placement of these ports is critical. To begin a routine laparoscopic procedure, a 10-mm incision is made in the inferior aspect of the umbilicus, and the abdominal wall is grasped and elevated. A Veress insufflation needle is inserted through the incision. Penetration of the peritoneum by the needle is felt as a definitive relief of resistance to passage of the needle. The needle is directed cephalad at an angle of about 30 degrees. The viscera are closely approximated to the abdominal wall until the peritoneal vacuum is broken by entry of air; thus care is required to prevent injury upon initial penetration. Entry into the peritoneal cavity is verified by one of several tests, although none are infallible (see Chapter 5). Alternative Veress needle insertion sites or open Hassan laparoscopy may be necessary if there are adhesions from previous procedures. The open laparoscopic technique utilizes a larger initial incision to directly visualize introduction of the first cannula. To provide a seal around the cannulas following introduction, a purse-string suture or a Hassan cannula can be used (see Chapter 2).[37, 38]

Following introduction of the Veress needle the peritoneal cavity is distended with approximately 3 to 4 L of carbon dioxide. Intra-abdominal pressure is carefully monitored and not allowed to exceed 15 mm Hg. Once a sufficient pneumoperitoneum is established, a 10-mm trocar allowing endosurgical access for most devices is inserted through the infraumbilical in-

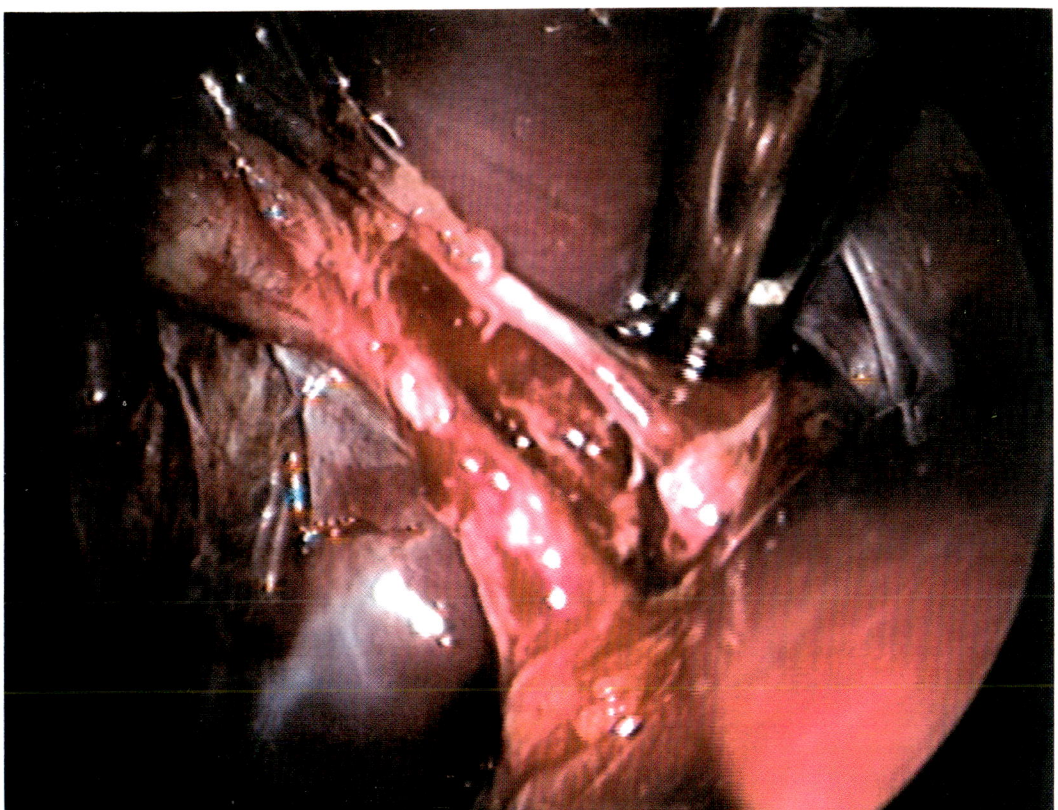

FIG 6–4.
Isolated cystic duct and artery.

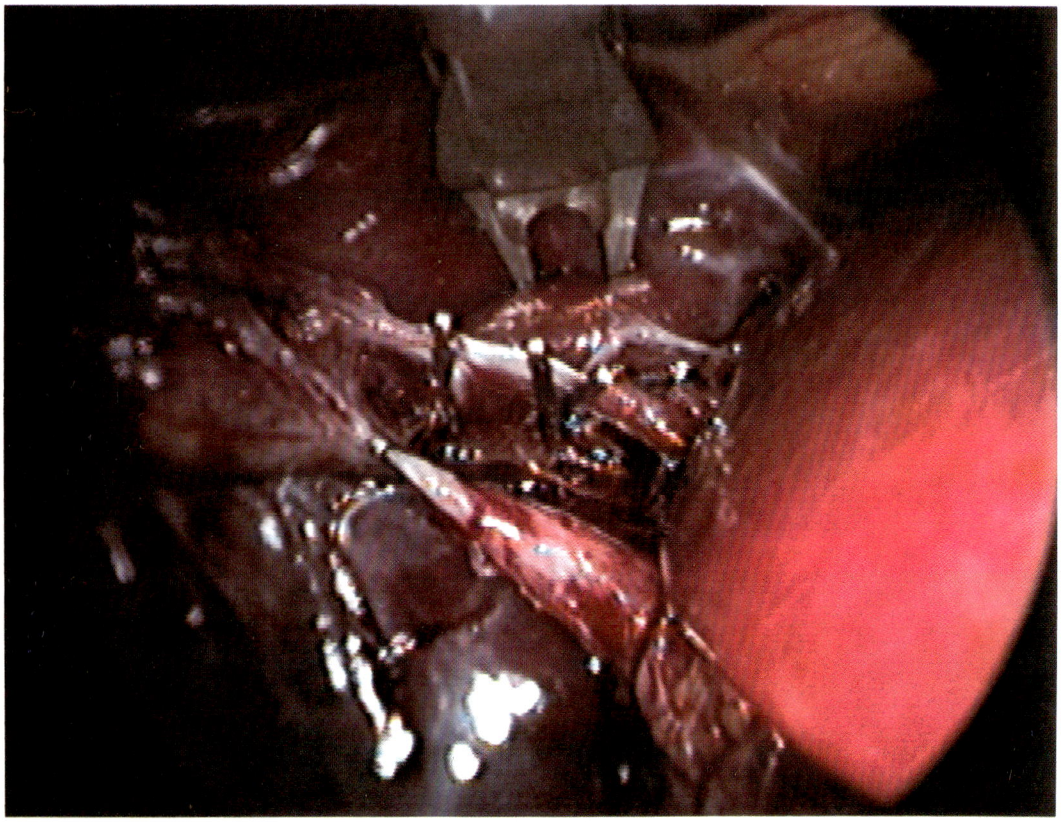

FIG 6–5.
Cystic duct and artery clipped.

cision. The trocar is removed, and a 10-mm laparoscope is inserted through the cannula and connected to a video camera. Three additional cannulas are inserted under direct vision. Placement of the ancillary ports is governed by abdominal cavity geometry and the presence of adhesions. The conventional sites are along a line two finger-breadths below and parallel to the right coastal margin: a 10-mm cannula just to the right of the midline, a 5-mm cannula at the midclavicular line, and a 5-mm cannula at the anterior axillary line (Figs 6–1,B and 6–2). These cannulas are inserted by using laparoscopic visualization through the umbilical port to avoid injury to intra-abdominal organs. The cannulas are inserted into the peritoneal cavity perpendicular to the skin surface. Care is taken to ensure adequate space between the cannulas to enable free intraperitoneal manipulation of the devices.

During the procedure, the surgeon may stand at either the right or left side of the patient. We prefer that the surgeon be positioned on the right side, retract the gallbladder through the most caudad-lateral port with the left hand, and perform the operation through the midclavicular port with the right. The assistant surgeon stands on the patient's left side, retracts the liver through the medial cranial port with the right hand, and manipulates the camera with the left (Fig 6–2). Alternatively, the surgeon may stand to the left of the patient and operate through the cranial-medial port. In this senario the assistant obtains exposure of the gallbladder via the two right lateral ports. A third person is usually required to operate the videocamera. This role is often best performed by the beginning laparoscopic surgeon.

Gallbladder dissection is initiated by passing an atraumatic grasping forceps through the lateral port to retract the gallbladder laterally and superiorly (Fig 6–3). Blunt forceps are inserted through the midclavicular port, and the cystic duct and artery are dissected free from surrounding peritoneum and fatty areolar tissue (Fig 6–4). The principle of traction and countertraction is used in order to facilitate blunt dissection. Cranial traction on the gallbladder fundus and lateral tension on Hartman's pouch at the cystic duct junction are the essential vectors. The tissues surrounding the cystic duct and artery are dissected with an instrument placed through the midclavicular port by teasing the overlying peritoneum and fatty-areolar tissue of Calot's triangle. Subsequent lateral and inferior traction on the gallbladder exposes the anterior aspect of the duct, while medial and ventral (lifting toward the anterior abdominal wall) traction exposes the posterior aspect. Initial dissection should be started on the inferolateral aspect of the cystic duct at its junction with the gallbladder neck to avoid injury to the common bile duct. Following isolation of a segment of cystic duct adequate to perform intraoperative cholangiography, a surgical clip is applied to the duct through the upper medial

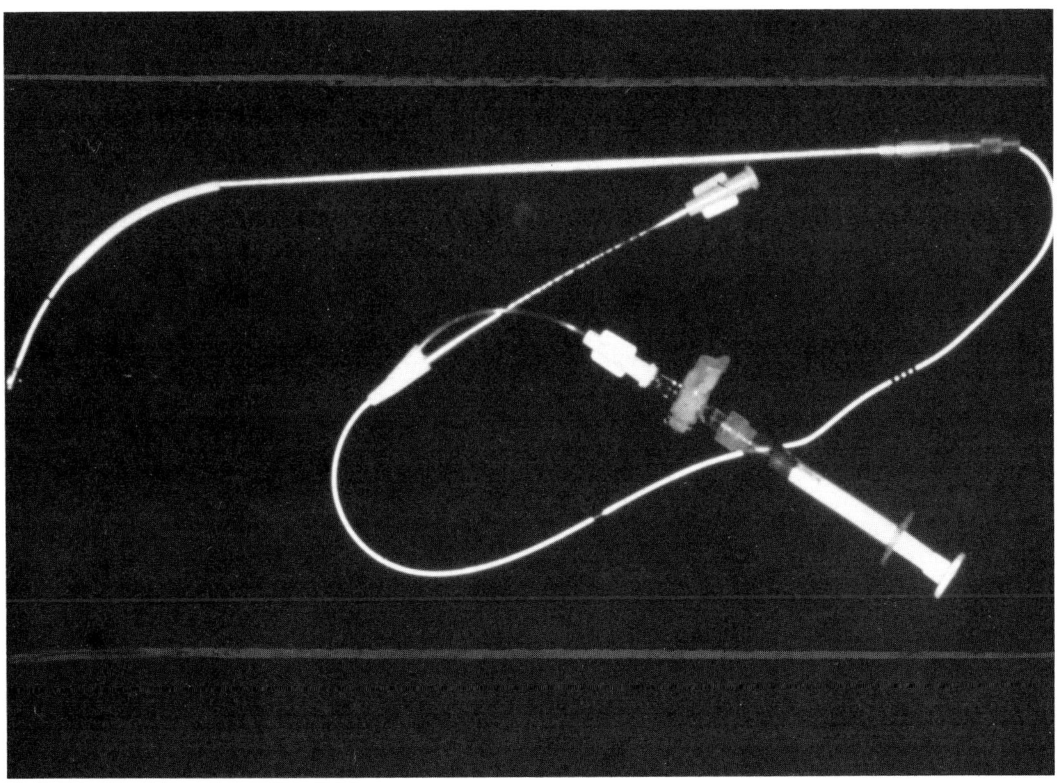

FIG 6–6.
Endosurgical cholangiography catheter (Arrow Co, Reading, Pa) that is introduced in the cystic duct over a guidewire. A balloon tip holds the catheter in position following placement.

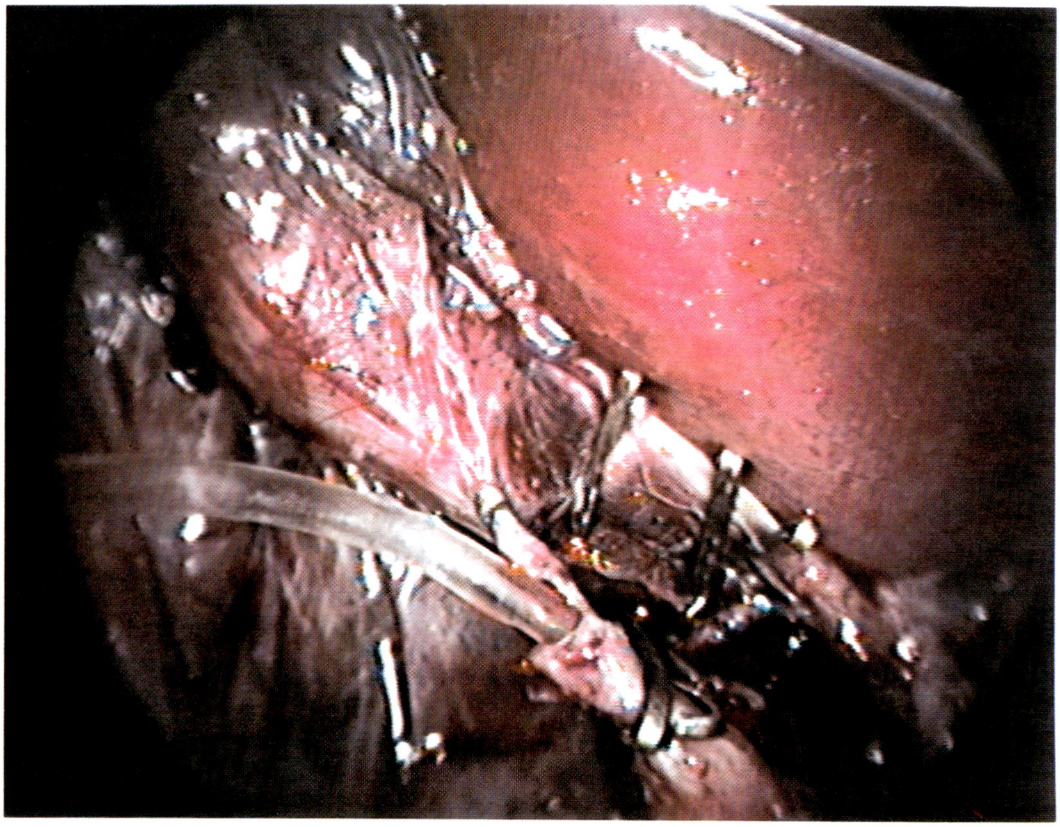

FIG 6–7.
Cholangiogram catheter in the cystic duct that is secured by nonocclusive clips.

port at the junction with the gallbladder neck. Comparing the lengths of the cystic duct to the size of the dissecting instrument provides the surgeon with a linear gauge in deciding whether an adequate length of cystic duct has been exposed. If the cystic artery has also been identified and isolated at this point, it is also clipped (Fig 6–5).

Cholangiography is performed by inserting a catheter through an incision in the cystic duct made with dissecting scissors. We prefer a soft 42-in., 5F pediatric feeding tube with the tip cut at a bevel for safe atraumatic introduction. There are also commercial catheters available for endosurgical cholangiography (Fig 6–6). The cholangiogram catheter is introduced through the surgical cannula via a 3-mm guiding sheath or specially designed forceps. Following placement of the catheter it is anchored in place by using an incompletely occlusive surgical clip (Fig 6–7). After the cholangiogram is completed (Fig 6–8), the cystic duct is doubly clipped and divided. The ability to perform cholangiography increases with surgeon experience.[39] At this point the cystic artery is usually dissected free from surrounding tissues, clipped, and divided (Fig 6–9). The surgeon should be cognizant of the wide variability in the biliary arterial anatomy. Of particular concern is the frequent appearance of separate anterior and posterior branches of the cystic artery, which is not generally appreciated in an open procedure. It is to be emphasized that if the anatomy is not apparent, the procedure should be converted to an open approach.

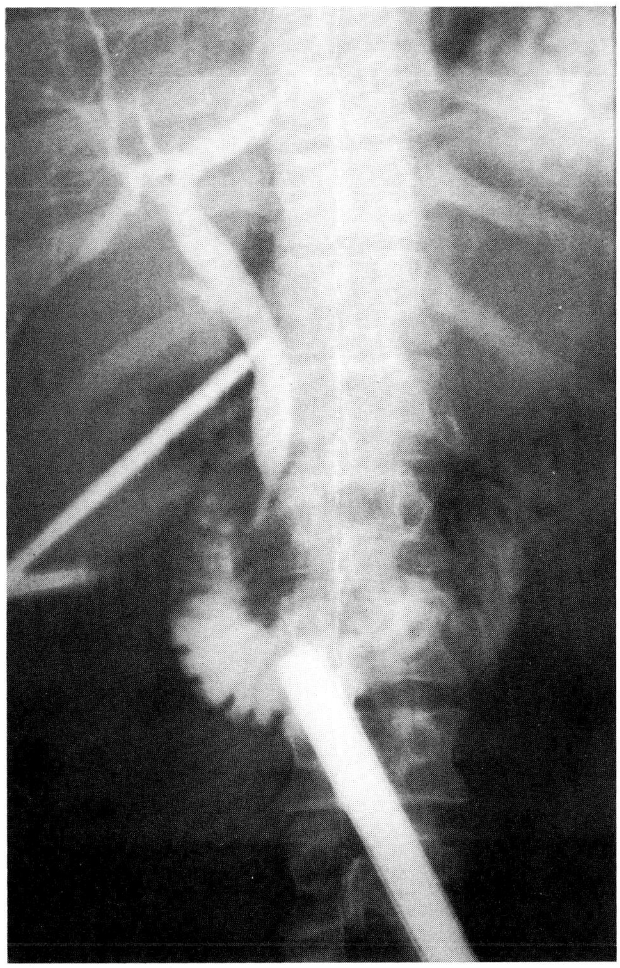

FIG 6–8.
A cholangiogram obtained during the procedure demonstrates laparoscopic instruments in the operative field.

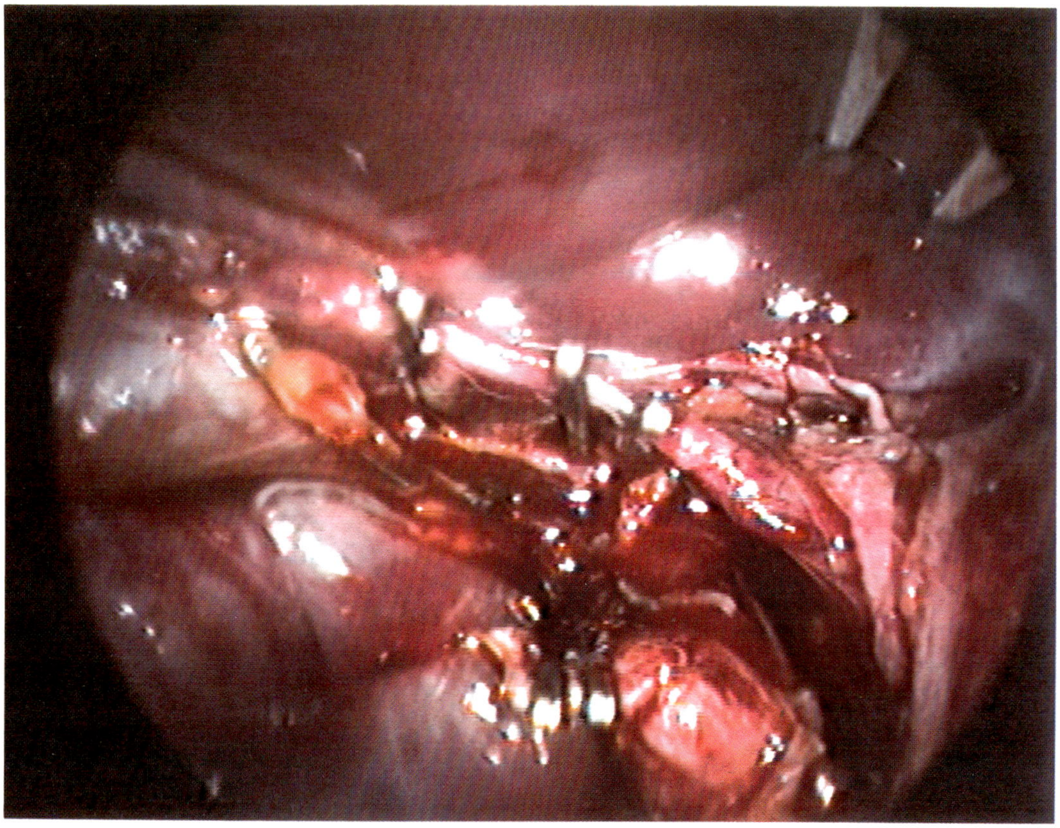

FIG 6–9.
Divided cystic duct and a cystic artery clipped prior to division.

The gallbladder is dissected from the liver bed by using either a laser or electrocautery for hemostasis. Electrocautery coagulates well and is satisfactory for dissection in virtually all circumstances. Tissue planes may be obscured due to the blanching and charring effects of the cautery. Smoke production is increased when cautery is used in hemostasis and dissection. Electrical burns of the bowel have been reported from unsuspected arcing of the current. Depth of tissue injury is greater with electrocautery, so difficult hepatic bleeding is better controlled with electrocautery.

The lasers most commonly used are the potassium titanyl phosphate (KTP)/yttrium-aluminum-garnet (YAG) with a bare fiber and the Nd:YAG with either a sapphire tip or a sculptured fiber. Sapphire tips are expensive, stay hot, may break, have a tendency to collect carbon deposits, and carry a risk of air embolism from hyperinsufflation. Sculptured fibers do not have to be cooled with high-flow nitrogen, are less expensive, and remain hot for only a short time. For these reasons, they are replacing sapphire tips for the delivery of Nd:YAG laser energy. Because of their highly reflective surface the fibers rapidly become hotter as the energy increases. At high energy density, cutting is improved, but coagulation may be compromised. By decreasing the energy and working in the near contact mode, coagulation is facilitated. The KTP/YAG laser system uses a bare fiber to deliver the energy. It cuts well on contact, and it coagulates well on near-contact because of the beam divergence and scatter. No "backstop" is necessary because the light energy quickly dissipates over a short distance. The ability to cut and coagulate without adjusting the power of the laser makes for a faster dissection. If deeper coagulation is needed, the machine can easily be switched to the YAG mode. Regardless of the mode of energy selected for the endosurgical procedure an electrocautery unit should always be available in the operating room.

Gallbladder removal commences at the neck of the gallbladder and progresses toward the fundus along the areolar plane between the gallbladder and the liver (Figs 6–10 to 6–12). By retracting the gallbladder neck laterally and alternatively superiorly or inferiorly the peritoneal attachments on either side of the gallbladder are exposed and divided. It is mandatory to stay in the plane between the gallbladder and liver to avoid bleeding from the liver or perforation of the gallbladder. If the gallbladder is perforated, dissection is continued for several millimeters to free the edges around the perforation. This area is then grasped with the dissecting forceps, and the perforation is closed with a clip or Endoloop. Calculi are subsequently retrieved from the peritoneal cavity. Throughout the dissection, bleeding points should be controlled with the laser or electrocautery as encountered. A saline irrigation channel built into the laser cannula or cautery wand facilitates identification and coagulation of

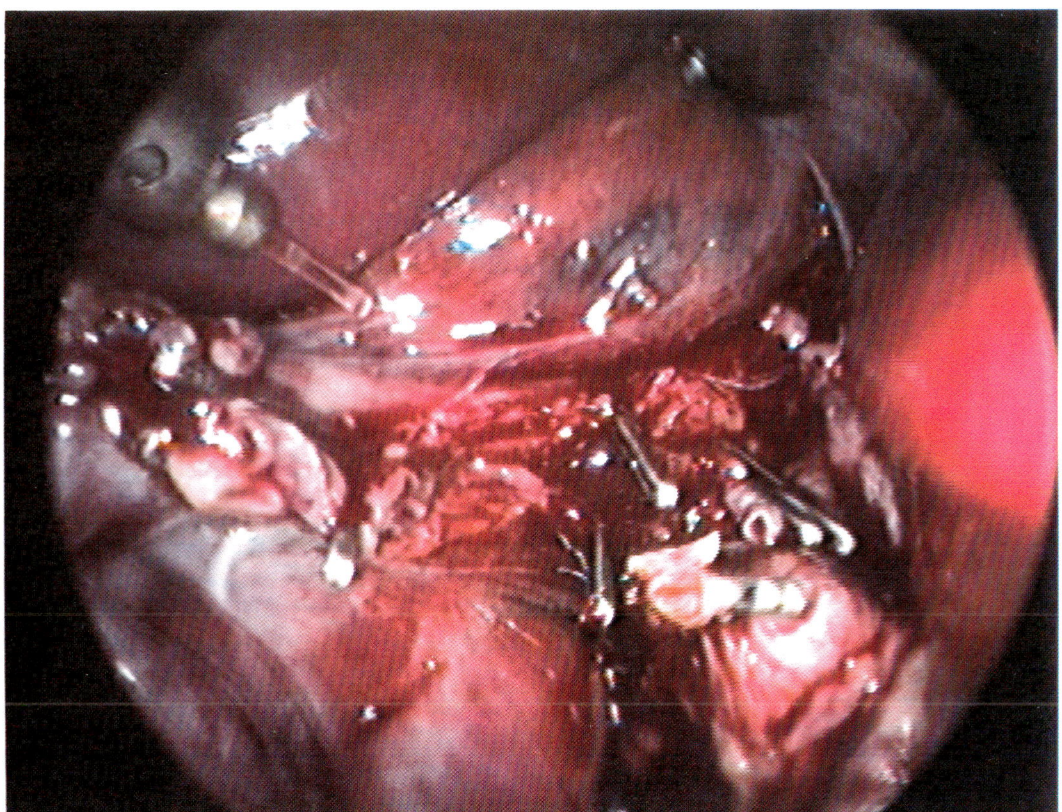

FIG 6–10.
Laser dissection started at the apex of the gallbladder fossa.

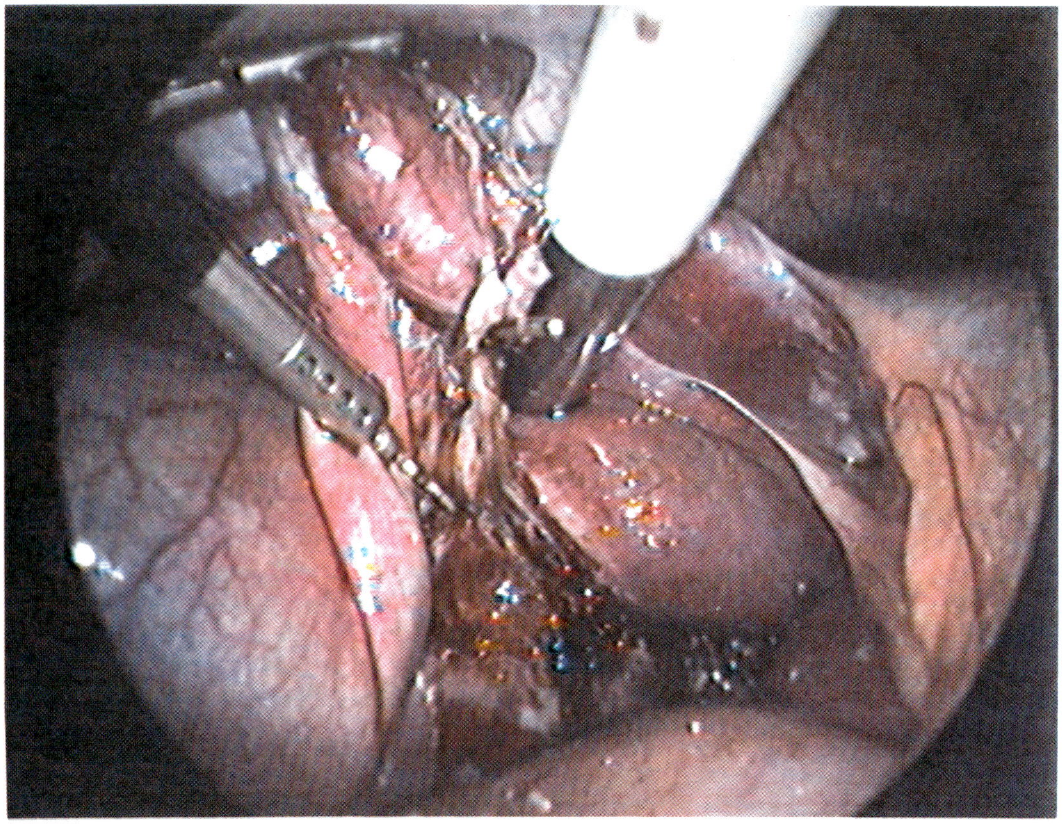

FIG 6–11.
Laser dissection continued along the gallbladder bed.

vessels. Prior to detaching the gallbladder from Glisson's capsule it is retracted cephalad into the right subphrenic space, and the gallbladder bed and porta hepatis are meticulously inspected for hemostasis and bile leaks.

After the gallbladder has been dissected from the liver, it is held by a lateral retraction grasper. The laparoscope is moved to the upper midline port, and the gallbladder neck is transferred to a forcep passed through the umbilical port. The gallbladder is pulled into the umbilical cannula, and the cannula is removed from the abdomen by bringing the neck of the gallbladder through the umbilical incision (Fig 6–13). The fundus of the gallbladder is decompressed through an opening in the apex outside of the abdomen (Fig 6–14) and the organ removed (Fig 6–15). To facilitate removal of the gallbladder, calculi may need to be removed or crushed with blunt curved clamps. Occasionally the umbilical fascial incision is extended to expedite removal.

Following removal of the gallbladder, the laparoscope is again repositioned through the umbilical port, the liver bed (Fig 6–16) is inspected and irrigated, and hemostasis is ensured. We rarely use drains, but if indicated they are inserted through the 10-mm upper medial cannula and exit the peritoneal cavity via a lateral 5-mm port. The cannulas are removed sequentially, with each abdominal wall tract inspected for hemostasis. Before removing the final cannula, the residual carbon dioxide is liberated from the abdominal cavity. The umbilical wound fascia is approximated with a 1–0 polyglactin 910 (Vicryl) suture, the skin incisions are closed with absorbable subcuticular sutures, and steristrips are applied.

Postoperative Care

The nasogastric tube and Foley catheter, if used, are usually removed immediately following the procedure. A clear-fluid diet is begun and the intravenous line removed when the patient is fully awake. Nausea, shoulder pain, and crampy abdominal pain are not unusual.[21, 24, 25] Caution should be taken to ensure removal of subphrenic carbon dioxide to minimize diphragmatic irritation. Oral or intramuscular narcotics and nonsteroidal analgesics are given as needed for pain control. Perchlorperazine (Compazine) or scopolamine dermal patches (Transderm Scop) can be used for nausea. Scopolamine is avoided in elderly patients because they may become disoriented. Most patients can be discharged within 36 hours. They are advised to not drive for several days but are usually not restricted in any other way. Patients are re-examined 1 week postoperatively and usually allowed to resume full activity. No postoperative blood tests are obtained unless indicated.

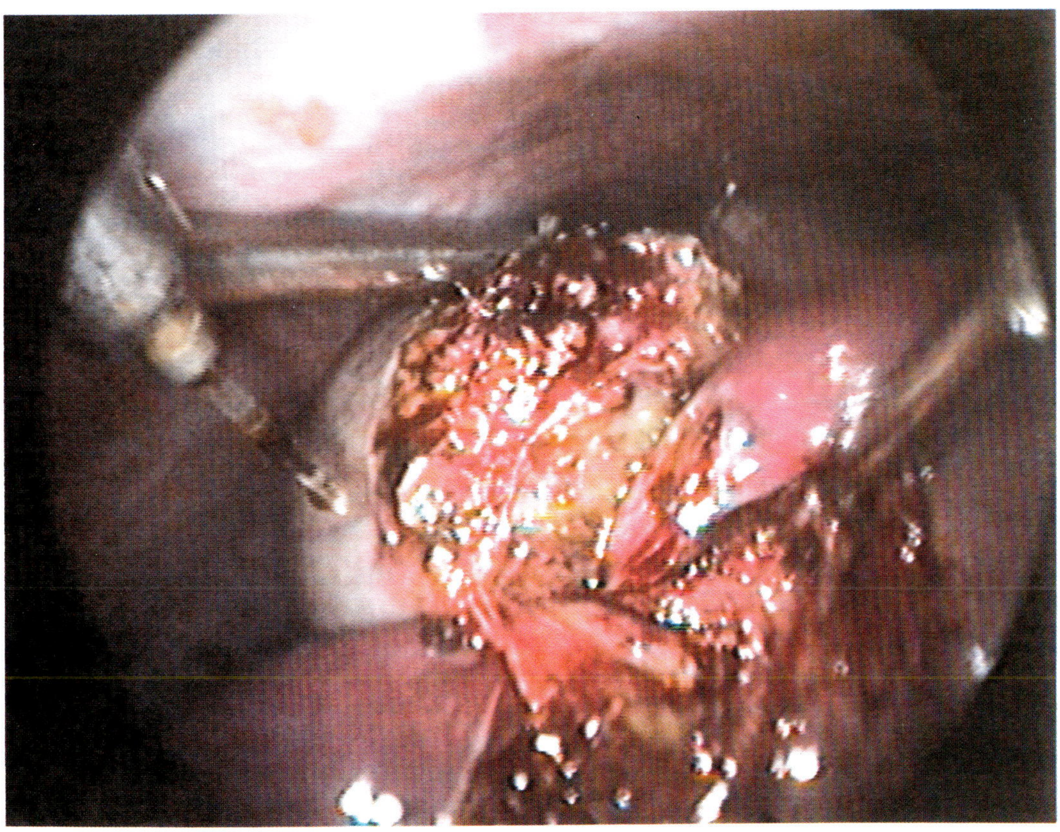

FIG 6–12.
Dissection nearly completed with the gallbladder retracted upward over the liver beneath the diaphragm.

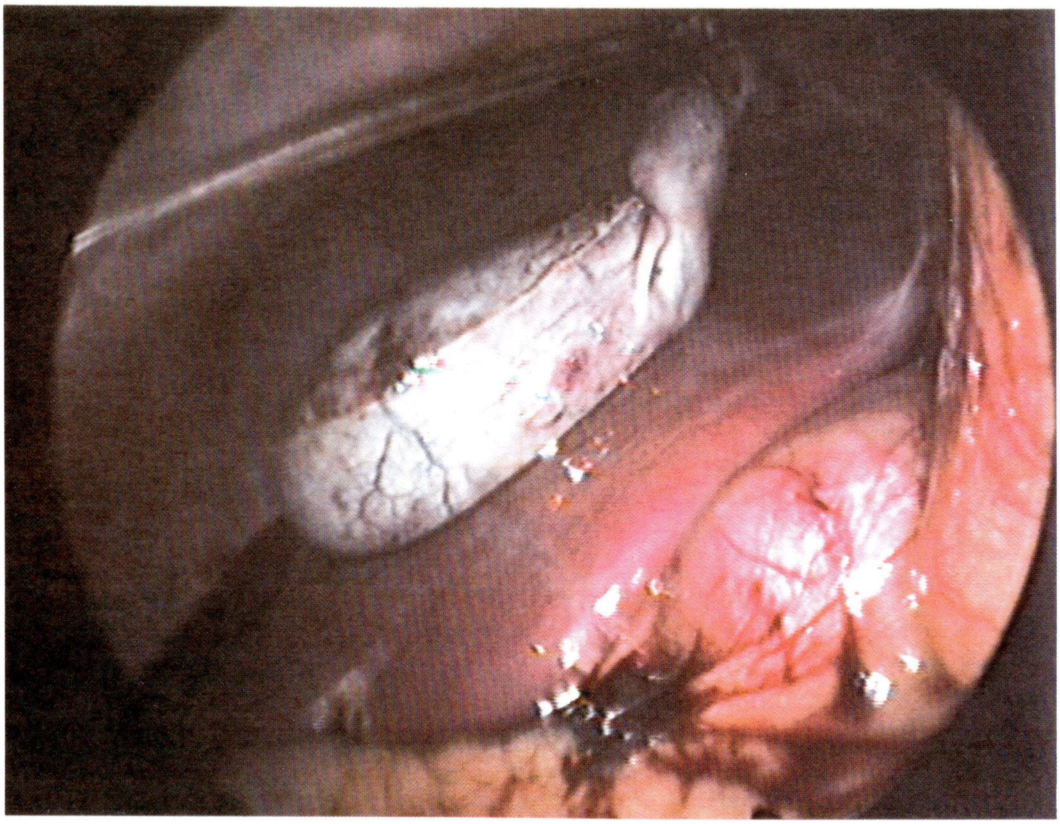

FIG 6–13.
Neck of the gallbladder passed through the umbilical incision.

SPECIAL CONSIDERATIONS

Choledocholithiasis

Patients with no dilatation of the biliary tree on ultrasound and normal liver function test results have a low incidence of common bile duct stones.[37] Patients suspected or documented as having common bile duct stones may be evaluated with endoscopic retrograde cholangiopancreatography (ERCP) and the stones removed via endoscopic papillotomy either preoperatively or postoperatively.[40–42] If unsuspected stones are found during operative cholangiography, some may be removed by irrigation, Fogarty catheter, or basket extraction through the cystic duct. Small ($\leq$0.4 mm) stones usually pass spontaneously. Choledochoscopes that can be inserted over a guidewire through the 5-mm endosurgical operating port are currently being developed. In the interim, flexible ureteroscopes, pediatric bronchoscopes, or angioscopes provide ductal visualization and may be helpful in stone extraction. Other developing alternatives include the destruction of stones with laser lithotripsy. If a stone is known to contain a predominance of cholesterol, it can also be dissolved transhepatically with monoctanoin. Stones that remain postoperatively may be removed through endoscopic papillotomy or via the percutaneous transhepatic route.

Our preference is to remove the ductal stones laparoscopically when they are encountered, if feasible. Some surgeons advocate conversion to conventional open cholecystectomy with common bile duct exploration upon detection of multiple ductal calculi. With the variety of therapeutic approaches to choose from, particularly when the ductal system is not dilated, we prefer avoidance of traditional common bile duct exploration because of the associated risk of stricture formation. The authors are aware of unpublished reports of endosurgical placement of a traditional T-tube following common bile duct exploration.

Unusual Encounters

Recently, one of the authors (M.V.) closed a cholecystoduodenal fistula by using laparoscopic surgery. Management of complicated biliary problems such as this demand expert technical skill of the surgeon as well as sophisticated instrumentation.

COMPLICATIONS

Complications due to removal of the gallbladder are thought to be comparable or less than with traditional open cholecystectomy. Data, however, are limited at present. It is essential for

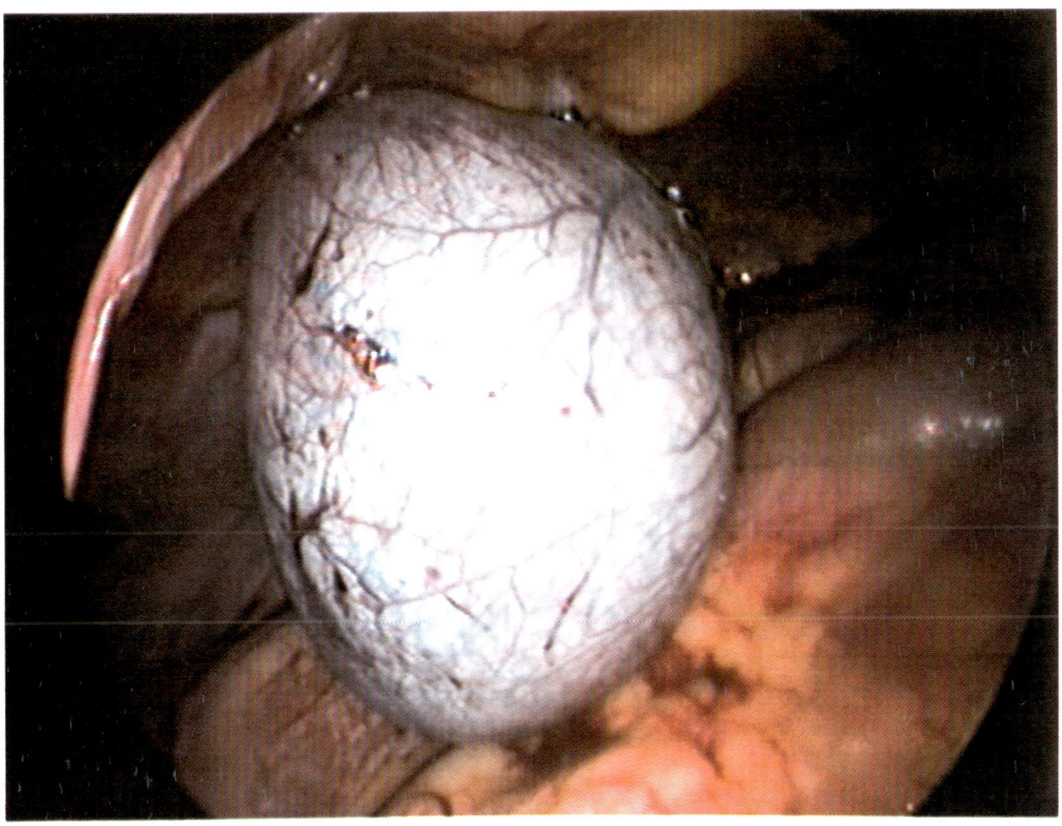

FIG 6–14.
Gallbladder removal continues.

the surgeon to be familiar with problems inherent with laparoscopy (see Chapter 8) as well as those unique to biliary surgery. It is also imperative that the surgeon recognize that there is a learning curve to endoscopic surgical procedures. Thus, appropriate patient selection and surgeon credentialing with adherence to established principles of laparoscopic surgery will minimize technical misadventures.

Because the incisions are smaller, wound infection and incisional hernia rates should decrease. Adhesions rarely form after laparoscopy, and therefore postoperative bowel obstructions may be less. Pneumonia, deep venous thrombosis, pulmonary emboli, and cardiovascular events may also decrease as patients have improved respiratory function and greater mobility in the immediate postoperative period.

CLINICAL RESULTS

During our first 100 laparoscopic cholecystectomies, complications included 1 umbilical wound cellulitis that resolved with antibiotic therapy, 1 myocardial infarction from which the patient recovered without further problems, and 2 readmissions for pain. The readmissions

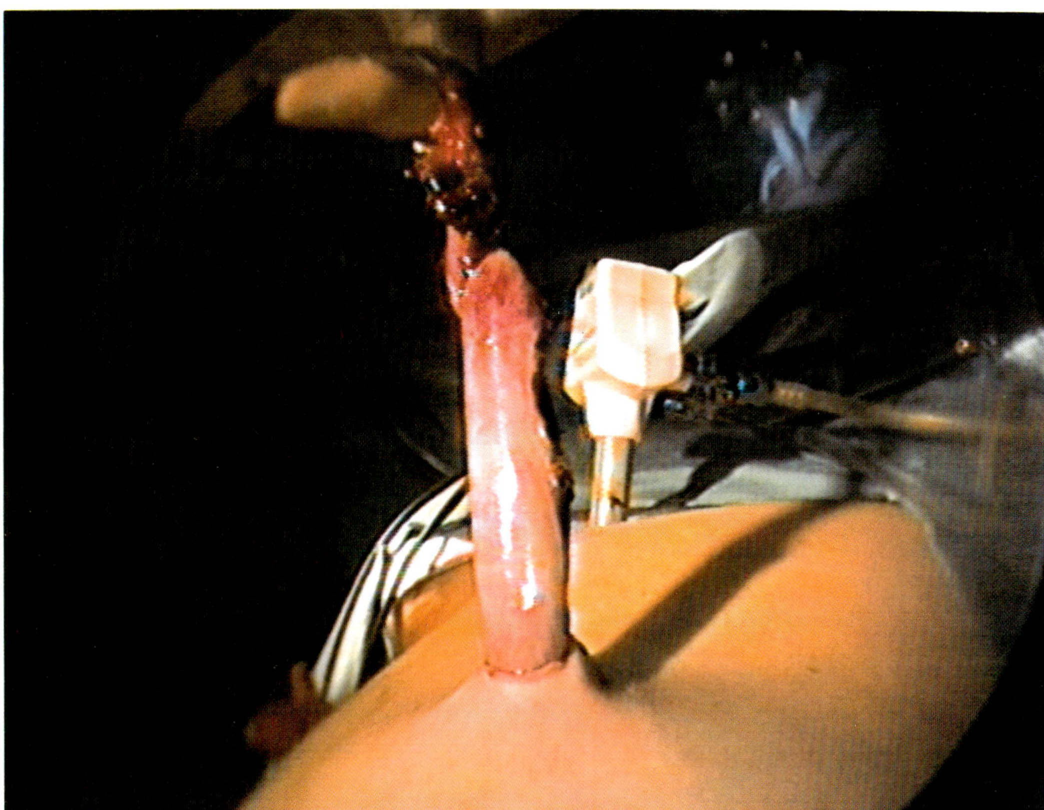

FIG 6–15.
Gallbladder removal following decompression of the fundus.

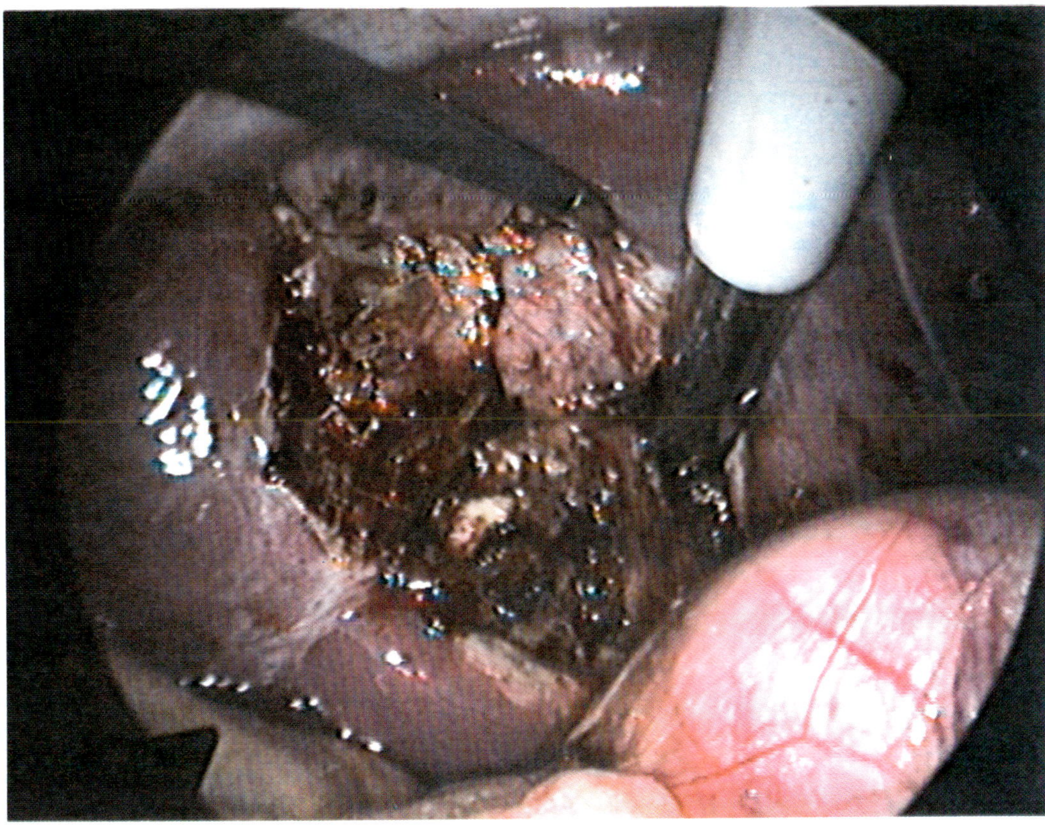

FIG 6–16.
Liver bed following removal of the gallbladder.

included 1 overnight stay and 1 additional day of hospitalization. The conversion rate of laparoscopic procedures to open cholecystectomy was 4%: 2 for bleeding and 2 for gangrenous gallbladders. All common duct stones that were encountered were successfully removed by ERCP.

REFERENCES

1. Hermann RE: The spectrum of biliary stone disease. *Am J Surg* 1989; 158:171–173.
2. McSherry CK: Cholecystectomy: The gold standard. *Am J Surg* 1989; 158:174–178.
3. Way LW: Trends in the treatment of gallstone disease: Putting options into context. *Am J Surg* 1989; 158:251–253.
4. Schoenfeld IJ, Lachin JM: The National Cooperative Gallstone Study Group. Chenodiol (chenodeoxycholic acid) for dissolution of gallstones: A controlled trial of efficacy and safety. *Ann Intern Med* 1981; 95:257–282.
5. Salen G: Gallstone dissolution therapy with ursodiol: Efficacy and safety. *Dig Dis Sci* 1989; 34:395–435.
6. Pitt HA, McFadden DW, Gadaez TR: Agents for gallstone dissolution. *Am J Surg* 1987; 153:233–246.

7. Thistle JL, May GR, Bender CE, et al: Dissolution of cholesterol gallbladder stones by methyl tert–butyl ether administered by percutaneous transhepatic catheter. *N Engl J Med* 1989; 320:633–639.
8. Made E: Dissolution of bile duct stones. *Am J Surg* 1989; 158:248–250.
9. Sue SO, Taub M, Pearlman J, et al: Treatment of choledocholithiasis with oral chenodeoxycholic acid. *Surgery* 1981; 90:32.
10. Sauerbruch T, Delius M, Paumgartner G, et al: Fragmentation of gallstones by extracorporeal shock waves. *N Engl J Med* 1986; 314:818–822.
11. Sackmann M, Delius M, Sauerbrauch T, et al: Shock-wave lithotripsy of gallbladder stones: The first 175 patients. *N Engl J Med* 1988; 318:393–397.
12. Haskin PH, Teplick SK, Sammon JK, et al: Monoctanoin infusion and stone removal through the transparenchymal tract: Use in 17 patients. *AJR* 1987; 148:185–188.
13. Geisinger MA, Owens DA, Meany TF: Radiologic methods of bile duct stone extraction. *Am J Surg* 1989; 158:222–227.
14. Chapman WC, Stephens WM, Williams LF Jr: Principles of biliary extracorporeal lithotripsy: Technical considerations and clinical implications. *Am J Surg* 1989; 158:179–183.
15. Vanderpool D, Jones RC, Oleary JP, et al: Biliary lithotripsy. *Am J Surg* 1989; 158:194–197.
16. Moody FG Jr, Amerson JR, Berci G: Lithotripsy for bile duct stones. *Am J Surg* 1989; 158:241–247.
17. Dempsey DT, Contreras C, Milner R, et al: Percutaneous ablation of gallstones. *J Surg Res* 1990; 49:116–120.
18. Lee PH, Hopkins TB, Howard PJ: Percutaneous cholecystolithotomy, *Urology* 1989; 33:37–39.
19. Dubois F, Icard P, Berthelot G, et al: Coelioscopic cholecystectomy: Preliminary report of 36 cases. *Ann Surg* 1990; 211:60–62.
20. Reddick EJ, Olsen DO, Daniel TF, et al: Laparoscopic laser cholecystectomy. *Laser Med Surg New* 1989; 7:38–40.
21. Reddick EJ, Olsen DO: Laparoscopic laser cholecystectomy. *Surg Endosc* 1989; 3:131–133.
22. Rubio PA, Rowe G, Freste JR: Endoscopic laser cholecystectomy. *Houston Med* 1989; 5:124–126.
23. Velez MA, Roys G, Ryan JJ: Laparoscopic cholecystectomy. *Contemp Surg* 1991; 38:11–20.
24. Peters JM, Ellison EC, Innes JT, et al: Safety and efficacy of laparoscopic cholecystectomy. *Ann Surg* 1991; 213:3–12.
25. Zucker KA, Bailey RW, Gadacz TR, et al: Laparoscopic guided cholecystectomy. *Am J Surg* 1991; 161:36–44.
26. Gracie WA, Ransohoff DF: The natural history of silent gallstones: The innocent gallstone is not a myth. *N Engl J Med* 1982; 307:798–800.
27. Walsh DB, Eckhauser FE, Ramsburgh SR, et al: Risk associated with diabetes mellitus in patients undergoing gallbladder surgery. *Surgery* 1982; 91:254–257.
28. Abramowitz M (ed): Laparoscopic cholecystectomy in *The Medical Letter. Med Lett* 1990; 32:115–116.
29. Phillips E, Daykhovsky L, Carroll B, et al: Laparoscopic cholecystectomy. *J Laparoendosc Surg* 1990; 1:3–15.
30. Hassler PC, Hill DS, Detorie FM, et al: High accuracy of songographic recognition of gallstones. *AJR* 1981; 136:517–520.
31. Cooperberg PL, Burhenne HJ: Real-time ultrasonography: Diagnostic technique of choice in calculous gallbladder disease. *N Engl J Med* 1980; 302:1277–1279.
32. Crade M, Taylor JW, Rosenfield AT, et al: Surgical and pathologic correlation of cholecystosonography and cholecystography. *AJR* 1978; 131:227–229.
33. Soderstrom RM: Safeguards in laparoscopy. *Contemp OB/GYN* 1978; 11:95–107.
34. Fishburne JI Jr: Anesthesia for laparoscopy: Considerations, complications and techniques. *J Reprod Med* 1978; 21:37–40.
35. Dye M, MacDonald A, Smith G: The bacterial flora of the biliary tract and liver in man. *Br J Surg* 1978; 65:285.

36. Strachan CJL, Black L, Powis SJAA, et al: Prophylatic use of cephazalin against wound sepsis after cholecystectomy. *Br Med J* 1977; 1:1254.
37. Hasson HM. Open laparoscopy: A report of 150 cases. *J Reprod Med* 1974; 12:234–238.
38. Copeland C, Wing RR, Mulka JF: Direct trocar insertion at laparoscopy. *Obstet Gynecol* 1983; 62:655–659.
39. Phillips EM, Berci G, Carroll B, et al: The importance of intraoperative cholangiography during laparoscopic cholecystectomy. *Am Surg* 1990; 12:792–795.
40. Thorbjarnarson B: *Surgery of the Biliary Tract.* Philadelphia, WB Saunders Co, 1982, pp 121–181.
41. Sivale MV: Endoscopic management of bile duct stones. *Am J Surg* 1989; 158:228–240.
42. Cameron JL: Retained and recurrent bile duct stones: Operative management. *Am J Surg* 1989; 158:218–221.

Chapter 7

Endosurgical Abdominal and Thoracic Procedures: Current Status and Future Perspective

Miguel Velez, M.D.

Stanley R. Klein, M.D.

"Less invasive surgery" is appealing from several perspectives. Patients actively pursue high-technology surgical methods because they produce less pain, have a diminished postoperative recovery period, and leave a more esthetic result. In addition, third-party payers are supportive of new surgical approaches that reduce hospital costs and stay as well as diminish postdischarge disability. Hospital and health care organizations aggressively market the availability of new technologies to attract patients and advertise related available services. In all regards, this enthusiasm must be tempered by careful comparisons to established procedures to document benefits, complications, and indications before adoption into routine surgical practice.

This chapter reviews the current literature and our experience in the application of new endoscopic surgical instrumentation and approaches to the management of several common surgical conditions. This review is intended to demonstrate the potential of these methods and to highlight future developments. Endoscopic gynecologic considerations are not discussed.

LAPAROSCOPIC APPENDECTOMY

Isolated reports of appendectomy were recorded in the 18th century, with Reginald Fitz being credited with the first description of appendicitis as a clinical and pathologic entity requiring surgical therapy.[1] Acute appendicitis is the most common acute abdominal surgical disease; it occurs at all ages but most frequently in the second and third decades of life.[2]

Operative mortality for nonperforated appendectomy should be less than 0.1%.[2,3] In contrast, perforated appendicitis has an operative mortality of about 2% and a substantially higher morbidity.[2–4] It is estimated that 5% of tubal infertility in the United States may result from perforated appendicitis.[4,5] Early diagnosis is now being emphasized as a method to reduce the approximate 20% overall incidence of perforated appendicitis and obviate the associated serious sequelae.[3,6] Currently, clinical judgment yields an accurate diagnosis of acute appendicitis in fewer than 85% of patients.[2,4,6]

Improved accuracy of diagnosis is being approached from several perspectives. High-resolution ultrasonography is most effective for delineation of appendiceal or tubal abscess (85% to 90%) but not in confirming acute nonperforated appendicitis.[7] A barium enema, although safe, can be deceptive and falsely negative.[8] Nuclear medicine studies have reported a positive predictive value of 76% and a negative predictive value of 97% but do not distinguish acute appendicitis from other local inflammatory conditions.[9] These studies are also not appropriate in pregnancy.[9,10] A computed tomographic (CT) scan is rarely justified but may be helpful in an ambiguous clinical picture where other modalities were not helpful.[10]

Currently, preoperative clinical observation and evaluations combined with postoperative recovery result in a 4-day average hospitalization.[2–4,6] In addition, the abdominal incision requires 3 to 4 weeks to heal, and this is a major portion of the expense and disability incurred by the patient. Laparoscopy has been utilized as an adjunctive procedure to verify early acute appendicitis and reduce the negative appendectomy rate.[11,12] Consequently, laparoscopic appendectomy has the potential to reduce costs by decreasing the number of adjunctive tests ordered, the length of hospital stay, and recuperative time.[13–15]

Laparoscopic appendectomy was first described by Semm in 1983.[16] Adoption of the technique in the United States was initially inhibited by a lack of laparoscopic instrumentation and reluctance of the general surgical community to evaluate the potential of this approach. Initial studies have suggested that conventional appendectomy incisions produce more pain and disability than do laparoscopic puncture sites and that exploration of the abdomen, especially the pelvis, is more effectively carried out through the laparoscope than a small, right lower–quadrant abdominal wall incision.[17,18] If the appendix is normal, early laparoscopy facilitates definitive diagnosis and institution of appropriate therapy for other intra-abdominal conditions mimicking acute appendicitis (e.g., pelvic inflammatory disease, inflammatory bowel disease, Meckel's diverticulitis). In addition, it in no way precludes open surgery for appropriate management of an encountered problem (e.g., sigmoid diverticulitis).[17–19]

Controversy exists as to whether a normal appendix should be removed. Early appendicitis may not be obvious to gross visual inspection, and subsequent episodes of abdominal pain may raise the possibility of appendicitis.[18–20] For these reasons we prefer to perform incidental appendectomy unless otherwise contraindicated. The morbidity of laparoscopic removal of a normal appendix appears to be minimal.[16–20]

Patient Preparation and Operative Technique

Patient preparation is identical to that for conventional open appendectomy including antibiotic administration and sterile field draping. The procedure is initiated by insufflating the abdomen and inserting a 10-mm cannuala/trocar unit at the inferior edge of the umbilicus.

Introduction of the 10-mm endoscope follows, and inspection of the lower abdomen and pelvis is methodically performed. To perform an appendectomy or other procedure or enhance exploration, ancillary endosurgical cannula(s) are introduced under direct laparoscopic vision. In acute appendicitis, a 5-mm cannula is inserted in the suprapubic area and a 10-mm port at McBurney's point.

To begin the procedure, the appendix is grasped and extended, when possible, to expose the mesoappendix (Fig 7–1). The mesoappendix is dissected and the vessels clipped and divided. Following mobilization of the appendix, ligating loops are inserted through the suprapubic port and placed so that one is at the base of the appendix and one approximately 1 cm distally. The appendix is then divided and removed through the 10-mm port. In the future, the EndoGIA stapler will greatly facilitate this procedure (see Fig 2–21). The appendiceal stump is then cauterized but not inverted into the cecum. The procedure is completed by irrigating the operative field, and drains are inserted if necessary. Necrotic debris or suppurative appendices may be placed in a sterile rubber or plastic receptacle (e.g., steam-sterilized condom) that is passed via the 10-mm port to expedite removal and prevent wound contamination.

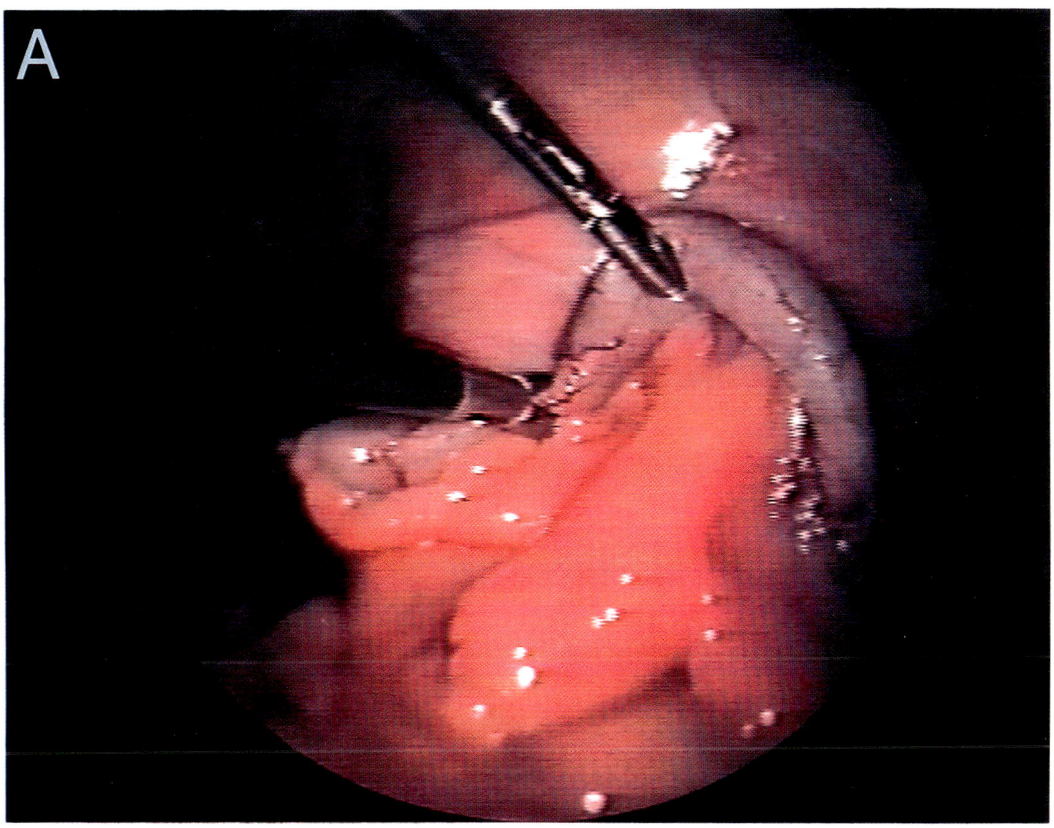

FIG 7–1.
Laparoscopic appendectomy. **A,** appendix grasped and mobilized; **B** (p. 120), appendix elevated to expose the mesoappendix; **C** (p. 120), initial dissection to expose vessels for ligation; **D** (p. 121), division of avascular tissue with the laser; **E** (p. 121), dissection continued to the base of the appendix; **F** (p. 122), endoloops applied, **G** (p. 122), appendix excised.

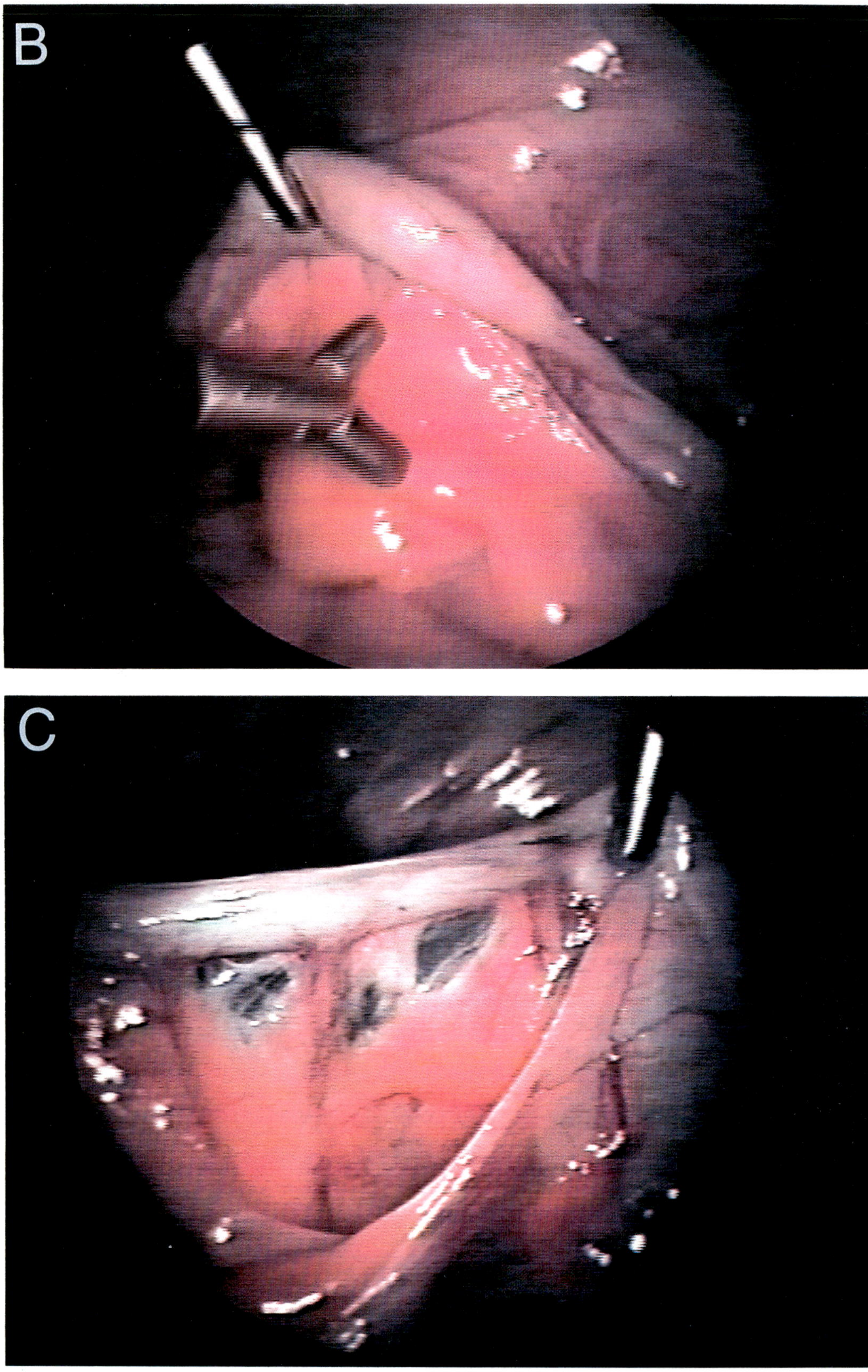
B
C

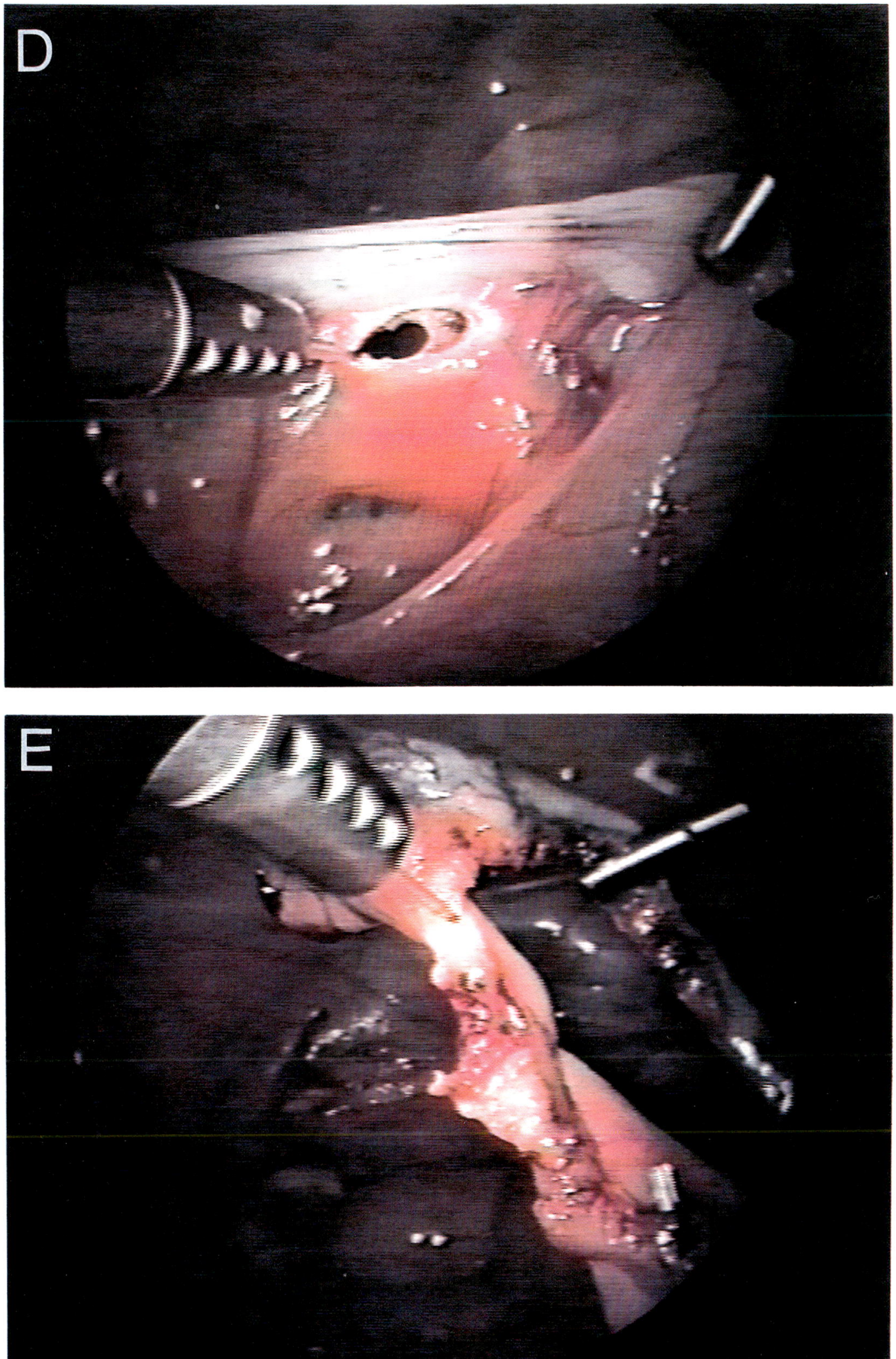
D
E

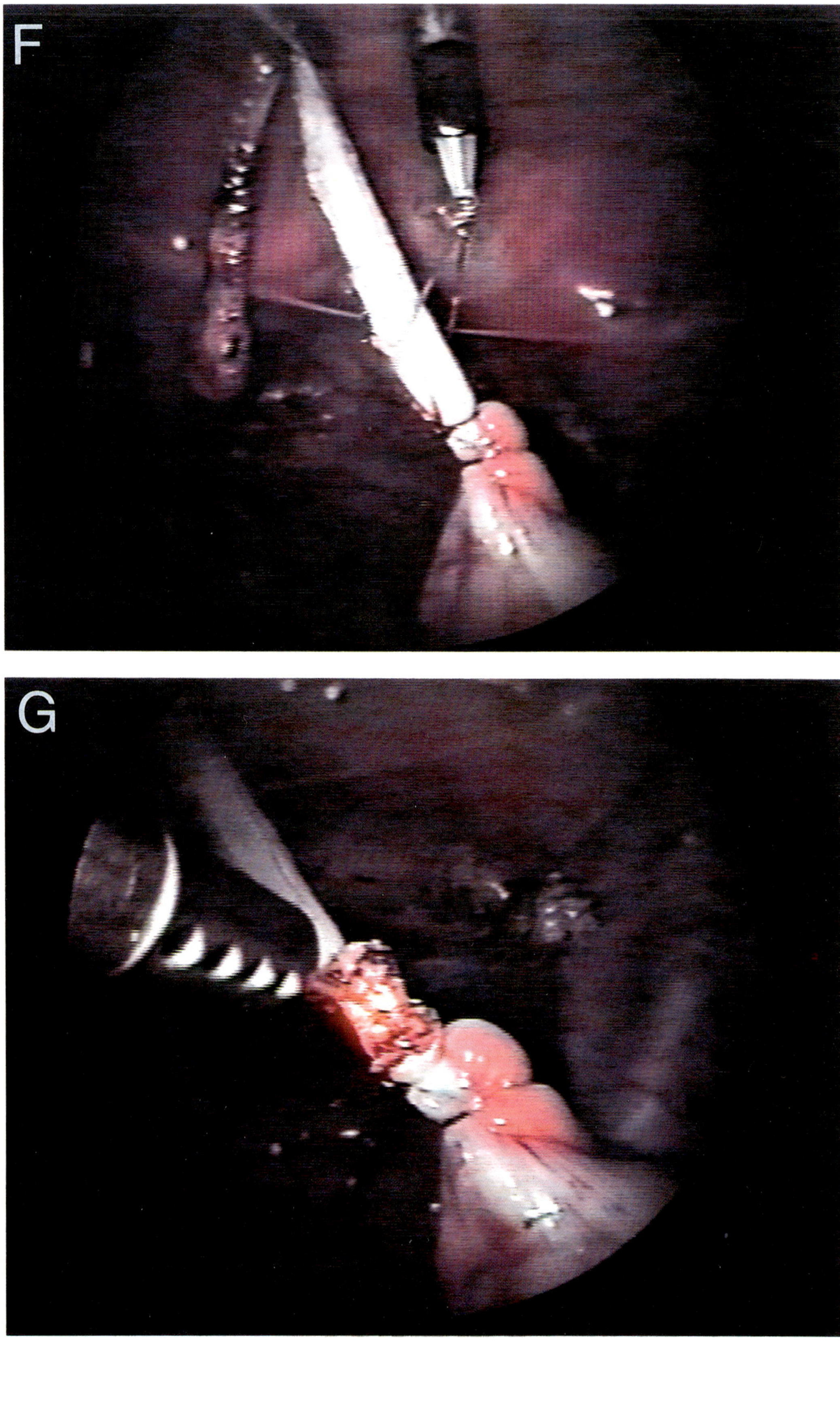
F
G

LAPAROSCOPIC ADHESION LYSIS

Treatment of chronic abdominal pain thought to be due to adhesions is a controversial subject. Laparotomy has had limited success because of associated morbidity and recurrence of adhesions. In the majority of instances attention to meticulous detail in order to minimize the extent and frequency of postoperative adhesion formation decreases their late sequelae.[21] Laparoscopic adhesion lysis may be helpful when pain is localized to a specific region, e.g., the pelvis or an incision scar. In patients with vague or diffuse abdominal pain, success is infrequent.[22] The technique of adhesion lysis is essential for the laparoscopic surgeon to master if he is going to operate upon patients with prior abdominal surgery.

Patient Preparation and Operative Technique

Preoperatively patients should receive mechanical and antimicrobial bowel preparation because of possible intestinal injury. Open laparoscopy is used to enter the abdomen, and all secondary ports are inserted under direct vision. Insertion of the Hassan cannula is performed as described in Chapter 5. Alternatively, a conventional cannula may serve as the primary en-

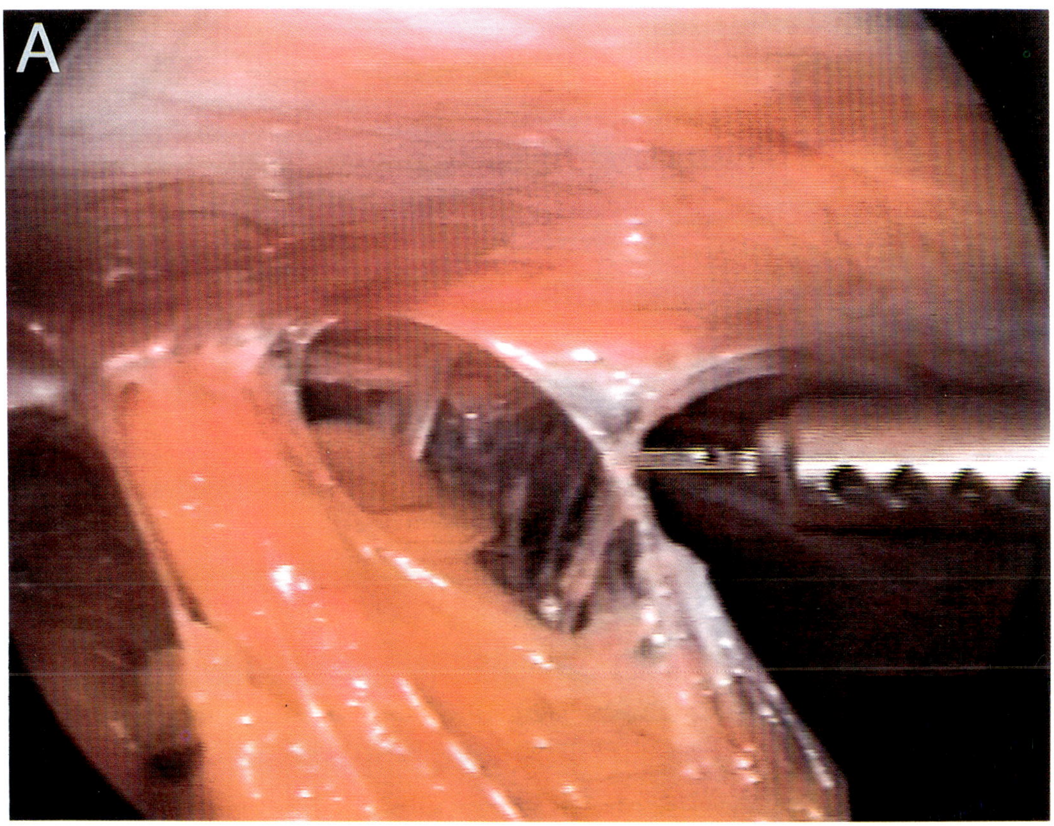

FIG 7–2.
Laparoscopic adhesion lysis. **A,** avascular adhesions before lysis with the KTP laser.

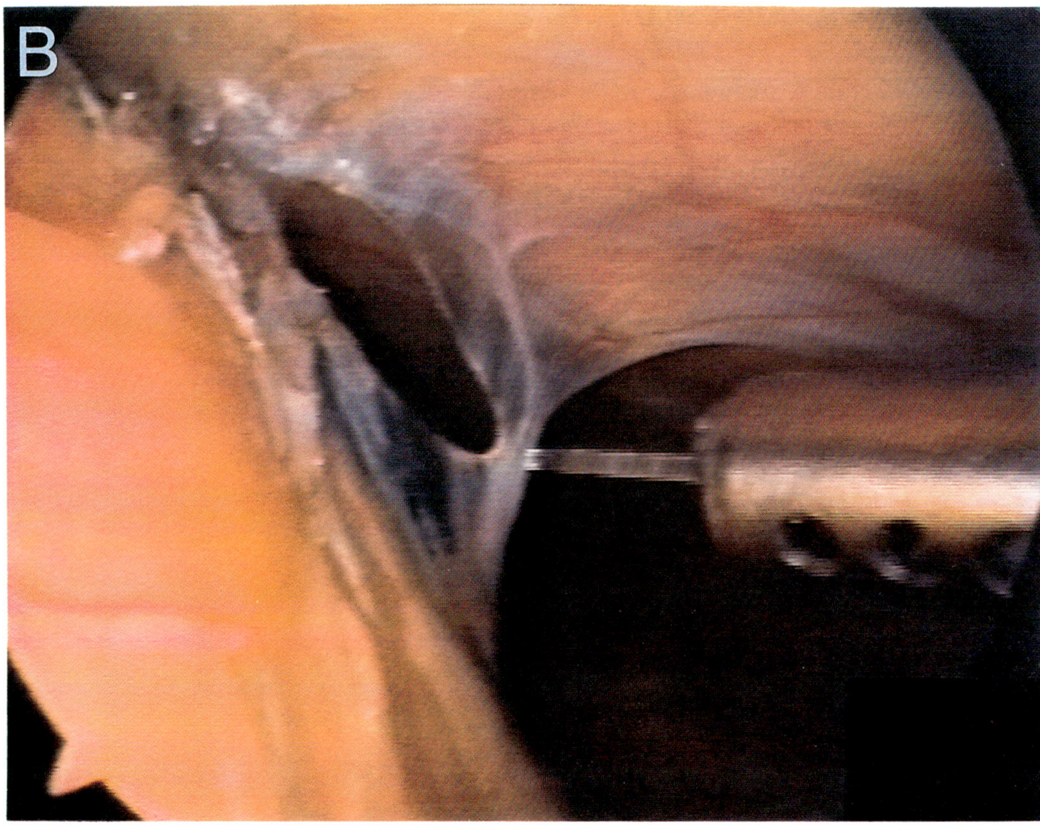

FIG 7–2 (cont.).
B, avascular adhesions following lysis with the KTP laser.

try site. A useful approach begins with a 1-cm incision being made in the inferior aspect of the umbilicus. The linea alba is identified, and the fascia is elevated with two Kocher clamps. A 5-mm incision is made, the 10-mm double-scoop forceps is inserted through a 10-mm cannula, and then the tips are passed into the abdominal cavity. The cannula is then guided over the forceps into the abdomen. Because of the small fascial opening, sutures are usually not necessary to preserve the pneumoperitoneum. In some cases, the incision is enlarged to visualize the peritoneal cavity, and a purse-string suture is then used to seal the fascia around the cannula. Following cannula insertion, insufflation is performed, and all secondary ports are inserted under direct vision. Lysis of avascular adhesions is best done with scissors. Vascular adhesions require hemostasis. Bleeding points should be controlled as encountered because they may be difficult to identify later in the procedure. Endoclips are excellent for control of larger vessels. Electrosurgery can lead to inadvertent injury to bowel due to electrical conduction via moist, gas-filled tissue. Bowel injury has been a particularly troublesome complication of electrocautery (see Chapter 2). In this situation some surgeons prefer laser coagulation, which avoids the electrical complications (Fig 7–2). For example, the potassium titanyl phosphate (KTP) laser at approximately 2 to 5 W is effective for dissection. At this level there is little tissue effect farther than 20 mm from the laser fiber.

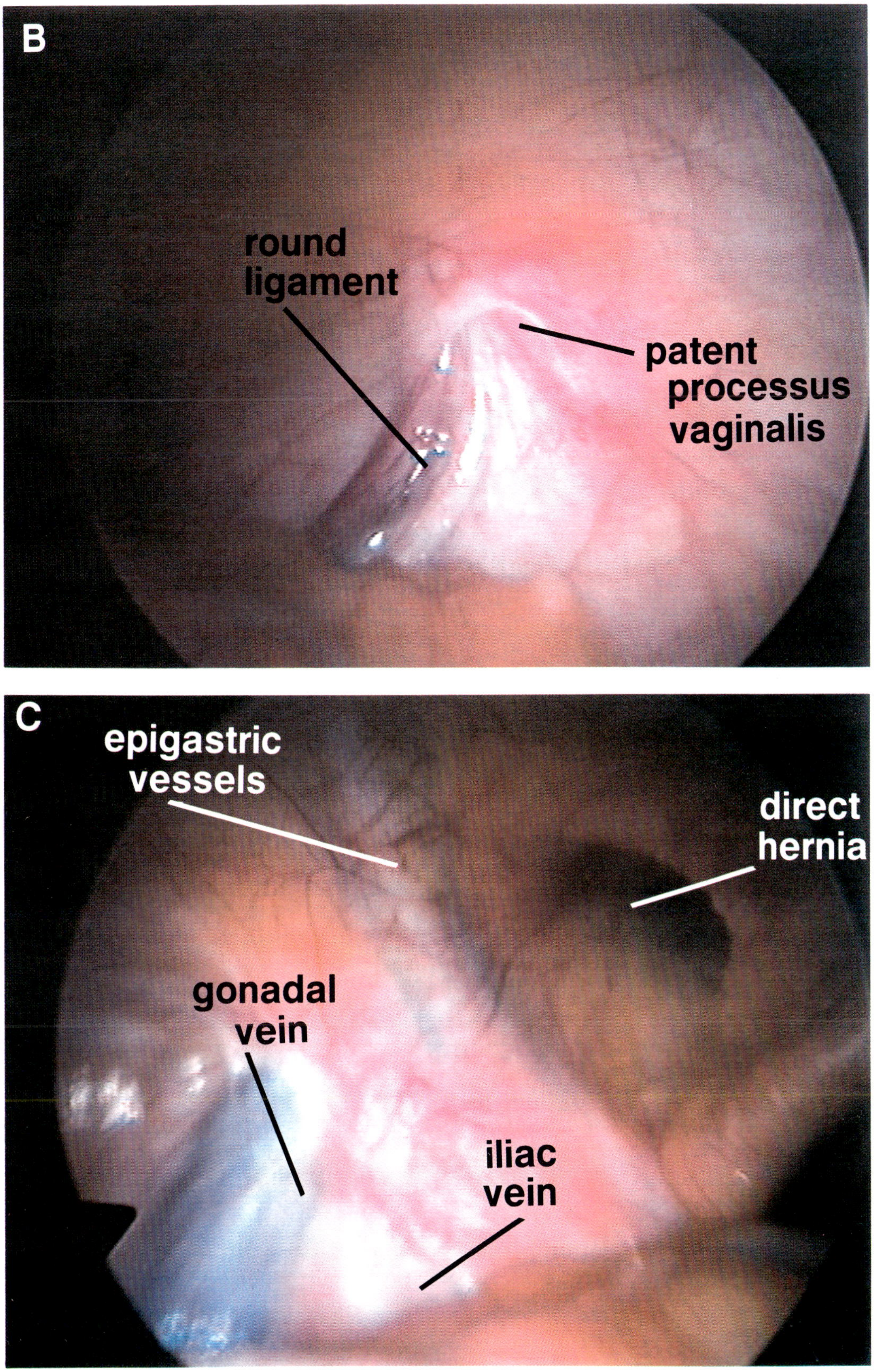
B
round
ligament
patent
processus
vaginalis
C
epigastric
vessels
direct
hernia
gonadal
vein
iliac
vein

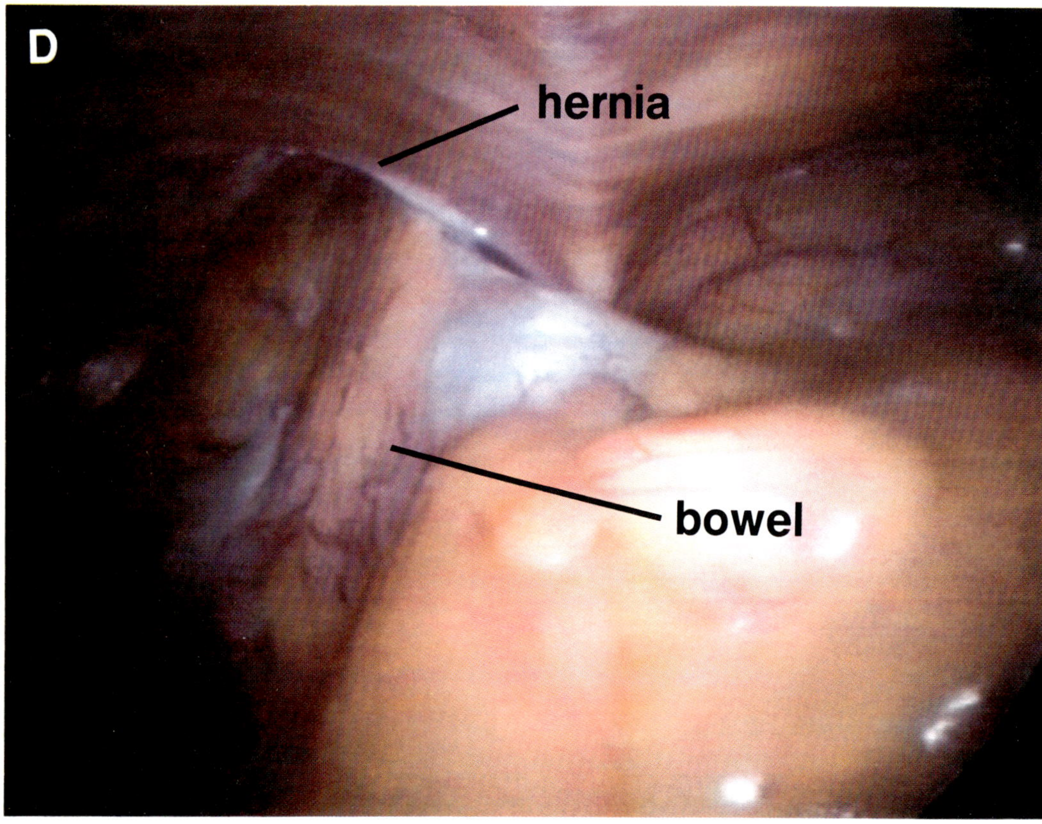

FIG 7–4 (cont.).
D, left inguinal hernia with an incarcerated bowel.

Additional Abdominal Endoscopic Procedures

As surgeons gain experience with laparoscopy and new instruments are developed, the diversity of endosurgical procedures is steadily increasing. Many promising reports are available to support continuing development and interest.

In selected instances, the magnitude of abdominal injury following trauma may be assessed laparoscopically and laparotomy avoided.[53, 54] Liver biopsy specimens can be safely harvested in patients who cannot have lesions localized by ultrasound or CT scan or in patients with a coagulopathy.[55, 56] Bleeding during a laparoscopic biopsy procedure can be controlled effectively with electrocautery when Tru-Cut needles are used to obtain specimens for histology and tissue assays.

Diagnosis can be established by laparoscopic inspection and biopsy samples in patients with suspected intra-abdominal metastasis not confirmed by noninvasive modalities.[57] The tissue obtained is useful to confirm a definitive diagnosis and to guide additional treatment such as chemotherapy or radiation therapy.

Cancer of the prostate is the second most common malignancy in men, most being adenocarcinomas.[58] Routes of dissemination of prostatic cancer are by direct extension to the pelvis, by lymphatic spread to the regional lymph nodes, and by metastasis to the skeleton.[58] Despite awareness and routine examination of the prostate, the majority of cases are not discovered before the tumor has spread (stage C and D lesions).[58] If a biopsy specimen of a suspicious prostate lesion is positive for carcinoma, further staging depends on bone and abdominal CT scans. Current techniques are limited for clinical staging because on many occasions retroperitoneal lymph nodes invaded by tumor are not apparent unless surgical exploration is performed.[58] Laparoscopic sampling of the obturator and iliac lymph nodes enables staging of metastatic disease while obviating open-procedure morbidity.[59] Favorable results when using this approach are being reproduced in studies in several centers.

Additional therapeutic procedures that show promising early results include vagotomy with and without pyloromyotomy for acid-peptic disease[60] and segmental gastric and bowel resection.[61, 62] Nephrectomies have been performed in humans, but because of the need to morsellate tissue to enable laparoscopic removal, histologic evaluation may be compromised.[63]

Treatment of varicoceles by laparoscopic methods has been performed. Varicoceles are abnormal venous tortuosities of the pampiniform plexus within the spermatic cord and have been associated with male infertility.[64] The incidence of varicocele in the general population

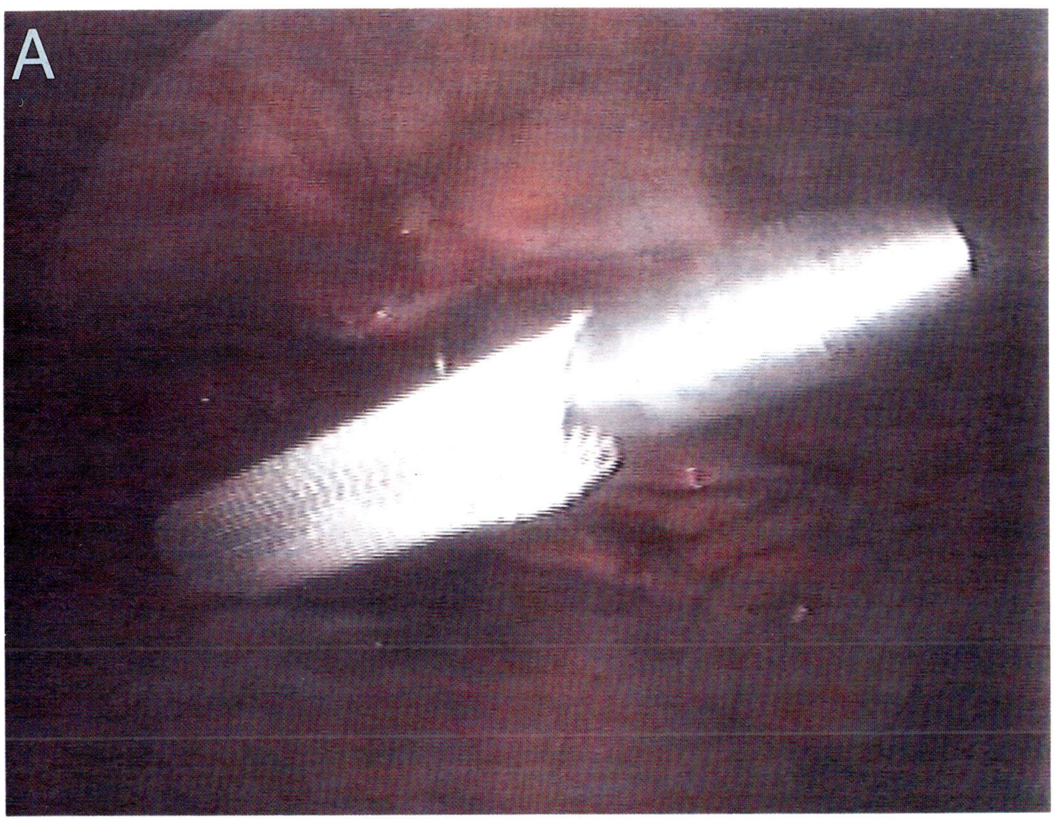

FIG 7–5.
Hernia repair by experimental mesh technique. **A,** rolled mesh introduction through the cannula; **B** (p. 132), mesh placed over the hernia defect after peritoneal flaps have been developed; **C** (p. 132), final placement of the prosthetic mesh. **D** (p. 133), mesh stapled to the inguinal floor with an experimental stapling device; **E** (p. 133), close-up view of a deployed staple. *Continued.*

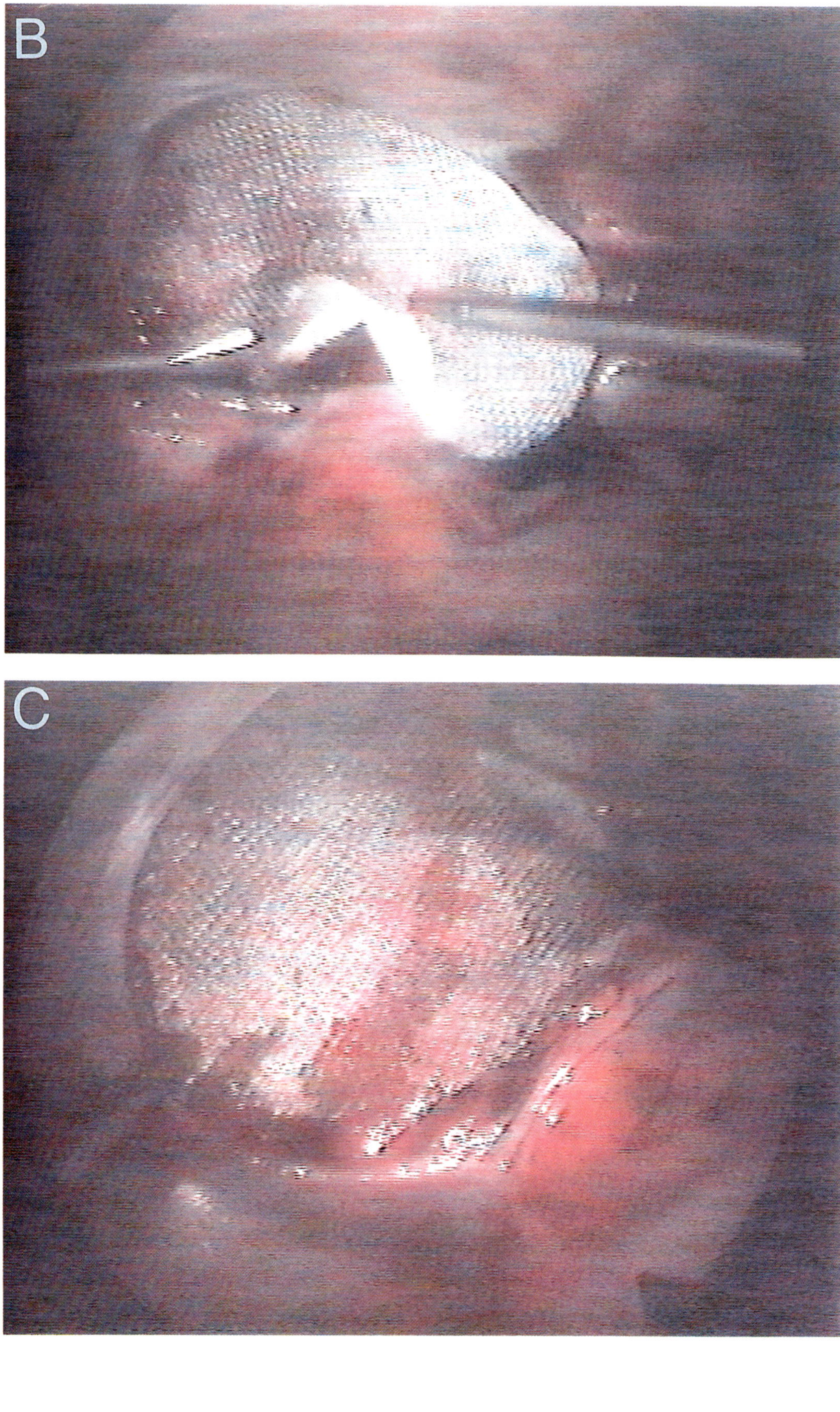
B
C

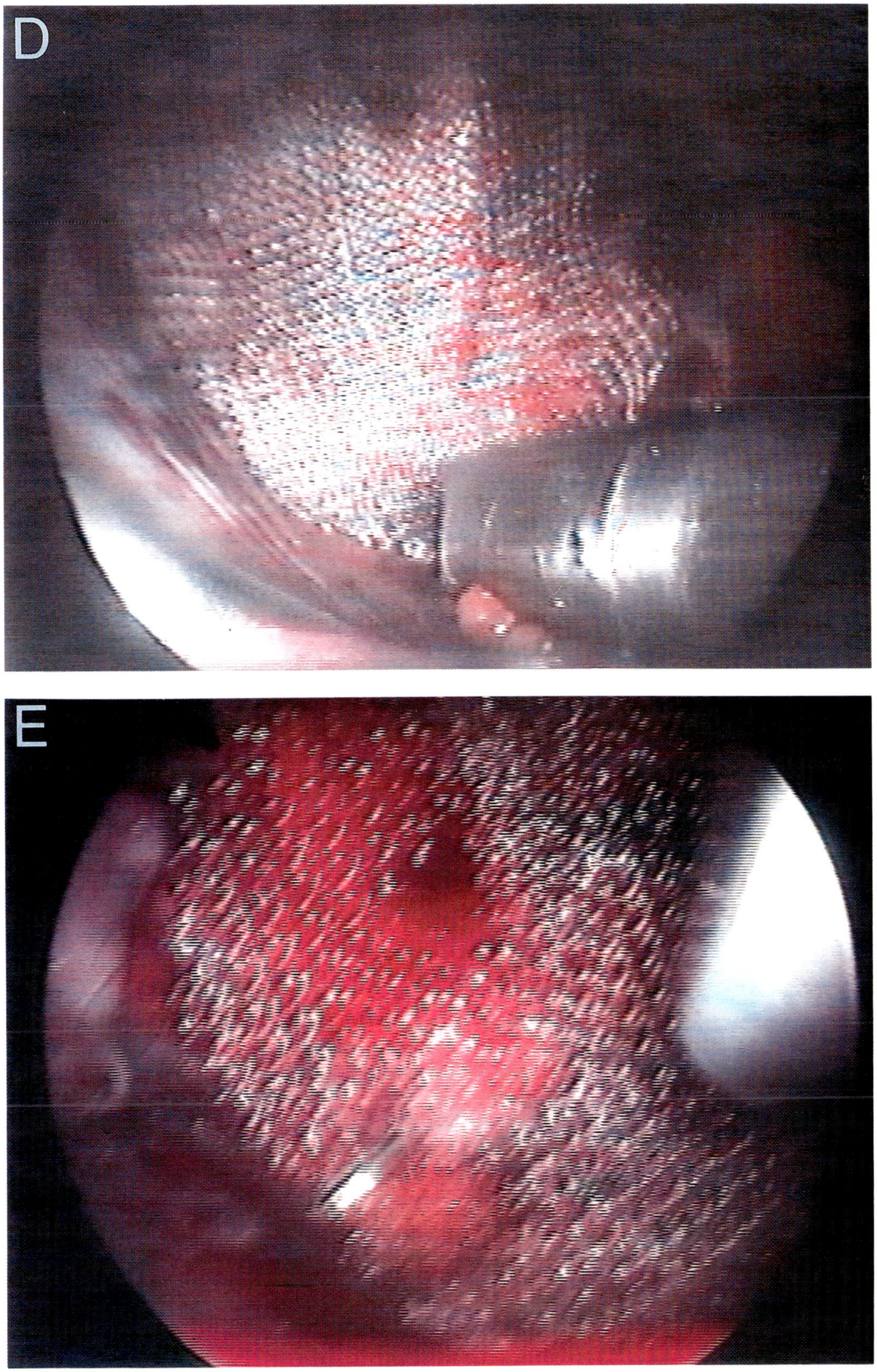
D
E

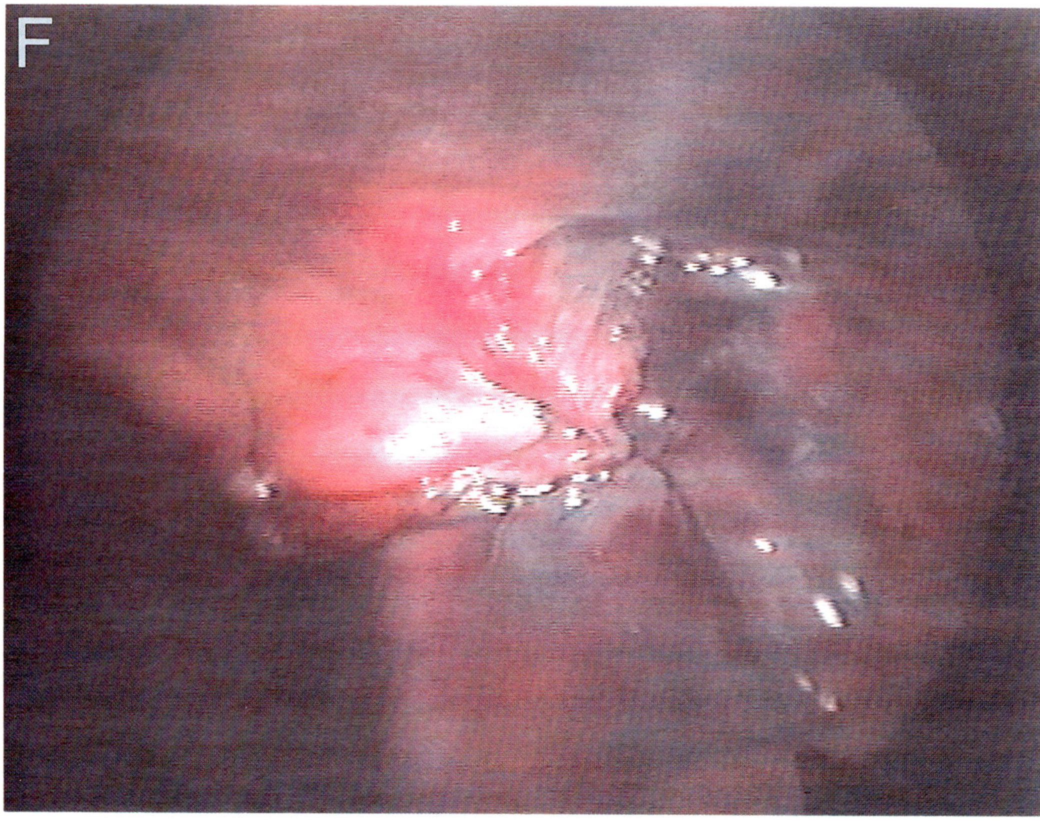

FIG 7–5 (cont.).
F, peritoneum closed over the mesh repair.

ranges from 10% to 20%.[64, 65] The majority of varicoceles occur on the left and are believed to be secondary to incompetence of the valvular structures of the internal spermatic vein. Recent appearance of the lesion on the right or in an older male should prompt further investigation prior to therapy.[65] Varicoceles are usually quite prominent. To evaluate the severity of the lesion, a patient should be examined in the upright position, first without and then with a Valsalva maneuver, to increase venous reflux. The major indication for repair of a varicocele is an attempt to correct abnormal semen quality, with less common reasons for repair being pain and cosmesis.[65, 66] Current management of a varicocele includes percutaneous occlusion[67, 68] of the internal spermatic artery and/or vein as well as surgical ablation.[69, 70] There are three distinct approaches to ligation of the internal spermatic vein: scrotal, inguinal, and retroperitoneal.[69] The scrotal approach is used infrequently because it is difficult to be certain that all of the numerous veins in the pampiniform plexus are ligated and since it is also possible to damage one or more of three arteries (spermatic, deferential, and cremasteric) that supply the testis and epididymis. The theoretical advantage of a scrotal incision is that all veins, even those that do not connect with the internal spermatic vein, can be ligated. The inguinal and the retroperitoneal approaches are both widely used and accepted.[69, 70] At present most large series reviewing the results of varicocele surgery show that about 75% of men will have improved semen quality.[67] Pregnancy rates after corrective surgery average 40%.[64, 66]

59. Gershman A, Daykhovsky L, Chandra M, et al: Laparoscopic pelvic lymphadenectomy. *J Laparoendosc Surg* 1990; 1:63–68.
60. Namir K: Endosurgical vagotomy. Personal communication.
61. Leahy PF: Endosurgical bowel surgery. Personal communication.
62. Leahy PF, Pennino RP, Hinshaw JR, et al: Minimally invasive esophagogastrectomy: An approach to esphagogastrectomy through the left chest. *J Laparoendosc Surg* 1990; 1:59–62.
63. Claman R: Endosurgical nephrectomy. Personal communication.
64. Coolsaet BL: The varicocele syndrome: Venography determining the optimal level for surgical management. *J Urol* 1980; 124:833–840.
65. Ivanissevich O: Left varicocele due to reflux: Experience with 4470 operative cases in 42 years. *J Int Cell Surg* 1960; 34:742–751.
66. Lipshultz L, Howards SS: Surgical treatment of male infertility, in Lipshultz L, Howards SS (eds): *Infertility in Males.* London, Churchill Livingstone Inc, 1983.
67. Getzoff Pl: Surgical management of male infertility: Results of a survey. *Fertil Steril* 1973; 24:553–557.
68. Seyferth W, Jecht E, Zeitler E: Percutaneous occlusion of the varicocele. *Radiology* 1981; 139:335–42.
69. Dubin L, Amelar RD: Varicocelectomy: 986 cases in a twelve year study. *Urology* 1977; 10:446–452.
70. Kaufman SL, Kadir S, Barth KH, et al: Mechanisms of recurrent varicocele after balloon occlusion or surgical ligation of the internal spematic vein. *Radiology* 1983; 147:435–443.
71. Pickett SL, Klein SR, Rajfer J: Endosurgical varicocelectomy: A preliminary report. Unpublished data.
72. Batata MA, Whitmore WF Jr, Chu FC, et al: Cryptorchidism and testicular cancer. *J Urol* 1980; 124:382–390.
73. Scorer CG, Farrington GH: *Congenital Deformities of the Testis and Epididymis.* London, Butterworth, 1971.
74. Gross RE, Jewett TC: Surgical experiences from 1222 operations for undescended testis. *JAMA* 1956; 160:634–643.
75. Job JC, Canlorbe P, Garagorri JM, et al: Hormonal therapy of cryptorchidism with human chorionic gonadotropin (hCG). *Urol Clin North Am* 1982; 9:405–412.
76. Hadziselimovic F: *Cryptorchidism: Management and Implications.* New York, Springer-Verlag NY Inc, 1983.
77. Koop CE: Technique of herniorraphy and orchidopexy. *Birth Defects.* 1977; 13:243–303.
78. Silber SJ: Microsurgery for the undescended testicle. *Urol Clin North Am* 1982; 9:429–441.
79. Silber SJ, Cohen R: Laparoscopy for cryptorchidism. *J Urol* 1980; 124:928–936.
80. Weiss RM, Seashore JM: Laparoscopy in the management of the nonpalpable testis. *J Urol* 1987; 138:382–384.
81. Pickett S, Klein SR, Rajfer J: Laparoscopic evaluation of gonads in the patient with ambiguous genitalia. Unpublished data.
82. Klein SR. Unpublished data.
83. Wakabayashi G. Personal communication.
84. Bloomberg AE: Thoracoscopy in perspective. *Surg Gynecol Obstet* 1978; 147:433–442.
85. Baumgartner WA, Mark JBD: The use of thoracoscopy in the diagnosis of pleural disease. *Arch Surg* 1980; 115:420–424.
86. DeCamp P, Moseley PW, Scott ML, et al: Diagnostic thoracoscopy. *Ann Thorac Surg* 1973; 16:79–86.

Chapter 8

Complications of Endoscopic Abdominal Surgery

Douglas Cavaye, M.D.

In the last two decades, the application and widespread acceptance of endoscopic surgery in the fields of urology and gynecology have provided many advantages to the patient and surgeon but brought with it a new set of complications associated with these so-called, minimally invasive techniques. With the recent application of endoscopic techniques to general surgical procedures, the complications associated with these newer techniques must be examined. Only by understanding the types and mechanisms of these problems can surgeons reduce the incidence of unwanted complications.

CLASSIFICATION

A clinically useful approach to the classification of complications is to consider the basic underlying mechanism. For this reason they are divided into general and patient-specific complications (Table 8–1).

GENERAL COMPLICATIONS

Anesthetic

Although it is possible to perform some diagnostic laparoscopic procedures under local anesthetic infiltration and sedation, certain problems may make the procedure uncomfortable for the patient and difficult for the surgeon. Lidocaine, 1% or 2%, infiltration prior to needle and trochar insertion, although mildly painful, is associated with an extremely low incidence of adverse reactions but should be avoided in patients with any known sensitivity to local anesthetics of the amide type. Systemic toxicity can occur if the recommended maximum dose is exceeded, i.e., 7 mg/kg body weight with epinephrine and 4.5 mg/kg without epinephrine. Despite good preoperative instructions, some patients are unable to relax and breathe satisfac-

TABLE 8–1.
Complications of Laparoscopic Surgery

General	Patient Specific
Anesthetic	Obesity
Needle insertion	Ascites
Pneumoperitoneum	Elderly
Trochar insertion	Organomegaly
Instrumentation	Abdominal hernias
Thermocoagulation	Diabetes
Laser	Clotting
Suction	Abdominal scars, adhesions

torily with pneumoperitoneum. It should also be noted that there is a substantial amount of discomfort associated with any manipulation of the parietal peritoneum and traction on the bowel or its mesentery.

If any more than a diagnostic laparoscopy is anticipated, regional or general anesthesia is usually indicated. Lumbar epidural anesthesia is suitable for pelvic and lower abdominal surgery, but when it is used for laparoscopic procedures, the patient must be warned that shoulder pain is common and that pneumoperitoneum may require a greatly increased respiratory effort. Despite these problems it is a very popular technique that is used in some centers in up to 50% of all patients undergoing a laparoscopic procedure.[1] In a series of patients receiving lumbar epidural as compared with general anesthesia for laparoscopy, the incidence of nausea and vomiting was reduced from 38% (general) to 4% (epidural).[2] However, because of the risk of regurgitation and aspiration associated with the increased intra-abdominal pressure, especially if Trendelenburg positioning of the patient is necessary, some centers always use endotracheal intubation and general anesthesia. Muscle relaxation is not a necessity for short-duration pelvic procedures but is preferred for more lengthy upper abdominal operations. General muscle relaxant anesthesia is therefore the most common choice for endoscopic general surgical procedures.

Needle and Trocar Insertion

Insertion of the pneumoperitoneum needle has the potential for serious complications because it carries with it the risks of inserting a sharp object into the patient's abdomen without the margin of relative safety provided by established pneumoperitoneum. The placement of the needle is crucial not only to prevent direct trauma to the abdominal contents but also because the pneumoperitoneum is instilled through this needle. Of 274 traumatic injuries reported in a recent Canadian survey on needle and trocar injuries in laparoscopy, 109 were due to the pneumoperitoneum needle, 104 due to the primary trocar, and 61 due to the secondary trocar.[3] Injuries occurred twice as often among those who experienced difficulty in inserting the needle ($P = .04$), and more injuries occurred among physicians who had not been trained in laparoscopy during their residency as compared with those who had been trained ($P = .041$). Although the double-lumen Veress needle reduces the risk of inadvertant perforation of mobile abdominal contents, it offers little or no protection to fixed structures.[4]

Vascular injuries, especially those involving the iliac vessels and aorta, constitute the most life-threatening complications of needle and trocar insertion and therefore warrant a detailed discussion. The incidence of major-vessel injury associated with needle and trocar insertion in reported series is between 0.07% and 0.7%.[5–8] The safety of perforating the abdominal aorta from a retroperitoneal approach has been proved by thousands of translumbar aortograms since extravasated blood is trapped in the tough periaortic connective tissue and the hole is plugged. However, the thin anterior peritoneal covering on the aorta and iliac arteries offers little or no protection. Since the reservoir of the peritoneal cavity allows large quantities of blood to escape undetected, several minutes may elapse before hemorrhage is recognized on the basis of altered vital signs.

The return of bright red arterial blood after needle puncture implies arterial injury and warrants taking steps to ensure that the abdomen may be opened rapidly while observation continues. The anesthesiologist should be alerted to the possible emergency and blood cross-matched. Any change in vital signs or expansion of the abdomen is an indication for immediate laparotomy. After opening the abdomen, large-vessel bleeding should be controlled with digital, manual, or sponge pressure. If prolonged arterial occlusion using vascular clamps is required, anticoagulation with heparin is advised to reduce the risk of distal thrombosis. In most cases, however, an expedient repair of the vessel can be achieved with minimal clamp time, and heparinization is not required. Large-vessel venous bleeding often occurs in poorly accessible areas but can be easily controlled with manual pressure. By maintaining strict adherence to caudal angulation when inserting the pneumoperitoneum needle, the incidence of life-threatening major-vessel injuries can be reduced[4,6] (Fig 8–1).

Abdominal wall vascular structures also may be injured, particularly if a large trocar is used.

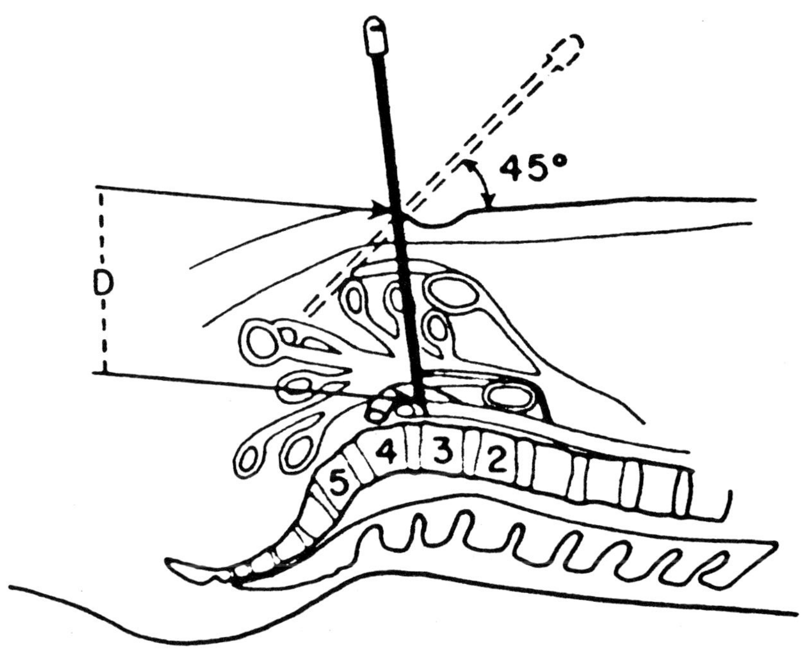

FIG 8–1.
Incorrect *(solid line)* and correct *(broken line)* techniques for insertion of the pneumoperitoneum needle. The distance between the anterior abdominal wall and the aorta *(D)* can be surprisingly short in thin patients, especially when downward pressure is applied to the needle during insertion. (From McDonald PT, Rich NM, Collins GJ, et al: *Am J Surg* 1978; 135:651–655. Used by permission.)

Inferior and superior epigastric arteries are medium-sized vessels with the potential for producing a large hematoma if lacerated by needle or trocar insertion.[9] Anterior abdominal wall hemorrhage during laparoscopy occurs at a rate of 0.25% to 6.0%,[10–12] and exploration may be required to control hemorrhage and evacuate the hematoma.

Other body wall structures such as a vesicourachal diverticulum (urachal sinus) may be damaged, and although less common than blood vessel injury, they produce a worrying postoperative problem.[13, 14] These rare vestiges of the obliterated allantois may be damaged by the trocar at surgery, but the diagnosis may not be made until the postoperative period because the bladder is usually drained before and during surgery. Fluid leaking from the umbilicus or suprapubic site should be cultured and compared with the patient's urine by biochemical analysis. The size of the trocar that caused the urachal injury and the communication of the defect with the bladder will determine the success of conservative management. Peritonitis requiring laparotomy has been reported,[14] and it is emphasized that the presence of umbilical discharge should alert the laparoscopist to the possibility of urachal anomalies.

Urinary bladder perforation can occur when there is difficulty in selecting a site for trocar insertion that results in carrying the route of entry too far caudally, especially if the bladder is full.[15] A noncatheterized bladder is more likely to be injured and has caused some centers to routinely catheterize and drain the bladder prior to any laparoscopic procedure. Bladder drainage via a urethral catheter and antibiotic coverage is usually sufficient treatment of these injuries since the defect is anterior and extraperitoneal in most cases.

Pneumoperitoneum

The physiologic disturbances created by installation of carbon dioxide gas have been described in a separate chapter of this book. The complications range from discomfort and increased respiratory effort in awake patients to pneumothorax, vagal arrest, and death.

Subcutaneous emphysema can occur if insufflation of gas continues despite high pressures in the system. This has been reported to occur when a faulty intra-abdominal pressure gauge resulted in high-pressure insufflation of gas with the needle tip in subcutaneous tissues.[16] Indeed, most cases of subcutaneous emphysema are caused by improper placement of the needle.[17, 18] Rarely, subcutaneous emphysema may occur in association with pneumomediastinum, pneumothorax, and pneumopericardium[19] (Fig 8–2).

Pneumothorax secondary to pneumoperitoneum was first recognized in the 1940s when pneumoperitoneum was a primary therapy for peritoneal tuberculosis. Published reports during this period were of right-sided pneumothoraces in all cases.[20] It is interesting to note that pneumothorax following laparoscopy has been reported to occur much more frequently on the left side.[21] Both CO_2 and N_2O pneumothoraces have been described, depending on which gas is used to create the pneumoperitoneum.[22] A number of hypotheses explaining the association of pneumothorax, pneumomediastinum, and pneumoperitoneum have been proposed. The most popular concepts are that air enters the retroperitoneal space and then dissects along the tissue planes to the mediastinum and pleural spaces or that air gains access to the mediastinum and pleural space via the tissue planes of the diaphragmatic hiatus[23] (Fig 8–3). Incomplete closure of embryonic connections between the pleura, peritoneum, and pericardium and congenital defects of the diaphragm are also believed to be associated with the development of this syndrome.[24] Whatever the exact mechanism is, the communication appears to allow gas to move from either cavity to the other without the generation of a major pres-

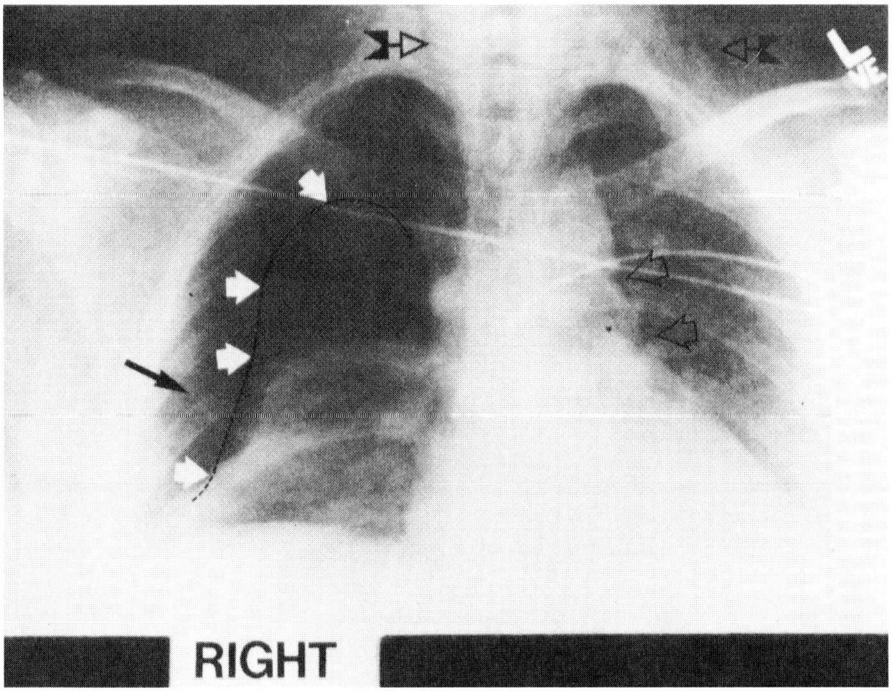

FIG 8–2.
Subcutaneous emphysema *(upper arrows),* pneumomediastinum *(left thoracic arrows),* and pneumothorax *(right thoracic arrows)* following diagnostic laparoscopy. In this case N_2O was used to produce the pneumoperitoneum. (From Batra MS, Driscoll JJ, Coburn WA, et al: *Anesth Analg* 1983; 62:1121–1123. Used by permission.)

sure difference. There have been a number of reports of pneumoperitoneum occurring secondary to pneumothorax, most frequently encountered with mechanical ventilatory support, even where ventilatory airway pressures have not been excessive.[25, 26]

There are a number of effects of increased intra-abdominal pressure produced by pneumoperitoneum. The alterations in lower esophageal sphincter tone are important because of the possibility of regurgitation and aspiration, although there is evidence that there may not be a clear confirmed pathophysiologic relationship.[27] Apart from the effects on large-vein venous return and changes in ventilatory work, increased intra-abdominal pressure is associated with changes in smaller systemic veins. Retinal hemorrhage has been reported following laparoscopy and is attributed to several factors that tend to increase the retinal venous pressure.[28] If a further pressure surge occurs, such as an involuntary Valsalva maneuver or a bout of coughing or vomiting, rupture of the retinal microcirculation becomes likely.[29] A defect in vision is noted by the patient only when the macula is involved. Since many patients may not volunteer information regarding a minor visual impairment following general anesthesia, retinal hemorrhage during laparoscopy may be more common than suspected.[28]

Carbon dioxide embolism association with laparoscopy is a rare event and occurs in 0.002% to 0.016% of all such procedures.[30–32] Fatal laparoscopic CO_2 embolism has been reported but is exceedingly rare.[33] Carbon dioxide is the insufflating gas of choice because of its high solubility in blood, capacity to be buffered by blood, and rapid excretion by the lungs. A typical case of major CO_2 embolism involves the insertion of the Veress needle and instilla-

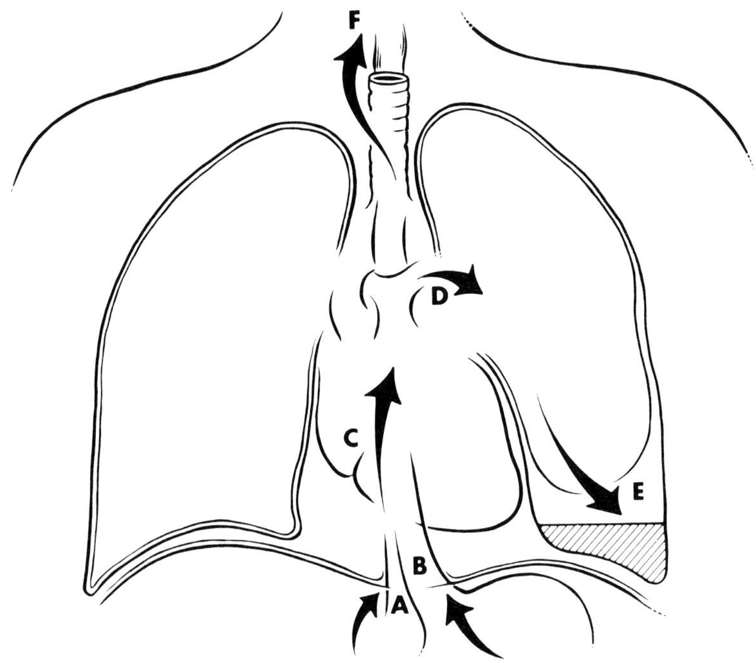

FIG 8–3.
Possible routes of gas tracking through one of the anatomic hiatuses *(A* and *B)* into the mediastinum *(C)*. The pneumomediastinum can then either rupture through the mediastinal pleura behind the root of the heart *(D)* into the pleural cavity and cause pneumothorax *(E)* or track into the tissues of the neck and cause subcutaneous emphysema *(F)*. (From Ramage AA, Singh M, Griffin JW Jr, et al: *J Clin Gastroenterol* 1986; 8:483–485. Used by permission.)

tion of gas with the pressure well below 20 mm Hg. Within 1 minute, heart sounds may change in character, typically assuming a "sloshing" nature.[34] This is usually associated with sudden, profound hypotension, cyanosis, tachycardia, and other cardiac dysrhythmias. Treatment of gas embolism consists of immediate cessation of the insufflation and placing the patient in the left lateral decubitus position.[35] The steep head-down position has also been advocated, but since the gas bubble may be found at the junction of the inferior vena cava and the right atrium, assumption of this position may cause the bubble to enter further into the cardiac chambers.[36] Discontinuing nitrous oxide, if in use, will allow 100% oxygen to be given but will not result in a reduction of the size of the CO_2 embolus, as is the case with an air embolus. This is due to the similarity of the solubilities of N_2O and CO_2, so there will not be significant diffusion of N_2O into or out of the CO_2 bubbles.[37] Hyperventilation will, however, increase CO_2 excretion. If these simple measures are not rapidly effective, a central venous catheter may be introduced for aspiration of the gas, although it has been shown that this technique was no more effective than the left lateral decubitus position in the treatment of induced air embolism in dogs.[38]

Cardiac arrhythmias associated with laparoscopy have been noted by several authors, but reports of asystole or life-threatening tachyarrhythmias are rare.[39] Vagally mediated cardiac arrest has been reported during a laparoscopic procedure, but insufflation of gas may not be directly associated with this phenomenon. In the reported case, the patient developed a rapidly progressing sinus bradycardia ending in asystole after the Veress needle was inserted and

500 mL of CO_2 was introduced. With the administration of 0.6 mg atropine intravenously and removal of the Veress needle, rhythm resumed after 20 seconds of asystole.[40] Further evidence for possible vagally mediated cardiovascular collapse during gas insufflation is given by reports of bradycardia and nodal cardiac rhythms in healthy young women undergoing laparoscopic sterilization procedures.[41] It is unclear whether these complications were directly related to gas insufflation or anesthetic pharmacologic technique.[42]

Instrumentation

By their very nature, surgical instruments are potentially dangerous. The normal eye-hand coordination required to successfully perform surgery is disrupted in laparoscopic procedures by the replacement of the surgeon's stereoscopic vision by a two-dimensional video monitor image. Apart from the alterations in three-dimensional visual guidance of the operators instruments, laparoscopic surgery may carry even greater risks because the tissue dissection and manipulation is performed at the end of a long instrument and the number of assistants may be limited.

Despite the improvements in safety of insertion of the trocar by the incorporation of an automatic safety shield and prior institution of pneumoperitoneum, problems may be associated with its removal. Herniation of bowel through the trocar site is rare and occurs in approximately 0.0025% of laparoscopies.[43] It was first described in 1968 in a patient who persistently coughed at the time of awakening from the general anesthetic.[44] Multiple cases of omental herniation through the infraumbilical incision site have also been noted.[45, 46] A review of the literature reveals that the onset of symptoms varied from 5 days to 7 weeks[45, 47] and that the cause of herniation was usually the patient coughing or gagging as the laparoscope was being removed. The presence of an umbilical hernia, coughing, and poor relaxation before sheath removal are factors that may facilitate herniation following laparoscopy.[45, 48] The possibility of a bowel obstruction should be entertained in any patient who develops or presents with symptoms and signs consistent with this diagnosis, regardless of the intervening period of time.[47] Techniques to reduce the probability of herniation include the use of smaller-diameter trocars ($<$11 mm) or the creation of a "Z" track by piercing the skin and fascia at different angles.[45]

More serious injuries can occur if pathologic conditions alter the anatomy or size of the abdominal contents, in particular, the solid organs. Splenic rupture has been reported as a complication of diagnostic laparoscopy for hepatosplenomegaly.[49] Because laparoscopy is now performed in many centers as an investigative procedure, i.e., in the diagnosis and management of gastrointestinal disease,[50] it is important to be aware of these possible complications. When dealing with patients with splenomegaly, especially those who have had previous abdominal surgery with possible adhesion formation, insufflation of gas and instrumentation must be carried out with extreme caution. When used as a diagnostic technique in a hepatology training program, laparoscopy has been shown to be safe despite the problems associated with organomegaly.[50] In this situation, it has been used to evaluate chronic liver disease, ascites, and the extent of intra-abdominal malignancy without a significant increase in the incidence of complications. If tense ascites is present, large-volume paracentesis can be performed as a preliminary step in the laparoscopy.[51] When performing routine laparoscopic liver and spleen biopsies, hemorrhage and bile leakage can occur. Fibrin sponge plugging of the biopsy site has been advocated as one technique to endoscopically control the leak.[52]

Bowel injury can be due to mechanical perforation or damage related to thermocoagulation, suction, laser, or mesenteric trauma. Mechanical perforation is a rare event, with an incidence of 0.06% to 0.3%.[7, 53–57] Inadvertent instrumental perforation of the bowel seems to have no correlation with the operator's experience, technical difficulty, or the patient's weight.[58, 59] It usually occurs during introduction of the primary trocar, especially when the gastrointestinal tract is dilated due to obstruction or through gaseous distension of the stomach. Bowel perforatíon is also more likely when there is adherence of the bowel to the abdominal wall from previous surgery or previous peritonitis.[12, 60] Laparotomy is usually required to repair the bowel and to effect adequate perioneal toilet, particularly if the large bowel has been damaged. Nonoperative management of a colonic perforation during laparoscopy by utilizing a tube colostomy, intravenous alimentation, and antibiotic therapy has been reported.[61]

Abdominal wall metastasis following diagnostic laparoscopy for abdominal malignancy can occur but is extremely rare. Metastatic seeding from ovarian adenocarcinoma and mucoid adenocarcinoma of the gastroesophageal junction has been reported[62, 63] (Fig 8–4). Cases have been described of neoplastic dissemination along the tract of needles or instruments used in several diagnostic or therapeutic procedures.[63] In the majority of these reports the primary tumor was adenocarcinoma, with the interval between the procedure and appearance of the metastasis ranging from 4 days to 5 years. During laparoscopy, ascitic fluid containing viable tumor cells can be introduced into the tract of one of the laparoscopic instruments. In the

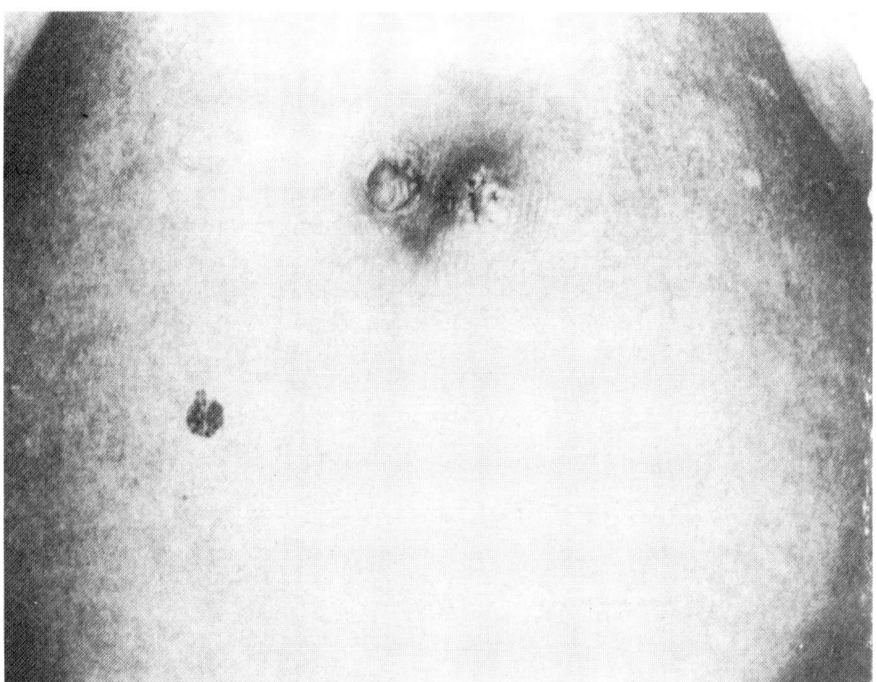

FIG 8–4.
Metastatic nodule of adneocarcinoma at the point of insertion of the trochar, adjacent to the umbilicus (frontal view). This was noticed 7 days following diagnostic laparoscopy in a patient with gastroesophageal adenocarcinoma and ascites. (From Cava A, Roman J, Gonzales Quentela A, et al: *Eur J Surg Oncol* 1990; 16:63–67. Used by permission.)

reported cases, the tumor seeding was first thought to be an inflammatory lesion or infection at the site of trocar insertion, before biopsy specimens confirmed the diagnosis of malignancy (Fig 8–5).

Bacteriologic contamination from dye or contrast injection during laparoscopy has been reported but seems to be exclusively related to salpingography in patients with pelvic inflammatory disease.[64] It does, however, demonstrate the ability to spread pathogenic microorganisms throughout the peritoneal cavity by using laparoscopic instruments.

Thermocoagulation

Unipolar or bipolar electrocautery devices are used routinely in all specialties of surgery. They present a set of complications common to their use in any setting, usually due to poor equipment or poor operator technique. Skin burns due to poor patient grounding, explosion of volatile gases or liquids, and electrocution of both staff and the patient have been described, but these are fortunately rare occurrences. In addition to these problems, there are reported cases of electrocautery injury during laparoscopy involving most intra-abdominal organs. Bowel and ureter burns are the clinically most important, and deaths have been reported following laparoscopic bowel burns in otherwise healthy young patients.[65]

In a review of 38 patients with unipolar cautery bowel burns, 33 of whom were known to have the injury at the time of laparoscopy, 27 did not require laparotomy.[66] Of the 6 who underwent formal exploration, only 2 were found to have a leaking perforation. Although the time from occurrence of the injury to onset of the symptoms varies from 18 hours to 14 days, most patients with unrecognized bowel injury present within 3 to 7 days with complaints of fever and abdominal pain. When perforation is known to have occurred or is discovered at surgery, the degree of thermal damage from unipolar cautery is much more extensive than would first appear. The crater itself is a small part of the devitalized tissue, with tissue damage

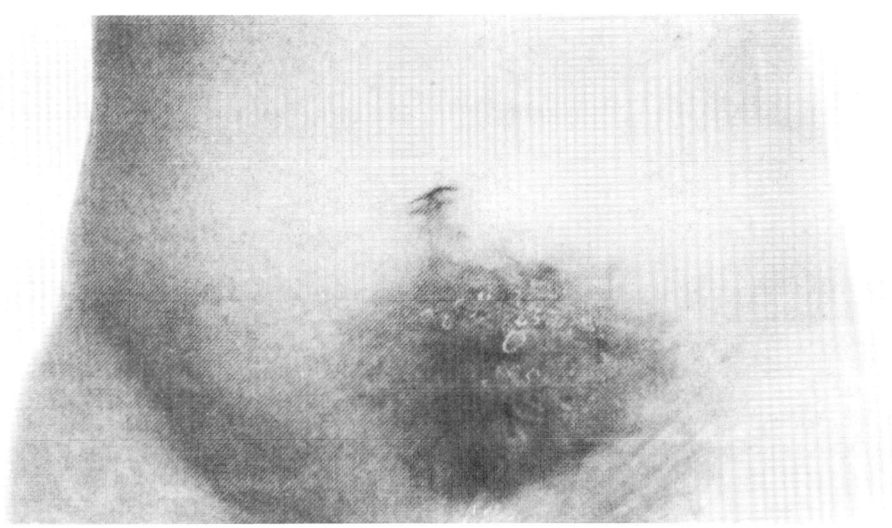

FIG 8–5.
Abdominal wall showing inflammatory tumor infiltration following diagnostic laparoscopy in a patient with ovarian adenocarcinoma. Infraumbilical and suprapubic trochars were inserted in this case. (From Stockdale AD, Pocock TJ: *Eur J Surg Oncol* 1985; 11:373–375. Used by permission.)

detectable up to 5 cm away from the burn site. This differs from the injury produced by bipolar cautery, where there is limitation of the extent of heating to the volume of tissue between the bipolar forceps. Burn injury to the ureter has been described but is extremely uncommon,[30] occurring in approximately 0.01% of laparoscopies performed. Complete transection has never been described, and most reports describe nonoperative management[12, 67] utilizing a combination of ureteric stenting, bladder catheter drainage, and antibiotic coverage.

Laser

When discussing the complications of laser use, it is important to consider both the dangers of laser light in general and the specific problems associated with its use in laparoscopic surgery. The general dangers and necessary precautions are discussed in a separate chapter in this book (Chapter 4). The use of laser energy to coagulate and cut tissue has both potential advantages and disadvantages over the use of electrocautery. With the use of lasers, there is no direct flow of current through the patient, and the extent of tissue damage is limited to a smaller area, particularly when compared with unipolar electrocoagulating devices. The current required to produce the laser light is very high, and most major accidents involving the medical use of lasers are due to electrocution of staff rather than inadvertent laser light exposure. The absolute necessity for an institutional, qualified laser safety officer and sound training of the surgeon operating the device cannot be overemphasized.

When light energy is emitted from a surgical laser device, it results in one of four effects; it is either absorbed, transmitted, scattered, or reflected. By a combination of absorption and scattering, the energy is able to produce its desired effects of coagulation or cutting. It must be understood that any laser light that does not interact with the chosen target, e.g., a small bleeding vessel, will continue on its path through the abdomen until it is absorbed, scattered, or reflected. Therefore, the desired effect on the original target, e.g., coagulation, will occur at the accidental target. This usually is recognized immediately, and therefore only a very short duration of laser energy is misdirected. When first using lasers during laparoscopic procedures, the surgeon may find it difficult to see the detail of the operative field when he puts on his laser safety glasses. This is because some of the glasses are made with necessary tints in the lenses that reduce the brightness and color definition of the video monitor image. It is advised that surgeons who plan to use the laser should try the glasses on during a noncrucial part of the procedure to familiarize themselves with the loss of definition they can expect. Higher-quality, more expensive safety glasses usually have less tinting in the lenses and are therefore preferrable for laparoscopic work.

Suction

Adequate suction can be a vital component of laparoscopic surgical procedures, especially when electrocautery or laser coagulation is being performed. Due to the closed confines of the peritoneal cavity, any smoke produced tends to remain airborne and obstruct the surgeon's view. Closed-loop continuous suction is available with modern equipment and does not generate high negative pressures. The use of the operating room wall suction units can produce higher negative pressures, and care must be taken when clearing the surgical field of blood, especially when operating near fragile or friable diseased tissues. Bowel injuries due to inadvertent suctioning have been reported,[57] and herniation of small bowel through the trocar site due to suction of the bowel into the trocar at the time of removal has resulted in an incarcerated hernia.[68]

PATIENT-SPECIFIC COMPLICATIONS

Obese Patient

Although these patients may be the very group who stand to gain the most from avoiding an open operation and the associated problems of an abdominal incision, they also present technical difficulties that may lead to major complications if not anticipated. The greatly increased thickness of the abdominal wall requires a longer pneumoperitoneum needle to avoid the possibility of subcutaneous emphysema or failed entry into the peritoneal cavity. The usual tacile and auditory aids that enable the surgeon to feel and hear the "pop" of the needle as it passes through the facial abdominal wall may be obliterated by the thick layer of insulating fat. In addition, once the needle is inside the peritoneal cavity, the hypertrophic omentum may engulf the needle tip and result in failed insufflation of the gas. The fatty deposits that occur in the abdominal wall and the omentum also occur in the bowel mesentery and throughout the ligaments and coverings of the abdominal organs. This acts as a mechanical obstruction to vision, particularly when the falciform ligament is very large, and may significantly prolong the procedure. Both the total amount and pressure of insufflated gas required to distend the abdominal cavity and counteract the weight of the compressing fatty mass of the abdominal wall may be increased. This can cause diffuse emphysema or may complicate a pre-existing pulmonary or cardiac condition already compromised by obesity.[69] In addition to the increased incidence of wound infection and incisional hernia in obese patients, the problems associated with laparoscopic surgery are related to the mechanical difficulty in maneuvering instruments and visualization of the operative field.

Ascites

Ascitic fluid can be drained prior to the laparoscopic procedure or evacuated once the pneumoperitoneum needle is in place. In either case, the fluid must be removed to allow adequate visualization. There is a degree of safety afforded the surgeon in an ascitic patient due to the separation of the parietal peritoneum and omentum due to the fluid. It must be remembered, however, that bowel will float on this fluid, and care must be taken, particularly since many of these patients have intra-abdominal malignancy that can tether the bowel loops to each other and to the abdominal wall. This results in a relative immobility or fixation of the bowel, and the loops do not slide away from the needle or trocar, as they tend to in a nonmalignant and noninflamed peritoneal cavity. The most common and troublesome complication of any abdominal procedure in an ascitic patient is the reaccumulation and leaking of fluid from the wound. Despite the small size and apparent firm closure of trocar sites, ascitic fluid may leak from the wound and present a persistent source of discomfort for the patient and route of entry for pathogenic microorganisms. In these cases, exploration and thorough suturing of the site of drainage should be undertaken, unless the patient is in the final stages of their disease and is not expected to survive more than a few weeks.

Elderly Patient

Age has not been shown to be an important factor in the occurrence of either minor or major complications in diagnostic laparoscopic procedures.[70] Despite the reduction in cardiopulmonary reserve in elderly patients, careful installation of pneumoperitoneum and gentle technique allow performance of diagnostic laparoscopy with no documented increase in the rate of complications as compared with younger patient cohorts. Such a confident statement cannot be made about the performance of more major laparoscopic surgical procedures in aged patients since many authors report an advanced age as an adverse factor.[57, 71] Complications that do occur, however, must be weighed against the problems associated with an abdominal incision and conventional surgery.

Organomegaly

Laparoscopy has been employed in a number of gastroenterology services since at least 1970 and has been an invaluable diagnostic tool.[10, 49] It has been performed to inspect and take biopsy specimens of diseased tissue in patients with chronic liver disease, primary and secondary liver tumors, and ascites of unknown origin and to help stage hematologic malignancies. In these settings, complications have been attributed to a combination of factors, including hepatosplenomegaly, bleeding tendencies, and the generalized poor condition of many of the patients. There is an increased incidence of complications in these groups that approaches 10% for minor and 2% for major complications, including abdominal wall hematoma, perforated hollow viscus, hemoperitoneum, bleeding from biopsy sites, and respiratory depression.[10] The presence of organomegaly without any of the accompanying problems outlined above is the exception rather than the rule. Therefore, it is the combination of an enlarged spleen and a clotting abnormality that renders the patient at risk rather than the splenic enlargement alone. When organomegaly is suspected or known to exist based on preoperative clinical examination or investigation results, the pneumoperitoneum needle and trocar should be placed a safe distance (at least 5 cm) from the edge of the organ while remembering the position of the bladder and other susceptible organs at all times.

Abdominal Hernias

The presence of a small or moderate-sized external, reducible hernia is not a contraindication to a laparoscopic procedure. Preoperative reduction and taping of the hernial orifice is recommended but may not be successful if the patient is obese or the hernial orifice is located at the base of a scaphoid hollow of the abdominal wall adjacent to a bony prominence. The sac may fill with gas at the time of pneumoperitoneum but usually empties at the conclusion of the operation, and the gas is reabsorbed by the peritoneum in the usual manner. Bowel may be driven into the hernial sac but, again, usually reduces at the conclusion of pneumoperitoneum. In the event that the hernia becomes irreducible and painful, the usual management of such a hernia applies. Large external abdominal wall hernias and diaphragmatic hernias can produce more serious complications and should be considered contraindications to laparoscopic surgery.[69]

Diabetes

Patients with diabetes mellitus suffer a number of well-known complications due to the systemic effects of their disease. In addition to problems associated with accelerated atherosclerosis, hyperglycemia, microangiopathic renal disease, and immunologic compromise, diabetics are at some specific risks related to laparoscopic surgery. Dramatic, life-threatening infections at the site of trocar insertion can occur but are exceedingly rare. Necrotizing fasciitis has been described in a diabetic patient undergoing a diagnostic laparoscopy[71] (Fig 8–6). The prevailing characteristic of the bacterial isolates is proteolytic toxin production by a single bacteria *(Streptococcus, Staphylococcus,* or *Pseudomonas)* or by the synergistic association of multiple bacteria (anaerobic bacteria including *Bacteroides* with facultative anaerobes). Because this complication is so rare, no specific precautions can be advised. Once the necrotizing process is established, however, wide and often repeated surgical debridement combined with prolonged appropriate antibiotic administration is necessary.

Clotting Abnormalities

The reported experience of diagnostic laparoscopy in patients with known coagulation problems has revealed an increased incidence of both minor and major complications.[10, 49] Because the majority of patients who undergo laparoscopic surgery do not have a formal clot-

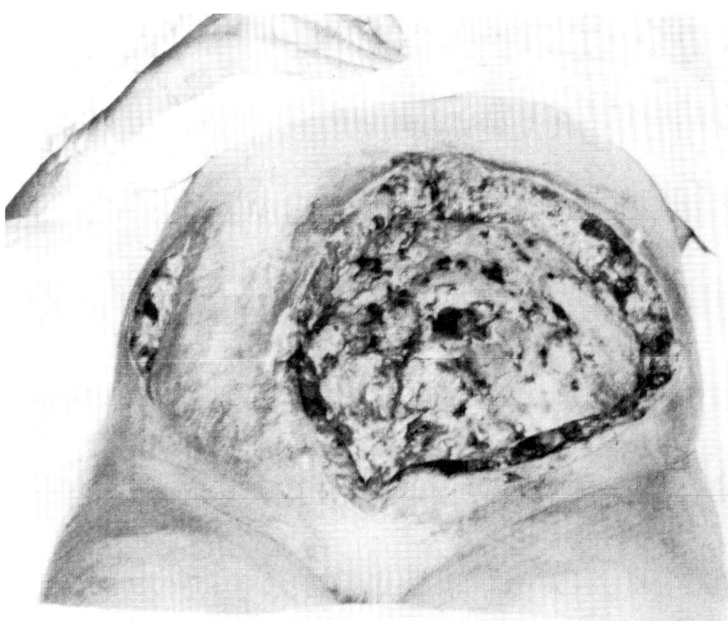

FIG 8–6.
Necrotizing fasciitis of the anterior abdominal wall following an uneventful diagnostic laparoscopy in an elderly diabetic patient. (From Sotrel G, Hirsch E, Edelin KC, et al: *Obstet Gynecol* 1983; 62(suppl):67–69. Used by permission.)

ting profile performed, there are no extensive published data to draw upon to advise strict practice guidelines. In patients with known hematologic disease who are undergoing invasive laparoscopic procedures, e.g., cirrhotics undergoing liver biopsy, a full coagulation screen is mandatory. Preparation for a laparoscopic operation is similar to the preparation for an open surgical procedure. An abnormal prothrombin time or platelet count less than $60{,}000/cm^3$ should be treated preoperatively or intraoperatively with appropriate fresh, frozen plasma or platelet replacements. Electrocautery or laser coagulation should be utilized during tissue dissection to maintain strict hemostasis, including the division of benign, avascular-appearing peritoneal adhesions. The fallback of "pack and wait" that is available to effect control of abnormally bleeding surfaces in open surgical wounds is not so readily available during a laparoscopic procedure. The use of a fibrin sponge or fibrin glue has been described as a technique to control troublesome bleeding.[52]

Abdominal Scars and Adhesions

Abdominal scars should alert the operator to the possibility of intra-abdominal adhesions. If a closed technique is planned, the needle and trocar sites should be at least 5 cm away from the scar(s). During insufflation of the gas, the abdomen should inflate symmetrically and easily, and the prehepatic dullness should disappear. Asymetric expansion or varying gas system pressures may indicate bowel perforation or loculated peritoneal pockets due to adhesions. If this occurs, an open laparoscopic approach may reduce the risks associated with repeated attempts to establish a satisfactory pneumoperitoneum. It is important to make a vertical infraumbilical incision and employ an experienced assistant who can accurately manipulate suitable retractors to provide adequate exposure. A focused spotlight is also a necessity when operating through the necessarily small incision.

REFERENCES

1. Mulroy MF: Regional Anesthesia: When, why, why not? in Wetchler BV (ed): *Outpatient Anesthesia. Problems in Anesthesia,* vol 2. Philadelphia, JB Lippincott, 1988, p 82.
2. Bridenbaugh LD, Soderstrom RM: Lumbar epidural block anesthesia for outpatient laparoscopy. *J Reprod Med* 1979; 23:85–88.
3. Yuzpe AA: Pneumoperitoneum needle and trochar injuries in laparoscopy—a survey on possible contributing factors and prevention. *J Reprod Med* 1990; 35:485–490.
4. McDonald PT, Rich NM, Collins GJ, et al: Vascular trauma secondary to diagnostic and therapeutic procedures: Laparoscopy. *Am J Surg* 1978; 135:651–655.
5. Katz M, Beck P, Tancer ML: Major vessel injury during laparoscopy: Anatomy of 2 cases. *Am J Obstet Gynecol* 1979; 135:544–545.
6. Baadsgaard S, Bille S, Egeblad K: Major vascular injury during gynecologic laparoscopy. A report of a case and review of published cases. *Acta Obstet Gynecol Scand* 1989; 68:283–285.
7. Riedel HH, Lehmann-Willenbrock E, Conrad P, et al: German pelviscopic statistics for the years 1978–1982. *Endoscopy* 1986; 18:219–222.
8. Phillips JM: Complications in laparoscopy. *Int J Gynecol Obstet* 1977; 15:157–162.
9. Pring DW: Inferior epigastric haemorrhage, an avoidable complication of laparoscopic clip sterilisation. *Br J Obstet Gynaecol* 1983; 90:480–482.
10. Youkey JR, Clagett GP, Rich NM, et al: Vascular trauma secondary to diagnostic and therapeutic procedures: 1974 through 1982—A comparative review. *Am J Surg* 1983; 146:788–791.

11. Lieberman BA: A clip applicator for laparoscopic sterilisation. *Fertil Steril* 1976; 27:1036–1037.
12. Loffer FD, Pent D: Indications, contraindications, and complications of laparoscopy. *Obstet Gynecol Surv* 1975; 30:407–427.
13. McLucas B, March C: Urachal sinus perforation during laparoscopy. *J Reprod Med* 1990; 35:573–574.
14. Yong L, Prabhakaran K, Lee YS, et al: Peritonitis following diagnostic laparoscopy due to injury to a vesicourachal diverticulum: Case report. *Br J Obstet Gynaecol* 1989; 96:365–368.
15. Georgy FM, Fetterman HH, Chefetz MD: Complication of laparoscopy: Two cases of perforated urinary bladder. *Am J Obstet Gynecol* 1974; 120:1121–1122.
16. Bard PA, Chen L: Subcutaneous emphysema associated with laparoscopy. *Anesth Analg* 1990; 71:100–106.
17. Hussain NH: Bilateral pneumothorax associated with laparoscopy: A case report of a rare hazard and a review of the literature. *Anaesthesia* 1973; 28:75–81.
18. Neuwirth RS: Recent experience with diagnostic and surgical laparoscopy. *Am J Obstet Gynecol* 1970; 106:119–121.
19. Pascual JB, Baranda MM, Taerrero MT, et al: Subcutaneous emphysema, pneumomediastinum, bilateral pneumothorax and pneumopericardium after laparoscopy. *Endoscopy* 1990; 22:59.
20. Stein HF: Complications of artificial pneumoperitoneum. *Am Rev Tuberc* 1951; 64:645–658.
21. Doctor NH, Hussain Z: Bilateral pneumothorax associated with laparoscopy. *Anesthesia* 1973; 28:75–81.
22. Batra MS, Driscoll JJ, Coburn WA, et al: Evanescent nitrous oxide pneumothorax after laparoscopy. *Anesth Analg* 1983; 62:1121–1123.
23. Murray DP, Rankin RA, Lackey C: Bilateral pneumothoraces complicating peritoneoscopy. *Gastrointest Endosc* 1984; 30:45–46.
24. Ramage AA, Singh M, Griffin JW Jr, et al: Hydropneumothorax following peritoneoscopy. *J Clin Gastroenterol* 1986; 8:483–485.
25. Glauser FL, Bartlett RH: Pneumoperitoneum in association with pneumothorax. *Chest* 1979; 66:536–540.
26. Altman AR, Johnson TH: Pneumoperitoneum and pneumoretroperitoneum. Consequences of positive end-expiratory pressure therapy. *Arch Surg* 1979; 114:208–211.
27. Jones MJ, Mitchell RW, Hindocha N: Effect of increased intra-abdominal pressure during laparoscopy on the lower esophageal sphincter. *Anesth Analg* 1989; 68:63–65.
28. Stow PJ: Retinal haemorrhage following laparoscopy. *Anaesthesia* 1986; 41:965–966.
29. Bolder PM, Norton ML: Retinal hemorrhage following anesthesia. *Anesthesiology* 1984; 61:595–597.
30. Chamberlain G, Carron-Brown J: *Gynaecological laparoscopy: The Report of the Working Party of the Confidential Enquiry into Gynaecological Laparoscopy.* London, Royal College of Obstetrics and Gynecology, 1978.
31. Phillips J, Kieth D, Hulka J, et al: Gynaecological laparoscopy in 1975. *J Reprod Med* 1976; 16:205–217.
32. Gomar C, Fernandez C, Villalonga A, et al: Carbon dioxide embolism during laparoscopy and hysteroscopy. *Ann Fr Anesth Reanim* 1985; 4:380–382.
33. Root B, Levy MN, Pollack S, et al: Gas embolism death after laparoscopy delayed by trapping in the portal circulation. *Anesth Analg* 1978; 57:232–237.
34. De Plater RMH, Jones IS. Non-fatal carbon dioxide embolism during laparoscopy. *Anaesth Int Care* 1989; 17:359–361.
35. Durant TM, Oppenheimer MJ, Lynch PR, et al: Body position in relation to venous air embolism: A roentgenological study. *Am J Med Sci* 1954; 227:509–520.
36. Nichols SL, Tompkins BM, Henderson PA: Probable carbon dioxide embolism during laparoscopy: Case report. *Wisconsin Med J* 1981; 80:27–29.
37. Shulman D, Aronson HB: Capnography in the early diagnosis of carbon dioxide embolism during laparoscopy. *Can Anaesth Soc J* 1984; 31:455–459.

38. Alvaran SB, Toung JK, Graff TE, et al: Venous air embolism: Comparative merits of external cardiac massage, intracardiac aspiration, and left lateral decubitus position. *Anesth Analg* 1978; 57:66–70.
39. Harris MNE, Plantevin OM, Crowther A: Cardiac arrythmias during anaesthesia for laparoscopy. *Br J Anaesthesiol* 1984; 56:1213–1217.
40. Doyle DJ, Mark PWS: Laparoscopy and vagal arrest. *Anaesthesia* 1989; 44:448.
41. Brantley JC, Riley PM: Cardiovascular collapse during laparoscopy: A report of two cases. *Am J Obstet Gynecol* 1988; 159:735–737.
42. Lip H, Delhaas E: Correspondence. *Am J Obstet Gynecol* 1988; 162:873. *Gynecology* 1974; 120:1121–1122.
43. Thomas AG, McLymont F, Moshipur J: Incarcerated hernia after laparoscopic sterilisation. *J Reprod Med* 1990; 35:639–640.
44. Fear R: Laparoscopy: A valuable aid in gynecologic diagnosis. *Obstet Gynecol* 1968; 31:297–302.
45. Bishop HL, Halpin TF: Dehiscence following laparoscopy: Report of an unusual complication. *Am J Obstet Gynecol* 1973; 116:585–586.
46. Corson SL, Bolognese RJ: Laparoscopy: An overview and results of a large series. *J Reprod Med* 1972; 9:148–157.
47. Sauer M, Jarette JC: Small bowel obstruction following diagnostic laparoscopy. *Fertil Steril* 1984; 42:653–654.
48. Schiff I, Naftolin F: Small bowel incarceration after uncomplicated laparoscopy. *Obstet Gynecol* 1974; 43:674–675.
49. Dancygier H, Jacob RA: Splenic rupture during laparoscopy. *Gastrointest Endosc* 1983; 29:63.
50. Phillips RS, Reddy R, Jeffers L, et al: Experience with diagnostic laparoscopy in a hepatology training program. *Gastrointest Endosc* 1987; 33:417–420.
51. American Society for Gastrointestinal Endoscopy: The role of laparoscopy in the diagnosis and management of gastrointestinal disease: Guidelines for clinical application. *Gastrointest Endosc* 1988; 34(suppl):30–31.
52. Dagnini G, Caldironi MW, Marin G, et al: Fibrin sponge plugging of hemorrhage from laparoscopic biopsy. *Gastrointest Endosc* 1985; 31:35–36.
53. Henning H: The Dallas report on laparoscopic complications. *Gastrointest Endosc* 1985; 31:104–106.
54. Ilter T, Bolukoglu MA, Musoglu A: Complication rates of diagnostic laparoscopy. *Gastrointest Endosc* 1986; 32:126.
55. Peterson HB, Hulka JF, Phillips JM: American Association of Gynecologic Laparoscopists 1988 membership survey on operative laparoscopy. *J Reprod Med* 1990; 35:587–589.
56. Phillips JM, Hulka JF, Peterson HB: American Association of Gynecologic Laparoscopists' 1982 membership survey. *J Reprod Med* 1984; 29:592–594.
57. Riedel HH, Lehmann-Willenbrock E, Mecke H, et al: The frequency of various pelviscopic (laparoscopic) operations, including complications rates—statistics of the Federal Republic of Germany in the years 1983–1985. *Zentralbl Gynakol* 1989; 111:78–91.
58. Thompson EH, Wheless CR: Gastrointestinal complications of laparoscopic sterilisation. *Obstet Gynecol* 1973; 41:669–676.
59. Penfield AJ: How to prevent complications of open laparoscopy. *J Reprod Med* 1985; 30:660–663.
60. Jordan JA, Edwards RL, Pearson J, et al: Laparoscopic sterilisation and follow up hysterosalpingogram. *J Obstet Gynaecol Br Commonw* 1971; 78:460–466.
61. Birns MT: Inadvertent instrumental perforation of the colon during laparoscopy: Nonsurgical repair. *Gastrointest Endosc* 1989; 35:54–56.
62. Stockdale AD, Pocock TJ: Abdominal wall metastasis following laparoscopy: A case report. *Eur J Surg Oncol* 1985; 11:373–375.
63. Cava A, Roman J, Gonzalez Quintela A, et al: Spontaneous metastasis following laparoscopy in gastric adenocarcinoma. *Eur J Surg Oncol* 1990; 16:63–67.
64. Pyper JD, Ahmet Z, Houang ET: Bacteriological contamination during laparoscopy with dye injection. *Br J Obstet Gynaecol* 1988; 95:367–371.

65. Peterson RB, Ory EW, Greenspan R, et al: Deaths associated with laparoscopic sterilisation by unipolar electrocoagulating devices, 1978 and 1979. *Am J Obstet Gynecol* 1981; 139:141–143.
66. Wheeless CR Jr: Gastrointestinal injuries associated with laparoscopy, in Phillips JM (ed): *Endoscopy in Gynecology.* Downey, California, American Association of Gynecologic Laparoscopists, 1978, pp 317–324.
67. Winslow PH, Kreger R, Ebbesson B, et al: Conservative management of electrical burn injury of ureter secondary to laparoscopy. *Urology* 1986; 27:60–62.
68. Hogdall C, Roosen JU: Incarcerated hernia following laparoscopy. *Acta Obstet Gynecol Scand* 1987; 66:735–736.
69. Saleh J: Complications, in Saleh J (ed): *Laparoscopy.* Philadelphia, WB Saunders Co, 1988, pp 253–266.
70. Orlando R, Lirussi F, Nassuato G, et al: Complications of laparoscopy in the elderly: A report on 345 consecutive cases and comparison with a younger population. *Endoscopy* 1987; 19:145–146.
71. Sotrel G, Hirsch E, Edelin KC: Necrotizing fasciitis following diagnostic laparoscopy. *Obstet Gynecol* 1983; 62(suppl):67–69.

Chapter 9

Cardiopulmonary Pathophysiology of Laparoscopy and Pneumoperitoneum

Fred Bongard, M.D.

Se-Yuan Liu, M.D.

Laparoscopy was originally introduced by Kelling in 1902 and has been employed with increasing enthusiasm in recent years.[1] Its great advantage is that it eliminates the need for celiotomy and potentially reduces the complications of fluid shifts, metabolic requirements of wound healing, and prolonged convalescence. Pneumoperitoneum produces its own unique set of physiologic cardiopulmonary alterations that will be of increased significance as laparoscopic procedures are used in sicker patients. This chapter will discuss the cardiopulmonary alterations and complications associated with laparoscopy and pneumoperitoneum.

RESPIRATORY PATHOPHYSIOLOGY

Gas Equilibria in Body Cavities

Laparoscopy requires peritoneal gas insufflation for successful completion. Carbon dioxide is usually employed, although nitrous oxide (N_2O) has been considered as an alternative when electrocautery is not required.[2] A discussion of respiratory alterations caused by peritoneal insufflation must include interactions between the instilled CO_2 and the blood-alveolar circuit.

Piiper noted that there are four types of gas cavities: (1) open ventilated cavities such as the lung, (2) open nonventilated cavities such as the paranasal sinuses, (3) closed rigid cavities such as the middle ear, and (4) closed collapsible cavities such as subcutaneous pockets.[3] Pneumoperitoneum most closely resembles the latter category. Once insufflation is complete, the movement of gas into or out of the cavity is determined by a combination of two factors: (1) diffusion of gas through the lining tissues (diffusion limitation) and (2) transport in the blood perfusing those tissues that line the cavity (perfusion limitation).[4]

When a cavity is filled with gas, movement across the lining membrane (flux) proceeds at a rate unique for the gas instilled until a steady-state concentration is reached or until all of the gas has been absorbed. If air is used, water vapor and carbon dioxide diffuse into the cavity until the partial pressures of each approach that in the lining tissues. The solubility of CO_2 and H_2O is so high that equilibrium is attained quickly.[4] When a metabolically inert gas such as nitrogen is used, oxygen achieves the same equilibrium and diffuses into the cavity along with water vapor and carbon dioxide. The final pressure of oxygen is that of the surrounding tissues, which is closely approximated by mixed venous blood.[4] If nitrogen (N_2) is used, its pressure in the cavity will be substantially higher than that found in the blood. If we assume that the patient is breathing room air, then the alveolar concentration of oxygen is approximately 101 mm Hg, while that of CO_2 is 40 mm Hg. At the tissue level, the partial pressure of oxygen is about 41 mm Hg, while it is 46 mm Hg for CO_2. The total pressure of respiratory gases in the tissues is therefore 54 mm Hg below what it is in the alveoli. If we assume that the PO_2 and the PCO_2 in the peritoneal cavity are the same as in the tissues lining the coelom, then the PN_2 in the cavity must be 54 mm Hg higher than that in the alveoli and in the arterial blood. This partial pressure gradient allows N_2 to leave the peritoneal cavity and enter the blood while at the same time increasing the partial pressures of the respiratory gases in the cavity. As the inspired oxygen concentration increases, so does the gradient for gas diffusion until at an FIO_2 of 1.0 the total gas pressure in tissue is approximately 610 mm Hg below atmospheric pressure.[5] Thus, regardless of the gases breathed or insufflated into a cavity, the equilibrium composition will be characterized by partial pressure differences that favor gas absorption from the cavity into the blood[4] (Fig 9–1).

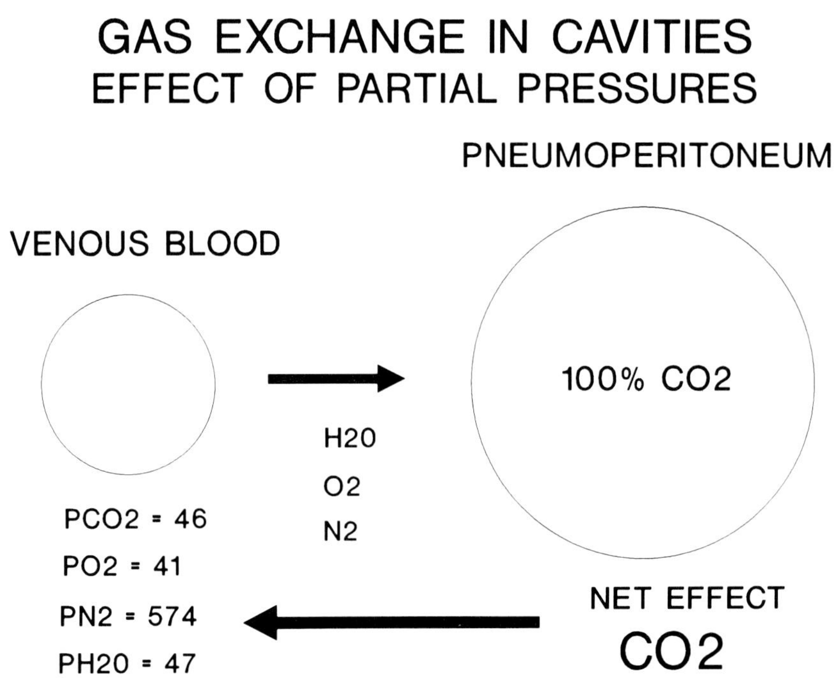

FIG 9–1.
A pictorial representation of partial pressures present during carbon dioxide pneumoperitoneum. Net movement of carbon dioxide out of the peritoneum is the primary effect.

An important additional consideration applies when CO_2 is used as the insufflating gas. Carbon dioxide is produced by metabolizing tissues and contributes to the overall equilibrium. Of the two respiratory gases, CO_2 has the higher solubility and is the first to equilibrate within tissue. Further, blood can carry more CO_2 than oxygen because of carbon dioxide's increased permeance. The outcome of this theoretical consideration is that since carbon dioxide diffuses so quickly and is transported so efficiently by blood, CO_2 diffusion from the peritoneum to the blood is usually far greater than its production, which makes local metabolic influences relatively unimportant in calculating total CO_2 flux.[4]

Respiratory Effects of Carbon Dioxide Insufflation

Carbon dioxide instilled into the abdominal cavity normally diffuses across the peritoneal surface to be carried away by flowing blood.[6] The blood CO_2 thus absorbed may either be eliminated by the lungs or stored, at least temporarily, in the body. The total body carbon dioxide storage capacity is near 120 L.[7] Storage capacity varies with the type of tissue and with its blood supply; bone is the largest reservoir.[8] Short periods of increased CO_2 that occur during a Valsalva maneuver probably involve only the blood and alveolar stores. Longer increases, typical of that associated with pneumoperitoneum, likely recruit visceral storage facilities such as skeletal muscle. Bone does not participate until a steady state is reached over the course of days or weeks. When multiple visceral sites are involved, the equilibrium established serves to lower the Pa_{CO_2}.

A series of equations derived by Seed and coworkers indicate that the rate of readjustment of the body stores to changes in carbon dioxide load is directly related to the rate of change of alveolar and mixed venous CO_2.[6] These, in turn, vary with CO_2 production (primarily insufflation), alveolar ventilation, cardiac output, and respiratory quotient. The implications for laparoscopy utilizing carbon dioxide–induced pneumoperitoneum are (1) the rate of increase in arterial CO_2 is related to the amount of CO_2 used during the procedure; (2) the elimination of such CO_2 is directly related to the minute ventilation and cardiac output of the patient during the procedure; and (3) the longer the duration of the pneumoperitoneum, the greater the utilization of peripheral storage facilities and the longer the duration of elevated arterial CO_2 after the procedure as these storage depots return to baseline levels.

Applications in Clinical Laparoscopy

Increased arterial partial pressure of carbon dioxide during pelvic laparoscopy was first noted over 30 years ago.[9–11] Alexander and Brown described 15 patients who underwent laparoscopy with carbon dioxide as the insufflating gas at 10 to 20 mm Hg pressure. Anesthesia was with nitrous oxide, oxygen, and halothane via a volume-limited ventilator that maintained a constant minute ventilation throughout the procedure. The average arterial carbon dioxide pressure following the induction of anesthesia before insufflation was 27.1 mm Hg but rose to an average of 35.7 mm Hg during the procedure (change, +8.6 mm Hg; $P < .001$). Similarly, arterial pH started at 7.47 and fell to 7.39 at the conclusion of laparoscopy. These patients were placed in a 15- to 20-degree head-down (Trendelenburg) position during the course of laparoscopy. Unfortunately, only two time points were recorded by these investigators, and the resolution of hypercapnia following desufflation was not discussed.

A number of anesthetic techniques have been tried to minimize the need for intubation and mechanical ventilation as well as reduce postoperative complications.[12] Concern arose early regarding the need for mechanical ventilation following insufflation. Increased Pa_{CO_2} and decreased pH, especially during halothane anesthesia, may lead to potentially serious cardiac arrhythmias. Desmond and Gordon reported 14 patients undergoing pelvic laparoscopy under halothane/oxygen/nitrous anesthesia. Ten were allowed to breathe spontaneously, while 4 were mechanically ventilated.[13] The investigators concluded that a "large amount" of the insufflated carbon dioxide was excreted through the lungs and that "it may be extremely hazardous to permit these patients to ventilate spontaneously." Hyperventilation to reduce the CO_2 burden was the best technique. Confounding this was the concern that insufflation would increase respiratory impedance through elevation of the diaphragm. This, in conjunction with cephalad movement of the viscera during Trendelenburg positioning, can lead to respiratory embarrassment. The decreased tidal volume thus produced would further elevate the arterial carbon dioxide in excess of that caused by diffusion and absorption across the peritoneum. The combination of these factors makes mechanical control of ventilation during laparoscopy desirable.

A similar study by Lewis and associates found significant variability between spontaneously breathing patients under halothane anesthesia in the extent of Pa_{CO_2} elevation during laparoscopy.[14] An average rise of 15 mm Hg was noted 12 minutes after insufflation, although some patients had exaggerated responses. One had a Pa_{CO_2} in excess of 100 mm Hg at 27 minutes *after* insufflation. The fact that arterial carbon dioxide tensions may remain elevated even after desufflation and completion of the procedure is in keeping with our understanding of carbon dioxide equilibrium between alveoli, blood, and soft tissue. The length of most pelvic laparoscopic procedures studied has been relatively short, typically less than 30 minutes. This is in contradistinction to the somewhat longer time required for laparoscopic cholecystectomy where average times are about 90 minutes, with more complicated dissections requiring up to 3 hours.[15] The duration of these general surgical procedures allows sufficient time for the uptake of CO_2 by soft tissue, especially skeletal muscle. Achievement of equilibrium by these stores after completion of the procedure and extubation of the patient raises concern for potential recovery room hypercarbia and implies that routine postoperative respiratory monitoring may be required (Fig 9–2).

Concerns about hypercarbia from CO_2 insufflation have led to an examination of alternate gases to induce pneumoperitoneum.[16] Some of the criteria for an ideal agent might include its being (1) nontoxic, (2) nonflammable, (3) colorless, (4) slowly diffusible (minimal solubility in tissue), (5) easily handled, and (6) inexpensive. Experimental studies with inert gases have been conducted, but little clinical information is available.[17] Nitrous oxide meets most of the listed criteria and has been investigated as an alternative to carbon dioxide. The advantages of nitrous oxide are that (1) it is available in every operating room, (2) its absorption does not directly increase arterial carbon dioxide tensions, and (3) its physical properties are favorable.

Alexander and Brown investigated the blood gas consequences of insufflation with nitrous oxide as compared with carbon dioxide.[10] Fifteen ventilated patients undergoing pelvic laparoscopy in the Trendelenburg position were assigned to each group. Insufflation pressures averaged 10 to 20 mm Hg. Overall, no significant increase in Pa_{CO_2} was noted in the nitrous oxide–treated group (−1.4 mm Hg), while those who received carbon dioxide experienced elevations of 8.6 mm Hg. Similar effects were observed for pH (−0.082 for CO_2 vs. +0.012 for N_2) and Pa_{O_2} (−24 mm Hg for CO_2 vs. −18 mm Hg for N_2O), although the changes in oxygenation were not significant. Since their initial study, several other investigators have obtained similar results.[2, 18] In spite of these initially favorable reports, nitrous oxide has not

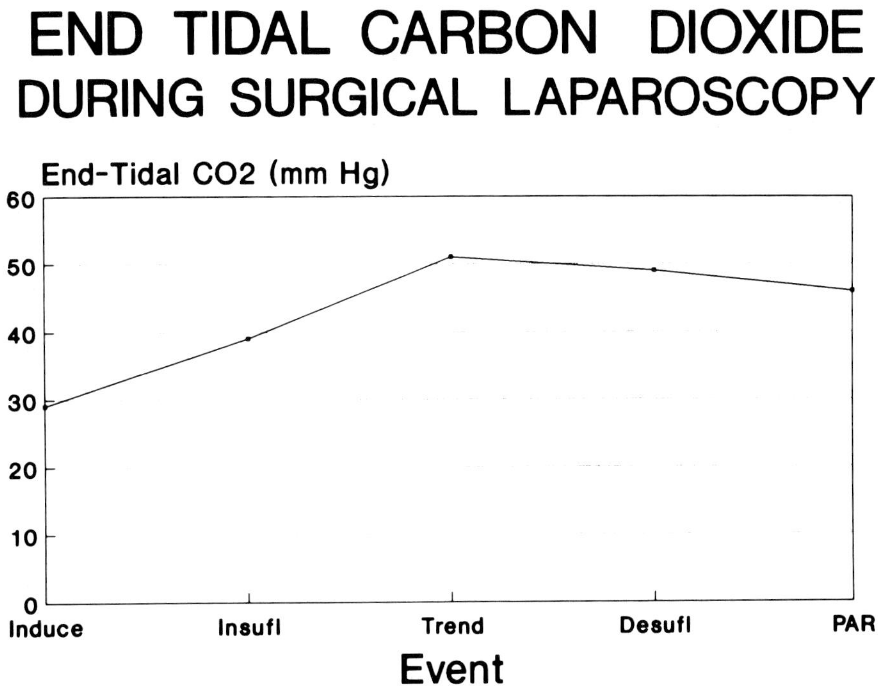

FIG 9–2.
End-tidal carbon dioxide concentrations observed in a young patient undergoing laparoscopic ligation of a varicocele. Overall length of the procedure was 2½ hours. Note that end-tidal CO_2 concentrations remained elevated after desufflation in the recovery room *(PAR)* (Trendelenburg position).

gained wide use in laparoscopy, partially because of concern that absorption from the abdomen might produce hypoxia. Studies thus far have failed to find this of clinical significance.[2] Another concern has been that nitrous oxide might cause prolonged postoperative distension. Again, this has not been borne out.[2] Perhaps of greatest concern is the fact that while nitrous oxide is not inflammable, it does support combustion and may be problematic when cautery is used. One of the criteria for selection of an insufflating gas in general surgical procedures is that it be absolutely stable with respect to thermal and electrical energy. For this reason, nitrous oxide is not advisable.

Respiratory Monitoring for Laparoscopy

Because of the potential for absorption of substantial quantities of carbon dioxide during lengthy laparoscopic surgical procedures, the need for monitoring of respiratory gases becomes important. Most patients receive supplemental oxygen as part of their anesthetic, with routine hemoglobin saturation monitoring via pulse oximetry. The simplicity, accuracy, and reliability of this technique has been reviewed extensively.[19]

Carbon dioxide monitoring can be accomplished either by routine arterial blood gases or by end-tidal CO_2 (P_{ETCO_2}) sampling. P_{ETCO_2} technology utilizes either infrared absorption or mass spectrometry to measure exhaled gas. The newer, more portable units sample through a sidestream adapter connected to the patient's endotracheal tube and anesthetic circuit. Gas is sampled at between 50 and 250 cc/min and conveyed to a small optical bench where the actual absorption is determined. Results are displayed both numerically and graphically so that trends over several hours can be analyzed. Graphic display of time trends is of particular importance since it may allow recognition of acute events such as CO_2 embolization. The units are portable and can be transported to the recovery room with the patient for continued monitoring if such facilities are not already available in that location. Recent advances in technique and catheter design allow reliable sampling of end-tidal CO_2 from nonintubated patients recovering from general anesthesia.[20]

Abnormalities in pulmonary ventilation and perfusion may cause differences between arterial blood gas determinations of CO_2 and those obtained by end-tidal monitoring. The two most important such physiologic conditions are increased dead-space ventilation and/or intrapulmonary shunt. Of the two, increased dead space produces the largest discrepancy in the arterial–end-tidal gradient ($Pa\text{-}Etco_2$). This gradient is typically 2 to 3 mm Hg, but may widen substantially as dead space increases.[21] Brampton and Watson studied the arterial to end-tidal carbon dioxide tension difference during laparoscopy in 25 patients, 12 of whom underwent pelvic laparoscopy under epidural anesthesia and the remainder of whom had the same procedure with a general anesthetic.[22] Overall, the $Pa\text{-}Etco_2$ gradient was 3.3 mm Hg, with the 95% confidence interval extending from 2.1 to 4.5 mm Hg. This excellent correlation is actually better than that reported for other operative procedures and did not vary with the type of anesthetic used. The use of capnometry is not limited to just the duration of the procedure since these patients will continue to excrete CO_2 from body stores after desufflation. Since many procedures are done in the short-stay setting, as described by Reddick and Olsen, more complete and reliable evaluation of the potential for discharge will be required.[15] Compounding this is the need for postoperative outpatient analgesia, which may have respiratory depression and CO_2 retention as a side effect.

Respiratory Complications of Laparoscopy

In addition to the expected physiologic alterations of decreased tidal volume, decreased functional residual capacity, and increased arterial carbon dioxide tension, respiratory complications may occasionally arise. Extension of retroperitoneal insufflating gas in a cephalad direction may cause pneumomediastinum and/or pneumothorax.[23] If a diaphragmatic, abdominal, or umbilical hernia is present, distension may force viscera through the hernia.

Carbon dioxide embolization is one of the best described cardiorespiratory complications and occurs with a frequency of less than a tenth of 1% in gynecologic procedures. Bruhl reported 15 such occurrences in a series of 113,253 (0.01%) pelvic laparoscopies under general anesthesia and in one of 63,845 laparoscopies for hepatic biopsy.[24] Deaths have been reported due to sudden cardiovascular collapse; they were presumed to have been caused by such emboli.[25–27] The proposed mechanism of entry is through veins of the abdominal wall that are accidentally punctured by the Veress needle. This scenario is most likely to occur in patients with previous operations in whom adhesions fix the vessels in relatively immobile positions to the abdominal wall. When gas enters in this way, it is rapidly transported to the right atrium and may form a type of "air lock" until the pumping action of the right atrium disperses the large bubble into a finer foam.[28, 29] If this fine layer of bubbles lodges in the pulmonary circulation, it can be manifested as pulmonary hypertension and right-heart strain.[29] Placement of the patient in the left decubitus position will minimize such effects but is generally not possible when a procedure is underway.[28]

Symptoms of carbon dioxide embolization may be minimal and include only the appearance of a new murmur. Platelet aggregation and resultant bronchospasm typically do not occur after CO_2 embolization.[30] However, if the episode is not recognized and CO_2 accumulation continues, oxygen will diffuse into and combine with the carbon dioxide bubbles, thus accentuating their effects and leading to cardiovascular collapse and death.[31] Early detection of such embolic episodes thus becomes of paramount importance. While esophageal or precordial Doppler can readily detect small amounts of intracardiac air, these are not used routinely during laparoscopy.[28] Shulman and Aronson described a patient with such an episode in whom capnometry was being used.[28] Their patient sustained a transient but significant rise in end-tidal CO_2 that was readily apparent when trend data were examined. The increased P_{ETCO_2} began a few seconds after the appearance of a precordial holosystolic murmur. Insufflation was stopped and the Veress needle withdrawn. No hemodynamic changes were noted, and the patient emerged from anesthesia without complication. Although not used in this patient, hyperventilation with oxygen forms a useful adjunct since it increases the excretion of carbon dioxide. The authors suggest that continuous monitoring of P_{ETCO_2} may be a useful way to evaluate not only CO_2 absorption from the abdomen but carbon dioxide embolization as well. Increased P_{ETCO_2} in association with a new murmur should arouse suspicion of such emboli.

CARDIOVASCULAR PATHOPHYSIOLOGY

Effects of Carbon Dioxide

The effects of carbon dioxide on the cardiovascular system are complicated by varying actions and responses on the different constituents. Many actions are in opposition to each other and, under different circumstances, may offset one another (Fig 9–3).

The direct effect of CO_2 on an isolated heart preparation results from pH changes and produces diminished myocardial contractility and heart rate.[32] The direct effect on systemic blood vessels results in vasodilatation. However, in the intact subject, the depressant action of CO_2 is counteracted by the stimulant effect of the sympathetic nervous system. Increased P_{ACO_2} stimulates chemoreceptors in the carotid body and aorta and also excites various subcortical centers in the hypothalamus, brainstem, reticular formation, and medulla, thereby resulting in an increase in concentrations of epinephrine, norepinephrine, angiotensin, and other vasoactive plasma peptides.[33] The sympathetic effects consist of increased cardiac contractility and rate as well as vasoconstriction of many of the peripheral vascular beds. Therefore, the overall circulatory effects of carbon dioxide in normal humans at rest are increased cardiac output and heart rate, elevation of systolic and diastolic blood pressures, and widening of pulse pressure.[34, 35] These changes are accompanied by a decrease in total peripheral vascular resistance.

At very high levels of P_{ACO_2} it is likely that cardiac output decreases and blood pressure declines, which may lead to death if allowed to persist for more than an hour.[36]

Multiple ventricular extrasystoles have been reported during acute hypercapnia, and the danger of ventricular fibrillation cannot be discounted. Arrhythmias caused by elevated P_{ACO_2} in anesthetized patients occur at catecholamine levels that are above normal but not high enough per se to cause arrhythmias. It therefore seems that these rhythm disturbances are caused in part by a direct action of carbon dioxide on the myocardium.[37]

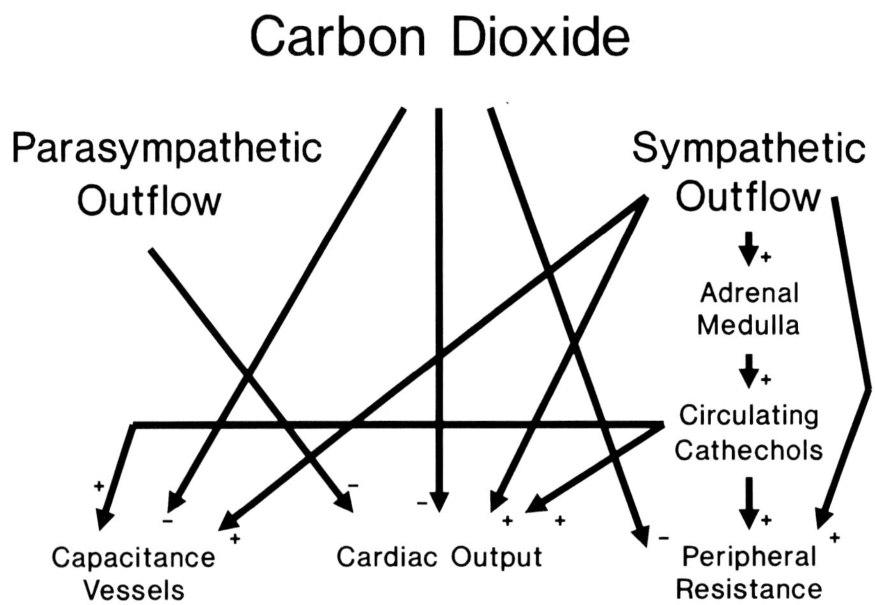

FIG 9–3.
A system diagram illustrating the overall effects of carbon dioxide on the cardiovascular system. Local negative effects may be offset by systemic sympathetic outflow. (Adapted from Nunn JF: The effect of changes in the carbon dioxide tension, in *Applied Respiratory Physiology,* ed 3. London, Butterworth & Co Ltd, 1987, pp 460–470.)

Intra-abdominal Pressure

Several factors contribute to circulatory instability during laparoscopy. The most important seems to be increased intra-abdominal pressure (IAP). Raised IAP hampers venous return by increasing venous resistance. Conversely, it also increases mean systemic pressure.[38] These two changes have opposite effects on venous return. The combined effect is thought to depend on the right atrial pressure prior to insufflation. At low or normal right atrial pressures, venous return is reduced with increased IAP. At high right atrial pressure, venous return is augmented by increased IAP.

Hodgson et al. found that when carbon dioxide is used to insufflate the peritoneal cavity to an IAP of 15 to 20 mm Hg, a rise in central venous pressure (mean value increased from 3.3 cm H_2O to 10.6 cm H_2O) and cardiac output (over 25%) occurred.[39] They postulated the mechanism to be transfer of blood from the abdominal viscera and inferior vena cava into the thoracic cavity, partly due to direct mechanical effect and partly due to enhanced sympathetic activity following the increase in $Paco_2$.[40] Kelman et al. also used CO_2 for insufflation and found a biphasic change in central venous pressure (CVP) and cardiac output.[41] The progressive increase in both CVP and cardiac output up to an IAP of 20 to 39 cm H_2O reversed when the later reached 30 to 40 cm H_2O. Another study from Denmark revealed a different result.[42] At maximum hemodynamic strain during laparoscopy with CO_2 insufflation, the stroke index and cardiac index were reduced by an average of 42% without significant changes in the heart rate or mean arterial pressure. Total peripheral resistance was markedly increased. The authors suggested that the hemodynamic depression of increased IAP was counteracted by surgical stimulation and by CO_2 absorption in "lightly anesthetized" patients. Marshall et al. used deeper anesthesia with 1% halothane and found that CO_2 insufflation up to 15 to 20 cm H_2O resulted in an increased heart rate and mean arterial pressure while cardiac output remained constant.[43] Following the administration of a beta-adrenergic blocker, cardiac output, mean arterial pressure, and heart rate all fell. They repeated the investigation with N_2O insufflation and found a clear reduction in cardiac output and stroke volume and only discrete increments in heart rate and total peripheral vascular resistance.[44] Apparently the local irritating effect of CO_2 and the effect of CO_2 absorption increased spontaneous ventilation and sympathetic activity, which counteracted the stroke volume reduction during elevated IAP.

Change of Body Position

Healthy active humans spend the greater part of their lives in the erect position, which can be considered the normal or "physiologic" state (equilibrium or homeostasis).[45] This stability can be threatened by prolonged bed rest, disease, and drugs (including anesthesia).

Before discussing the circulatory effects of changes in body position, the concept of the hydrostatic indifferent point (HIP) must be considered. This represents the transition zone in which intravascular pressures remain relatively constant and constitutes a natural reference point for hydrostatic shifts in the circulation.[46] At this point, the intravascular pressures and the vessel sizes are not affected by the hydrostatic forces in the circulation. The HIP is specific for any given posture. The effect of a change of posture on venous return to the heart and thus the cardiac filling pressures and cardiac output depends on the position of the HIP relative to the heart.

The head-down (Trendelenburg) position increases the intrathoracic and intracardiac blood volume and leads to an increased cardiac output. However, in patients with hypovolemic shock, the head-down position leads to a reduction of right atrial filling pressure, a slight increase in vascular resistance, and a drop in cardiac output.[47] A study of healthy, normovolemic subjects placed in a 15-degree head-down position showed only 1.8% central displacement of blood volume. This small volume shift was not enough to cause significant hemodynamic changes.[48] In normotensive subjects, the baroceptor reflex may be responsible for the stable cardiovascular status because the head-down position in normovolemic humans has been shown to increase CVP and cardiac output without increasing the heart rate or systemic vascular resistance.[49] Taylor and Weil found the Trendelenburg position to adversely affect both hypotension and cardiac output in patients with normovolemic shock.[50]

The reverse Trendelenburg position (head up) with an inclination of 10 to 15 degrees is usually used to facilitate exposure in patients undergoing laparoscopic procedures on upper abdominal organs. Cardiovascular alterations associated with this position consist of an increase in mean arterial blood pressure and systemic vascular resistance and a decrease in cardiac output. The heart rate is usually unchanged or increased only slightly.[45] The systolic blood pressure remains relatively constant, and changes in mean arterial pressure (may up to 18%) are largely the result of alterations in diastolic pressure.[51] Pulmonary vascular resistance can double on changing from the supine to the sitting position.[52] Left atrial pressure decreases significantly due to decreased intrathoracic blood volume. Right atrial pressure also decreases, but the change is usually less than on the left side due to compensatory increases in pulmonary vascular resistance.

Application in Clinical Laparoscopy

Cardiovascular changes during laparoscopy for gynecologic procedures have been studied extensively, although the results of these investigations are equivocal.[39, 41–44] Variations in anesthesic techniques and insufflation gases used (CO_2 vs. N_2O) may explain some of the inconsistencies.

Motew et al. studied ten women with intraperitoneal CO_2 insufflation.[16] The patients were anesthetized with 0.6% halothane in a 50% N_2O and 50% O_2 mixture. Arterial and central venous pressures were elevated with IAP up to 20 mm Hg. Further increases in IAP above 20 mm Hg were accompanied by depressions in CVP, systolic and pulse pressure, and cardiac output (Table 9–1). Lenz et al. studied stroke volume and cardiac output by using impedance cardiography in 24 patients undergoing laparoscopy.[53] The subjects were artificially ventilated with a mixture of 6 L of N_2O and 2 L of O_2. Insufflation of 4 to 5 L of CO_2 resulted in progressive falls of stroke volume and cardiac output.

Cardiovascular Monitoring for Laparoscopy

It has been noted that routine intraoperative cardiovascular monitoring (blood pressure, pulse rate, and the clinical assessment of peripheral circulation) gives inadequate indications of decreases in cardiac output in patients undergoing laparoscopy, even with decreases as much as 45%.[53] In view of the complicated circulatory effects of CO_2 insufflation, change in body position, and increased intraperitoneal pressure, measurement of cardiac output is desirable during laparoscopic procedures, especially when complicated lengthy operations requiring 2 to 3 hours are undertaken.[15] Although an invasive monitoring system is not indicated in relatively healthy patients, a noninvasive continuous-wave Doppler esophageal or suprasternal probe is an ideal alternative.[54, 55] Correlation of this technique with conventional thermodilution has been very good. Data trending using this technique is an added advantage. At present, insufficient information exists to set the criteria for such monitoring. Clearly, in healthy young patients without pre-existent disease in whom a routine procedure is planned, monitoring is probably not indicated. However, in older patients and possibly in those with hypertension or previous episodes of congestive failure, such monitoring becomes highly desirable. Doppler

TABLE 9–1.
Average Effects of Laparoscopy on Arterial Pressure, Central Venous Pressure, and Cardiac Output*†

			IAP‡ (mm Hg)		
	Control	Trendelenburg	20	30	Horizontal Deflated
Systolic blood pressure, mm Hg	101	105	118	110	112
Diastolic blood pressure, mm Hg	66	67	82	80	72
Central venous pressure, mm Hg	7.0	9.7	16.3	12.0	6.9
Cardiac output, L/min	4.7	4.5	4.5	4.3	4.7

*Adapted from Motew M, Ivankovich AD, Bieniarz J, et al: *Am J Obstet Gynecol* 1973; 115:1002–1012.
†Cardiovascular effects change after the insufflation pressure exceeds 20 mm Hg.
‡IAP = intrararterial pressure.

techniques are reproducible with greatest accuracy in experienced hands because changes in position of the probe and angle of insonation may alter the results obtained. The suprasternal probe may be taped in place and used as needed. It represents a simple way to detect potentially severe cardiovascular complications during a "minimally invasive" laparoscopic procedure.

Cardiovascular Complications of Laparoscopy

In addition to the cardiovascular effects of pneumoperitoneum, CO_2 absorption through the peritoneum, and changes in body position, acute cardiovascular collapse during laparoscopy has been reported.[56] Overdistension of the abdomen and peritoneal manipulation with resultant serious vasovagal reflex lead to marked bradycardia and hypotension. If recognized promptly and treated by atropine injection, recovery without sequelae is the rule.[16] Kelman et al. also reported a case of cardiac arrest that was successfully resuscitated during laparoscopy. He attributed the incident to be a result of carbon dioxide embolism. This condition has been discussed thoroughly in a previous section of this chapter.

Cardiac arrhythmias during laparoscopy using halothane anesthesia with spontaneous breathing have been reported with an incidence of up to 27%.[57] These arrhythmias are relatively benign. Ectopic beats with R-on-T phenomena or falls in blood pressure are uncommon.

REFERENCES

1. Kelling G: Uber Oesophagoskopie, Gastroskopie und Colioskopie. *Munchen Med Wochenschr* 1902; 49:21.
2. El-Minawi MF, Wahbi O, Sharawi M, et al: Physiologic changes during CO_2 and N_2O pneumoperitoneum in diagnostic laparoscopy. A comparative study. *J Reprod Med* 1981; 26:338–346.
3. Piiper J: Physiologic equilibria of gas cavities in the body, in Fenn O, Rahn H (eds): in *Handbook of Physiology,* vol 2, *Respiration.* Washington DC, American Physiological Society, 1965, pp 1205–1218.
4. Loring SH, Butler JP: Gas exchange in body cavities, in Farhi LE, Tenney SM (eds): *Handbook of Physiology,* section 3—*The Respiratory System,* vol 4—*Gas Exchange.* Bethesda, Md, American Physiologic Society, 1987, pp 283–295.
5. Tobin CE, Van Liew HD, Rahn H: Reaction of the subcutaneous tissue of rats to injected air. *Proc Soc Exp Biol Med* 1962; 109:122–126.
6. Seed RF, Shakespeare TF, Muldoon MJ: Carbon dioxide homeostasis during anesthesia for laparoscopy. *Anaesthesia* 1970; 25:223–231.
7. Farhi LE, Rahn H: Gas stores of the body and the unsteady state. *J Appl Physiol* 1955; 7:472.
8. Farhi LE, Rahn H: Dynamnics of changes in carbon dioxide stores. *Anesthesiology* 1955; 21:604.
9. Baratz RA, Karis JH: Blood gas studies during laparoscopy under general anesthesia. *Anesthesiology* 1969; 30:463–464.
10. Alexander GD, Brown EM: Physiologic alterations during pelvic laparoscopy. *Am J Obstet Gynecol* 1969; 105:1078–1081.
11. Alexander GD, Noe FE, Brown EM: Anesthesia for pelvic laparoscopy. *Anesth Analg* 1969; 48:14–18.
12. Kenefick P, Leader A, Maltby R, et al: Laparoscopy: Blood-gas values and minor sequelae associated with three techniques based on isoflurane. *Br J Anaesth* 1987; 59:189–194.
13. Desmond J, Gordon RA. Ventilation in patients anaesthetized for laparoscopy. *Can Anaesth Soc J* 1970; 17:378–387.

14. Lewis DG, Ryder W, Burn N, et al: Laparoscopy—An investigation during spontaneous ventilation with halothane. *Br J Anaesth* 1972; 44:685–690.
15. Reddick EJ, Olsen DO: Outpatient laparoscopic laser cholecytectomy. *Am J Surg* 1990; 160:485–488.
16. Motew M, Ivankovich AD, Bieniarz J, et al: Cardiovascular effects and acid-base and blood gas changes during laparoscopy. *Am J Obstet Gynecol* 1973; 115:1002–1012.
17. Collins JM: Inert gas exchange of subcutaneous and intraperitoneal gas pockets in piglets. *Respir Physiol* 1981; 46:391–404.
18. Cameron E, Pocock J, de L Dear G, et al: Gas exchange in abdominal cavity during laparoscopy. *J R Soc Med* 1983; 76:1015–1018.
19. Tobin MJ: Respiratory monitoring in the intensive care unit. *Am Rev Respir Dis* 1988; 138:1625–1642.
20. Bongard FS, Wu Y, Lee TS, et al: Accuracy of capnography in nonintubated patients. *Anesthesiology,* in press.
21. Fletcher R: Arterial to end-tidal CO_2 tension differences. *Anaesthesia* 1987; 42:210–211.
22. Brampton WJ, Watson RJ: Arterial to end-tidal carbon dioxide tension difference during laparoscopy. *Anaesthesia* 1990; 45:210–214.
23. Sivak BJ: Surgical emphysema: Report of a case and review. *Anesth Analg* 1964; 43:415–417.
24. Bruhl W: Complications of laparoscopy and liver biopsy under vision: The results of a survey. *German Med Monthly* 1967; 12:31–32.
25. Root B, Levy MN, Pollack S, et al: Gas embolism death after laparoscopy delayed by trapping in the portal circulation. *Anesth Analg* 1978; 57:232–237.
26. Ivankovich AD, Albrecht RF, Zahed B, et al: Cardiovascular collapse during gynecological laparoscopy. *Ill Med J* 1974; 145:58–61.
27. McKenzie R: Laparoscopy. *N Z Med J* 1971; 74:87–91.
28. Shulman D, Aronson HB: Capnography in the early diagnosis of carbon dioxide embolism during laparoscopy. *Can Anaesth Soc J* 1984; 31:455–459.
29. Yacoub OF, Cardona I, Coveler, et al: Carbon dioxide embolism during laparoscopy. *Anesthesiology* 1982; 57:533–535.
30. Clark CC, Weeks DB, Gudson JP: Venous carbon dioxide embolism during laparoscopy. *Anesth Analg* 1977; 56:650–652.
31. Stauffer HM, Durant TM, Oppenheimer MJ: Gas embolism. *Radiology* 1956; 66:686–692.
32. van den Bos GC, Drake AJ, Noble MIM: The effect of carbon dioxide upon myocardial contractile performance, blood flow, and oxygen consumption. *J Physiol (Lond)* 1979; 287:149–161.
33. Staszewska-Barezak J, Dusting GJ: Importance of circulating angiotensin II for elevation of arterial pressure during acute hypercapnia in anesthetized dogs. *Clin Exp Pharmacol Physiol* 1981; 8:189–210.
34. Rasmussen JP, Dauchot PJ, De Palma RG, et al: Cardiac function and hypercarbia. *Arch Surg* 1978; 113:1196–1200.
35. Lin YC, Shida KK, Hong SK: Effects of hypercapnia, hypoxia, and rebreathing on circulatory response to apnea. *J Appl Physiol* 1983; 54:172–177.
36. Nunn JF: The effects of changes in the carbon dioxide tension, in *Applied Respiratory Physiology,* ed 3. London, Butterworth & Co Ltd, 1987, pp 460–470.
37. Price HL: Effects of carbon dioxide on the cardiovascular system. *Anesthesiology* 1960; 21:652–663.
38. Kashton J, Green JF, Parsons EQ, et al: Hemodynamic effects of increased abdominal pressure. *J Surg Res* 1981; 30:249–255.
39. Hodgson C, McCelland RMA, Newton JR: Some effects of the peritoneal insufflation of carbon dioxide at laparoscopy. *Anaesthesia* 1970; 25:382–390.
40. Prys-Roberts C, Kelman GR, Greenbaum R, et al: Circulatory influences of artificial ventilation during nitrous oxide anesthesia in man. II. Results: The relative influence of mean intrathoracic pressure and arterial carbon dioxide tension. *Br J Anaesth* 1967; 39:533.

41. Kelman GR, Swapp GH, Smith I, et al: Cardiac output and arterial blood gas tension during laparoscopy. *Br J Anaesth* 1972; 44:1155–1162.
42. Johannsen G, Andersen M, Juhl B: The effect of general anesthesia on the haemodynamic events during laparoscopy with CO_2 insufflation. *Acta Anesthesiol Scand* 1989; 33:132–136.
43. Marshall RC, Jebsen PJR, Davie IT, et al: Circulatory effects of carbon dioxide insufflation of the peritoneal cavity for laparoscopy. *Br J Anaesth* 1972; 44:680–684.
44. Marshall RC, Jebsen, Davie IT, et al: Circulatory effects of peritoneal insufflation with nitrous oxide. *Br J Anesth* 1972; 44:1183–1187.
45. Gauer OH, Thorn HL: Postural changes in the circulation, in Hamilton WF, Dow P (eds): *Handbook of Physiology,* set 2, vol 3. Washington, DC, American Physiological Society, 1965, pp 2409–2439.
46. Coonan TJ, Hope CE: Cardio-respiratory effects of change of body position. *Can Anaesth Soc J* 1983; 30:424–437.
47. Sibbald WJ, Paterson NAM, Holliday RL, et al: The Trendelenburg position: Hemodynamic effects in hypotensive and normotensive patients. *Crit Care Med* 1979; 7:218–224.
48. Bivins HG, Knopp R, dos Santos PAL: Blood volume distribution in the Trendelenburg position. *Ann Emerg Med* 1985; 14:641–643.
49. Zippe C, Bruchard KW, Gann DA: Trendelenburg versus PASG application in moderate hemorrhagic hypoperfusion. *J Trauma* 1985; 25:923–932.
50. Taylor J, Weil MH: Failure of the Trendelenburg position to improve circulation during clinical shock. *Surg Gynecol Obstet* 1967; 124:1005–1010.
51. Ward RJ, Danziger F, Bonica JJ, et al: Cardiovascular effects of change of posture. *Aerospace Med* 1966; 37:257.
52. Fournier P, Mensch-Dechene J, Ranson-Bitker B: Effect of sitting up on pulmonary blood pressure, flow, and volume in man. *J Appl Physiol* 1979; 46:36–40.
53. Lenz RJ, Thomas TA, Wilkins DG: Cardiovascular changes during laparoscopy: Studies of stroke volume and cardiac output using impedance cardiography. *Anaesthesia* 1976; 31:4–12.
54. Kumar A, Minagoe S, Thangathurai D, et al: Non-invasive measurement of cardiac output during general anesthesia by continuous wave doppler esophageal probe: Comparison with simultaneous thermodilution cardiac output (abstract). *Anesthesiology* 1985; 63:68.
55. Freund PR, Padavich CA: A comparison of cardiac output techniques: Transesophageal doppler versus thermodilution cardiac output during general anesthesia in man (abstract). *Anesthesiology* 1985; 63:191.
56. Arthure H: Laparoscopy hazard. *Brit Med J* 1970; 4:492.
57. Scott DB: Some effects of peritoneal insufflation of carbon dioxide at laparoscopy. *Anesthesia* 1970; 25:590.

Chapter 10

Gastrointestinal Endoscopy: Diagnosis and Therapy of Hollow Organs

Cuong C. Nguyen, M.D.
David E. Fleischer, M.D.

Despite its long history dating back to the late 1860s with Kussmaul's attempt to examine the stomach with a straight, rigid metal tube,[1] gastrointestinal (GI) endoscopy has really blossomed only in the last few decades (Fig 10–1). Owing to advances in optics, electronics, and material sciences, the entire GI tract is now accessible to the modern-day endoscopist who has at his disposal an impressive technical armamentarium that can establish the diagnosis and, in many cases, provide immediate therapy. This latter capability of therapeutic intervention is an integral part of the modern management of GI disorders and can significantly complement surgery.

The goal of the next two chapters is to present an overview of the utility of endoscopy in the diagnosis and treatment of GI disorders. They are divided in three major sections. The first section provides some background information that is necessary to understand and appreciate the endoscopic instruments. The second and third sections are devoted to the hollow-organ GI tract and the pancreatobiliary tract, respectively. Common entities will be mentioned, and emphasis will be placed on the therapeutic potentials.

BASIC ENDOSCOPIC INSTRUMENTATION

Currently there are two type of endoscopes available, fiber-optic and video endoscopes. Both of them are by-products of the advent of optical fibers, which allows direct examination of the GI tract by providing either a direct image or an electronic reproduction on the television monitor.

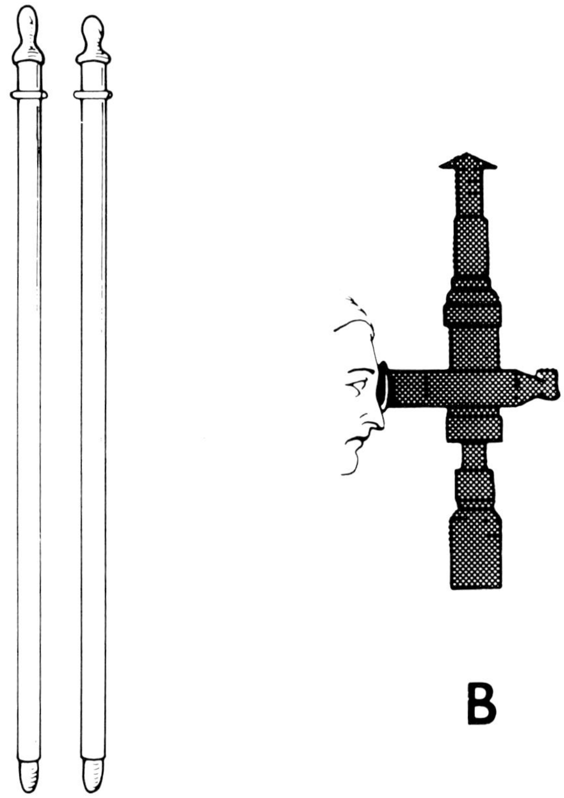

A

B

FIG 10–1.
Earlier version of an endoscope used in the 1800s.

PRINCIPLES OF FIBER OPTICS

That light could follow the curved path of a transparent medium such as water is nothing new, as first demonstrated by the British physicist John Tydall in 1870. However, it was not until the early 1950s that technology existed to propagate light through thin fibers of glass, a discipline now known as fiber optics.[2]

The basic tenet in fiber optics is the fact that at an interface between two transparent media, rays of lights are both transmitted and reflected. The angle at which light is transmitted into the adjacent medium is governed by Snell's law

$$n_1 \sin A = n_2 \sin B$$

where n_1 and n_2 are the material properties of the media and A and B are angles between the rays of light and the line perpendicular to the interface, as shown in Figure 10–2.

By applying Snell's law one can then determine the critical angle beyond which rays of light striking the interface between the glass fiber and an optically less dense medium will become totally internalized and propagate along the entire length of the fiber. Since the physical configuration of the glass fiber has no effect on the transmission of light, the fiber and hence the endoscope can then be made as flexible as the materials allow, thus giving rise to the modern flexible instruments.

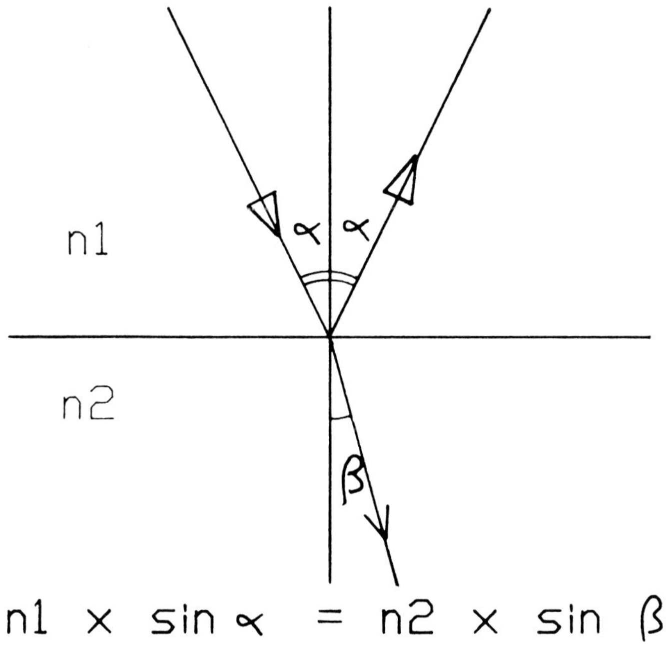

FIG 10–2.
Snell's law.

The first prototypic fiberscope was constructed by Hirschowitz in 1957,[3] but numerous refinements were necessary before flexible fiber-optic endoscopes started gaining widespread use in the late 1960s. Improved optical lenses and light delivery systems provided a better image, a wider field of vision, and a longer depth of field. Better materials and construction enabled a more manipulable distal tip and facilitated easier passage. When compared with the rather crude rigid instruments of previous decades, the fiber-optic endoscopes provide much more information and are better tolerated by patients.

With fiber-optic instruments, the endoscopist could readily diagnose many pathologic conditions, but documenting and sharing the information learned from the fiber-optic examination was rather difficult. There was no practical means to provide high-quality hard copies of the endoscopic images. However, in 1983, video endoscopy was introduced and made it feasible to record and transmit images with high resolution and acceptable cost.

PRINCIPLES OF VIDEO ENDOSCOPY

An application of quantum mechanics and solid-state electronics, video endoscopy is made possible by an invention from the Bell Laboratories known as the charge-coupled device (CCD). Mounted on the distal tip of the endoscope, the CCD is a light-sensitive solid-state sensor that utilizes Einstein's photoelectric effect to generate electrical charges proportional to the incident light (photons). This ability to generate charges is the inherent property of the CCD's silicon wafer grid, which changes its resistance according to the incoming light reflected off the object.

Once the charges are generated, they are periodically transported as isolated packets to the output device, which forms an analog electrical image of the object. The analog information is

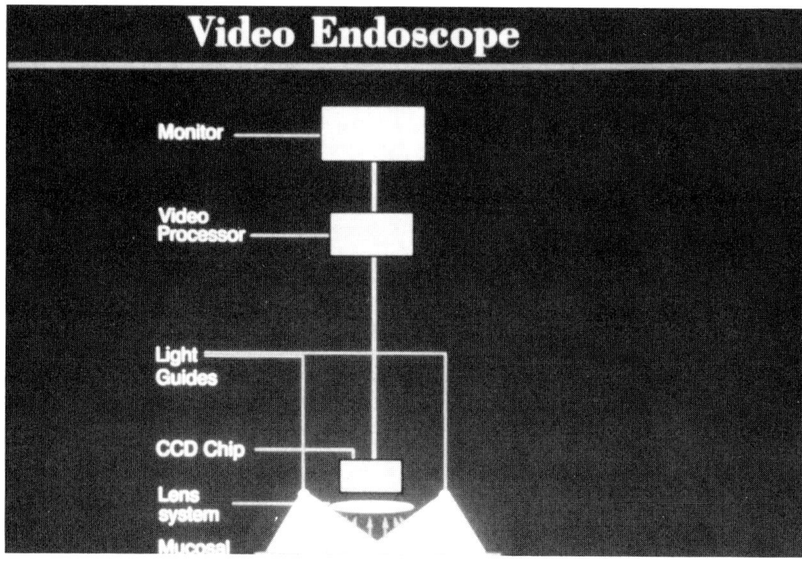

FIG 10–3.
Principle of videoendoscopy. A CCD captures light reflected off the subject. The electrical image is converted by a video processor to an image that can be projected on a monitor. *(Courtesy of Dr. Stanley Benjamin.)*

then converted by the video processor into the standard binary (digital) code. It is this digital information that allows easy storage and faithful reproduction of endoscopic images. Additionally, as digitized signal, images can be enhanced and analyzed by computers in techniques similar to those used in photos from aerospace satellites. Ultimately, the digital signal is converted by the video processor into analog information for synthesis of the image projected on a television monitor (Fig 10–3).

Improvement in computer capabilities and electronic circuitry have resulted in video endoscopes that produce images several times sharper than those of fiber-optic endoscopes. Better images and the capability to capture, store, and reproduce them have made video endoscopy the standard at most institutions.[4]

THE MECHANICS OF ENDOSCOPES

All endoscopes consist of two basic components: an aggregate of glass fibers, each measuring several micrometers in diameter, and a separate channel for the biopsy forceps, air insufflation, and water irrigation. Additionally, the fiber-optic endoscope has a series of optical lenses at the distal ends of the fibers to focus the light that illuminates and reflects off the subject. On the other hand, the video endoscope has the optical lenses to focus the illuminating light and, as mentioned above, the CCD to receive the photons. All these components are housed within a helical steel band with a waterproof plastic sheath on the outside. The whole construction is specially designed so that the endoscope is rigid enough to withstand the mechanical stress inherent to the many maneuvers of endoscopy, yet the endoscope's distal tip is sufficiently flexible to deflect in four different directions, left, right, up, and down.

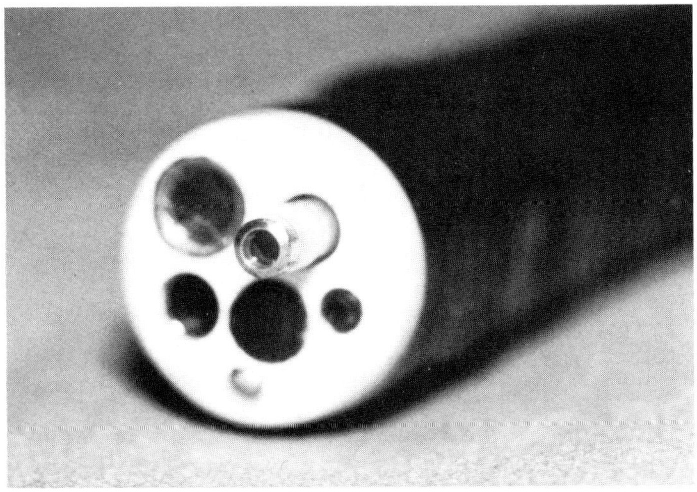

FIG 10–4.
Distal end of a two-channel therapeutic endoscope. Laser fiber is seen to protrude from one channel.

Advances in material sciences have enabled a reduction in the size of the optical fibers and therefore the size of the endoscopes. Since the glass fibers are smaller, more space is now available for a larger suction/biopsy channel or even a second channel. This type of endoscope is referred to as therapeutic endoscopes because they enable the use of therapeutic tools such as a heater probe, which normally would fill up the space within the regular-sized channel and greatly diminish any suction. This added feature of a second channel is extremely useful in situations such as GI hemorrhage where the endoscopist can apply suction to clear the field in one channel and at the same time be able to insert therapeutic tools in the other (Fig 10–4).

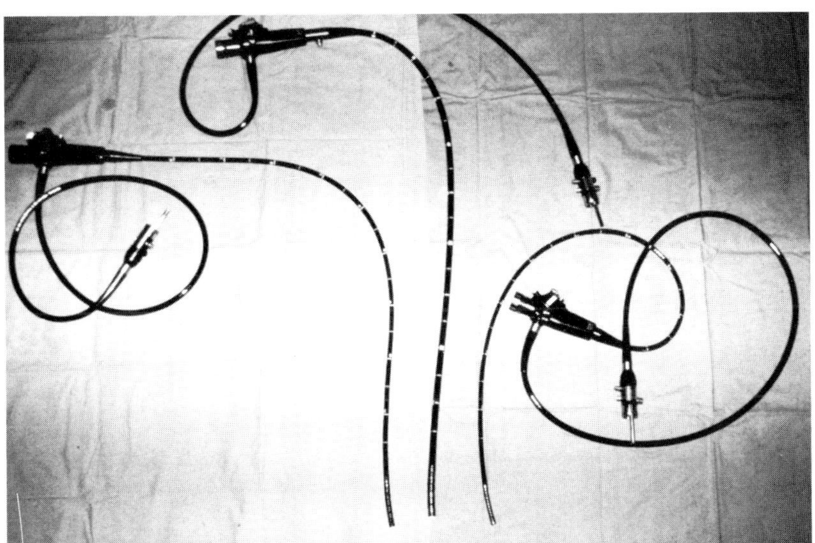

FIG 10–5.
Examples of three fiber-optic endoscopes of different diameters and lengths.

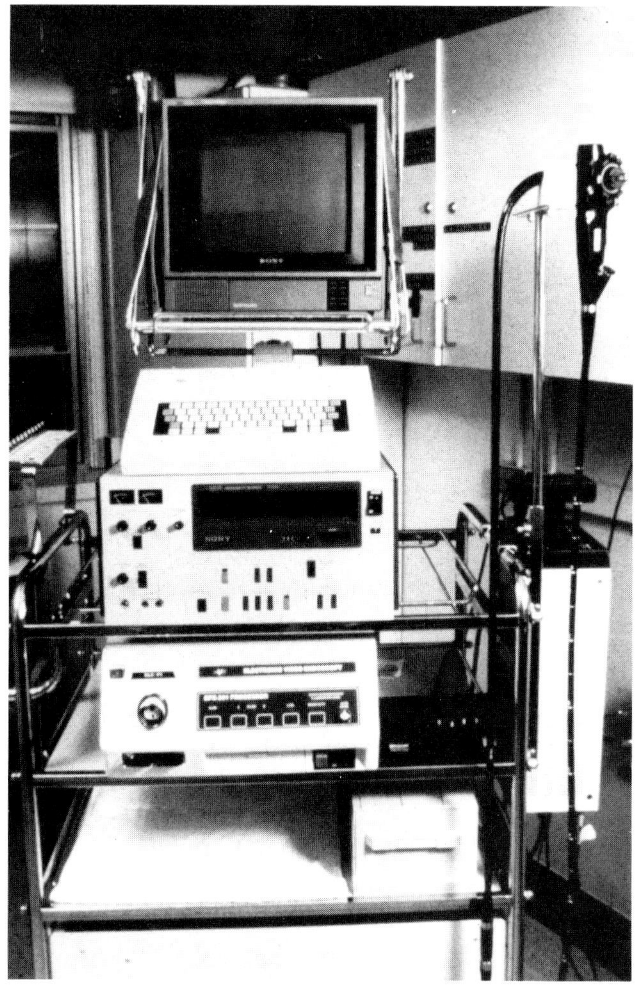

FIG 10–6.
Videoendoscopic system. The endoscope is hanging on the cart next to the other components. From *top to bottom:* monitor, keyboard, videotape recorder, and processor.

Due to the flexibility of the glass fibers, their distal ends can be placed at either the distal end or the side of the endoscope. When placed at the end of the instrument, the fibers will illuminate directly ahead of the instrument, thereby allowing forward viewing. Such forward-view endoscopes are used for routine upper GI endoscopy, sigmoidoscopy, and colonoscopy. On the other hand, light illuminating from the side of the endoscope provides visualization lateral to the instrument and is used in endoscopic retrograde cholangio-pancreatography (ERCP). These ERCP endoscopes are known as side-view duodenoscopes.

Currently, GI endoscopes are manufactured by several companies. Each type of endoscopes can be found in many lengths and sizes, with some variations in the operational features (Fig 10–5). Examples of some common endoscopes are listed in Table 10–1.

A fiber-optic unit is composed of a fiber-optic endoscope and a light source, whereas a complete video endoscopy unit consists of a videoscope; a video processor with a built-in light source, usually a 300-W xenon lamp; a keyboard for data entering; and a high-resolution television monitor (Fig 10–6). To capture images, most major gastroenterology endoscopy centers use a videotape player/recorder, a still video recorder/player that stores data on reusable video floppy disks, and a color dye-transfer thermal printer. Depending on the type of

TABLE 10–1.
Endoscope Types and Features

Type of Endoscope	Field of View (degrees)	Diameter (mm)	Length (mm)
Diagnostic upper	105	9.6	1,100
Therapeutic upper	105	11.4	1,100
Colonoscope	125	13.5	1,750
Sigmoidoscope	125	13.5	770
Side-viewing duodenoscope	90	13.0	1,250

setup and the accessories, such complete video endoscope systems can cost from $30,000 to $50,000.

UTILITY OF ENDOSCOPY IN THE GASTROINTESTINAL TRACT

For organizational purposes, the hollow GI tract is hereby defined as the alimentary canal that extends from the mouth to the anus, thereby excluding the pancreas and biliary tract. Diagnostic procedures and examples of common pathologic processes will be described first, and then therapeutic applications will be presented.

DIAGNOSTIC UPPER GASTROINTESTINAL ENDOSCOPY

The most common procedure in GI endoscopy, upper GI endoscopy, or esophagogastroduodenoscopy (EGD) involves examination of the mucosal surface of the esophagus, stom-

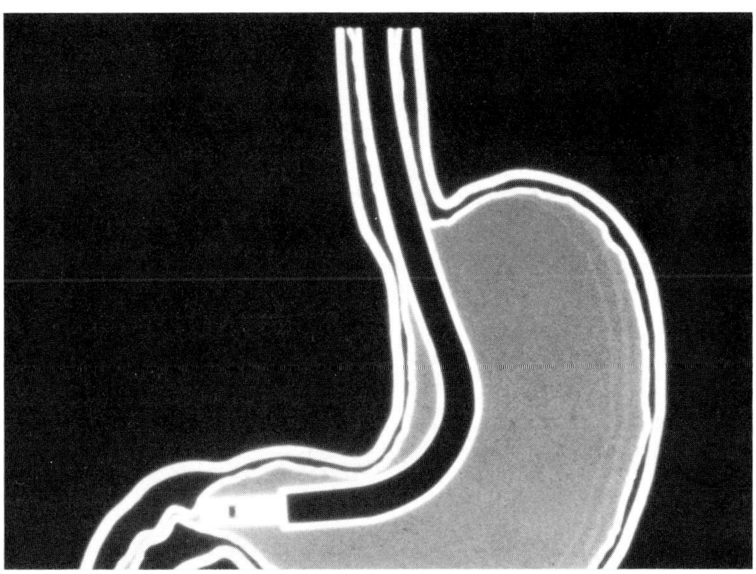

FIG 10–7.
Schematic view of endoscope advanced through the esophagus into the stomach.

ach, and proximal portion of the duodenum. Indications for EGD generally include dyspepsia refractory to medical conservative therapy, dysphagia, odynophagia, gastroesophageal reflux symptoms, GI bleeding, unexplained upper abdominal pain, and abnormal results of barium studies.[5]

The EGD procedure is relatively simple. After informed consent is obtained, the fasting patient is placed on a stretcher in the left lateral decubitus position. After dental appliances, if any, are removed, pharyngeal anesthesia is induced with local spraying of an anesthetic agent such as lidocaine. Conscious sedation then follows with intravenous administration of benzodiazepines and narcotics such as midazolam and meperidine. When sedation is sufficient for the patient to relax, the endoscope is gently advanced over the tongue and through a bite block and guided downward toward the upper esophageal sphincter. The patient is then asked to go through the motion of swallowing so that the cricopharyngeal muscles can relax so as to allow visualization of the esophageal lumen. The endoscope is slowly advanced under direct vision into the proximal portion of the stomach, antrum, pylorus, and the descending duodenum (Fig 10–7). The endoscope then is withdrawn into the stomach and is turned back on itself to form a U-shape to examine the cardia and fundus, which are not visible during the advancement phase of the examination. Subsequently, the endoscope is straightened, and withdrawal is continued into the esophagus and upper portion of the pharynx. A complete

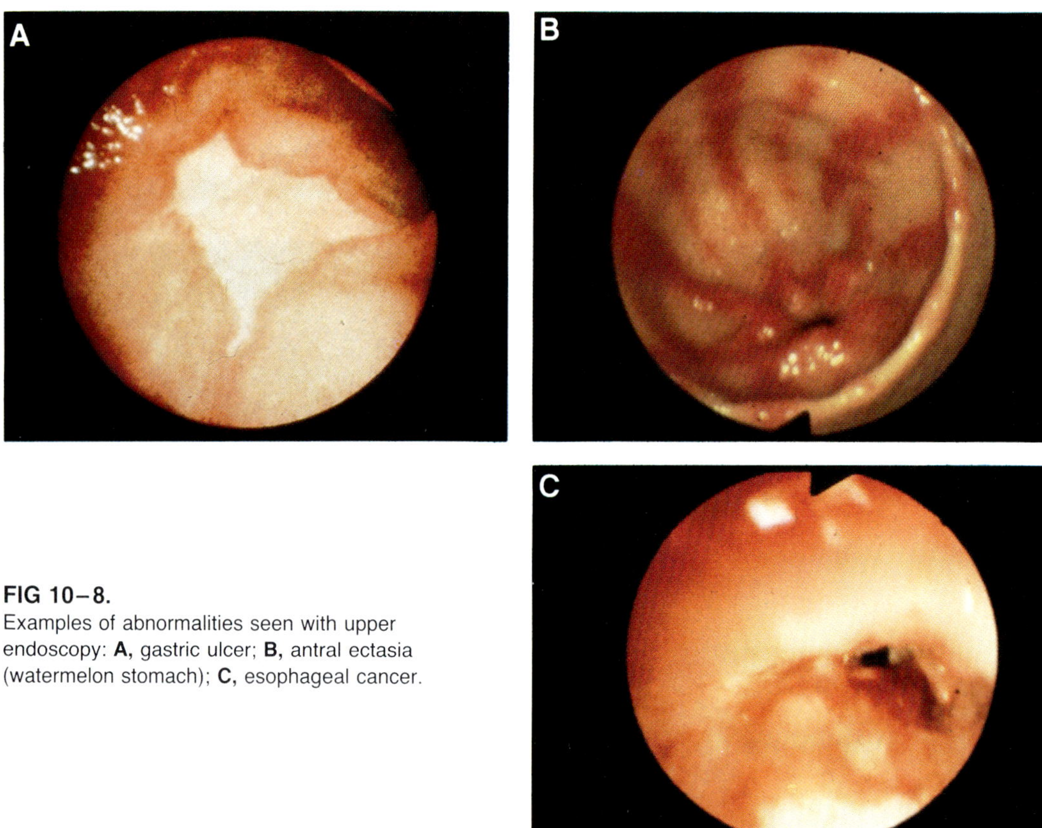

FIG 10–8.
Examples of abnormalities seen with upper endoscopy: **A,** gastric ulcer; **B,** antral ectasia (watermelon stomach); **C,** esophageal cancer.

diagnostic examination usually takes 10 to 15 minutes, and the patient will be kept in a recovery area until he awakens.

Diagnostically, upper GI endoscopy is most useful in detecting mucosal abnormalities such as peptic ulcer disease, esophagitis, gastritis, peptic ulcer disease, or malignancy (Fig 10–8,A–C). For these conditions, endoscopy is more sensitive than barium examination.[6] For example, the earliest changes in esophagitis such as mucosal edema and congestion are much more readily demonstrable endoscopically. Furthermore, endoscopy, but not radiography, allows for biopsy samples, which are used for a multitude of studies ranging from a urease marker test for on-the-spot diagnosis of *Helicobacter* gastritis to DNA analysis for tumor markers. By the same token, distinguishing a Mallory-Weiss tear from other mucosal lesions is easier with direct vision than with a barium swallow. Anatomic abnormalities such as esophageal diverticula, esophageal strictures, or duodenal deformities are easily seen by endoscopy. Vascular lesions such as esophageal varices, the ulcer of Dieulafoy, watermelon stomach (antral ectasia) (Fig 10–8,B), or Osler-Weber-Rendu telangiectasia are usually not seen on the barium examination, but they are well defined endoscopically, therefore obviating the need for invasive studies such as angiography.

In experienced hands, upper endoscopy as well as most endoscopic procedures are relatively safe, but complications do occur.[7] Just like other interventions, problems would most likely arise in the acute setting and/or the elderly populations. Medications for conscious sedation must be used judiciously, with continuous-pulse oximetry, sphygmomanometry, and electroencephalographic (EEG) monitoring becoming more of a norm. However, the most important variable of this equation is the endoscopy nurse, who must be well trained to ensure uncompromised respiration and to detect any early changes in patient's clinical status.[8]

In the largest survey in the United States, death resulting from upper endoscopy is only 6 per 100,000 cases, with the most common complication being aspiration or clinically insignificant arrhythmia. Perforation occurred in 3 of 10,000 cases.[9] The incidence of bacteremia is from 2% to 4%, but the actual number of reported case of endocarditis is quite rare.

THERAPEUTIC UPPER GASTROINTESTINAL ENDOSCOPY

Undoubtedly, upper GI endoscopy has made quite an impact on the diagnostic capability of modern-day medicine. Intraluminal lesions are readily identified, and therefore surgical/medical management can be expediently formulated. It is then only natural evolution for therapeutic maneuvers to develop. Indeed, every day, many patients benefit from the endoscopic therapeutic approach and can avoid open surgery.

FOREIGN-BODY REMOVAL

One of the first therapeutic interventions that endoscopy made possible was the removal of ingested foreign bodies in the upper GI tract. The domain now belongs to the GI endoscopist with a flexible endoscope instead of the otorhinolaryngologist with the rigid endoscope.

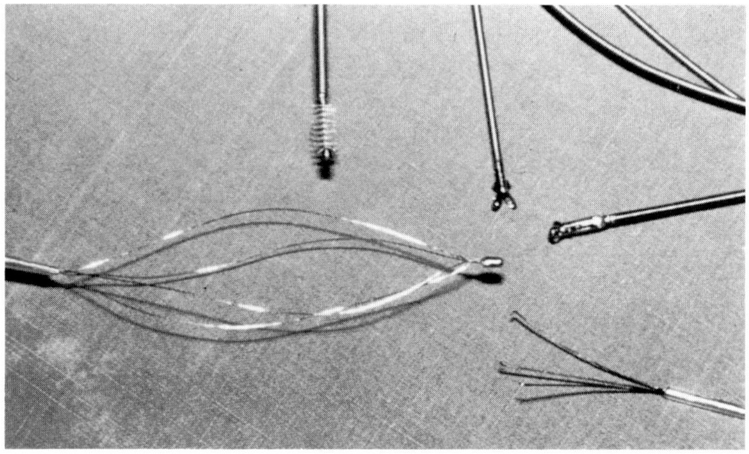

FIG 10–9.
Extraction devices include forceps, snares, baskets, and graspers.

Children, especially infants, the elderly with poor dentition, and the mentally retarded are at high risk for this problem.[10, 11] Any item can be ingested, with the size of the oral pharynx as the limiting factor. Up to 80% of foreign subjects may pass spontaneously,[12] but in the upper GI tract, some will be trapped at the cricopharyngeus, the aortic arch, the gastroesophageal junction, the pylorus, and the duodenal flexure. An impacted object at these locations can lead to hemorrhage, erosion, or perforation and therefore may need to be removed promptly.[13] A number of extraction devices are now available for this purpose, including rat-tooth forceps, wire snares, suture cutting forceps, baskets, and polyp removers (Fig 10–9).

Prior to endoscopy, soft-tissue x-ray films of the neck, chest x-ray films, and a flat plate of the abdomen to look for signs of perforation are necessary. A contrast swallow is also indicated in most instances. Figure 10–10,A shows a barium swallow demonstrating complete esophageal obstruction caused by meat impaction. An endoscopic view prior to removal is seen in Figure 10–10,B.

The technique is the same as in diagnostic endoscopy, with the exception that an overtube may be necessary in instances of sharp or long objects to prevent injury to the esophagus during the evacuation phase.[14, 15] A rehearsal prior to the actual procedure may be worthwhile.

After successful removal of the objects, patients must be re-examined endoscopically for any anatomic abnormalities such as unsuspected tumors or strictures. Tumors may require surgical resection, and esophageal strictures can, in certain situations, be dilated endoscopically.

DILATION OF BENIGN ESOPHAGEAL STRICTURES

Benign esophageal strictures can be caused by a number of conditions, with the majority due to reflux esophagitis, drugs, or prior nasogastric intubation.[16] Patients may benefit from a barium swallow to define the anatomy prior to the actual dilation. Upper endoscopy is then performed in the usual fashion, and a guidewire is then inserted through the biopsy channel

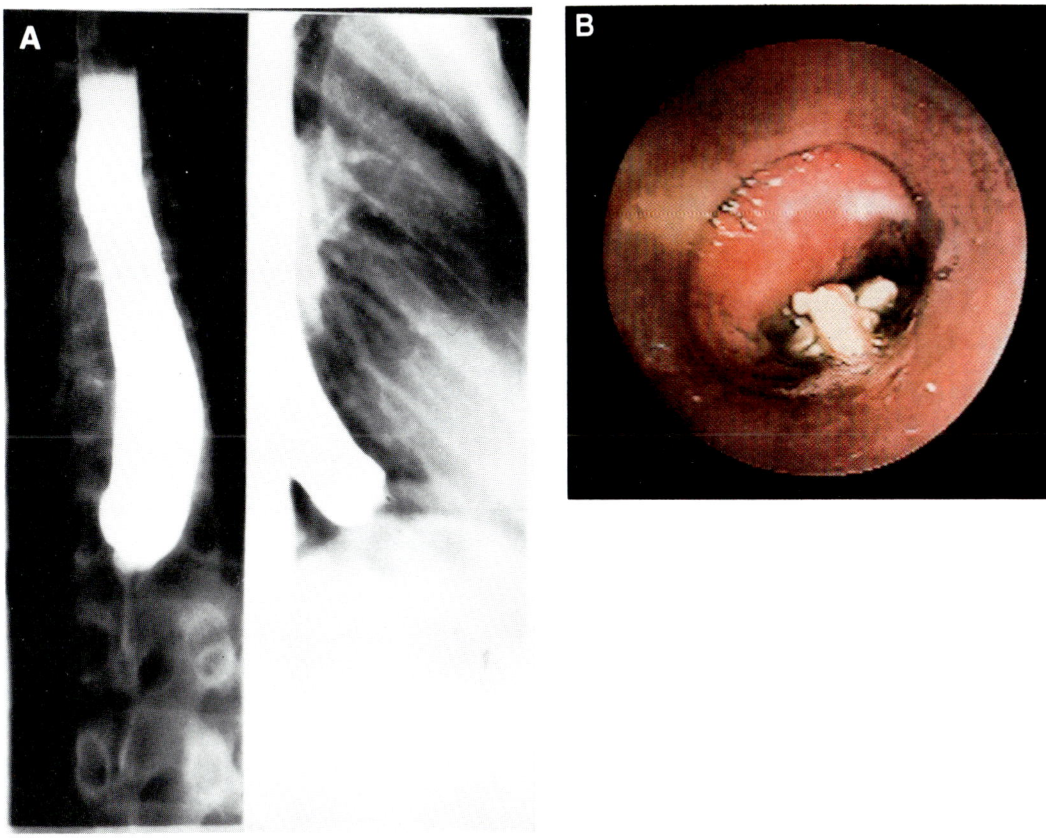

FIG 10–10.
A, barium swallow showing esophageal obstruction caused by meat. **B,** endoscope advanced through the overtube finds that the obstruction is caused by a piece of chicken.

into the antrum. The guidewire position must be verified and frequently rechecked during the procedure by fluoroscopy. Once the wire is in good position, the endoscope is removed, and a succession of polyvinyl dilators are passed over the wire (Fig 10–11). After a dilator with sufficient diameter has been advanced past the stricture, both the dilator and the wire are withdrawn, and endoscopy is repeated immediately to assess the results.[17]

An alternative method is to pass a balloon catheter via the biopsy channel and inflate it with the endoscope in place, thereby ensuring the correct position without the need for fluoroscopy (Fig 10–12). However, one prospective trial has shown that for esophageal strictures, the balloon does not provide adequate shearing force and therefore is less efficacious than bougie dilators.[18] The balloon dilator does have its usefulness in more distal strictures

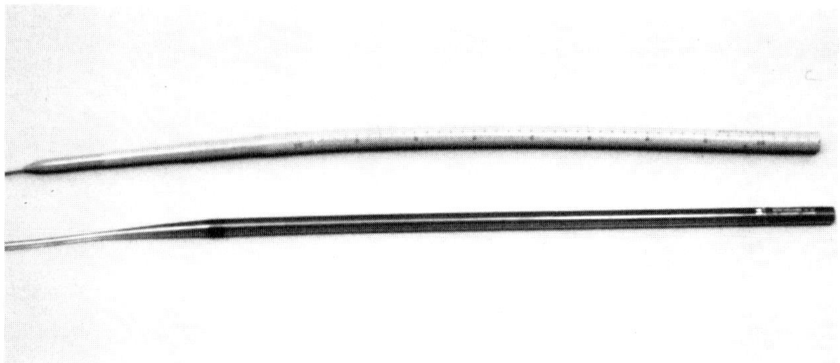

FIG 10–11.
Examples of two popular polyvinyl dilators.

such as those in the pylorus or duodenum or in patients who either cannot tolerate the mechanical dilators or have had previous perforations.

In patients who have simple, previously defined strictures, endoscopy is not required. Dilation can be carried out with tapered mercury-filled rubber dilators.

TREATMENT OF MALIGNANT ESOPHAGEAL STRICTURES

For those who have dysphagia due to malignancy and are not candidates for curative surgery or radiation therapy, three other endoscopic treatments are available for palliation purposes. These are laser ablation, stent, and percutaneous gastrostomy.

Laser Ablation of Tumor

Laser, or light amplification by stimulated emission of radiation, was first developed in 1960[19] and has numerous established applications in medicine. Lasers have since captured the fasci-

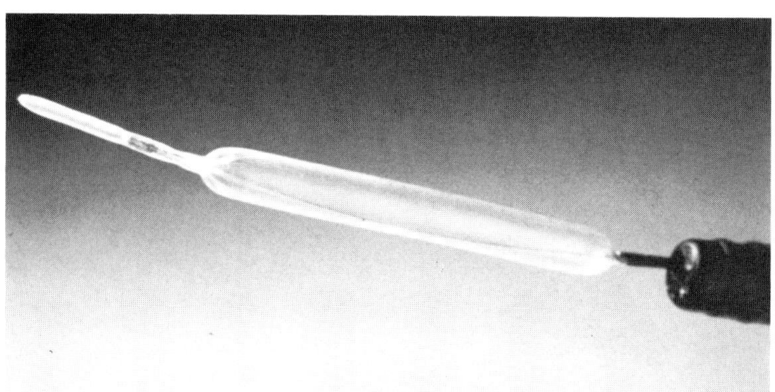

FIG 10–12.
Balloon dilator passed through an endoscope and inflated for dilation.

nation of many gastroenterologists due to the fact that lasing can be delivered at the precise location with predictable laser-tissue interaction. Detailed reviews of this subject have been published,[20, 21] and therefore only the basic principles are recounted here.

According to the classic Bohr atomic models, electrons revolve around the nucleus in separate orbits, with each orbit corresponding to a distinct energy level. Normally, electrons tend to reside at lower energy levels; however, they can absorb energy from light photons and use it to jump to a higher energy level. If the lower energy level is not completely occupied, the electrons will spontaneously return to the lower energy state and emit a photon whose wavelength is proportional to the energy difference between the two levels. Known as spontaneous emission, this process obeys Max Planck's equation of quantum mechanics:

$$E = \mathrm{hc}/l$$

where E is the energy of the photon, h is Planck's constant, c is the speed of light, and l is the wavelength.

To stimulate the emission, a photon of specific wavelength is imparted upon an excited atom and causes electrons to return to the lower energy level faster than they would spontaneously. The photons emitted by this process are of exactly the same wavelength, are in phase, and travel in the same direction as the incident photons. The same wavelengths of all the photons make the laser light monochromatic, the same phase produces coherence, and the same direction of travel enables low divergence.

When the material capable of producing the stimulated emission is enclosed between two parallel mirrors, reflection of photons by the mirror amplifies the reaction and creates a cascade of photons. Because one of the mirrors is partly reflective and partly transmitting, some of the photons are transmitted out of apparatus and form the laser beam (Fig 10–13).

Material used in this reaction can be a gas such as argon or CO_2 or solids such as Nd:YAG. By convention, lasers are named after the producing media.

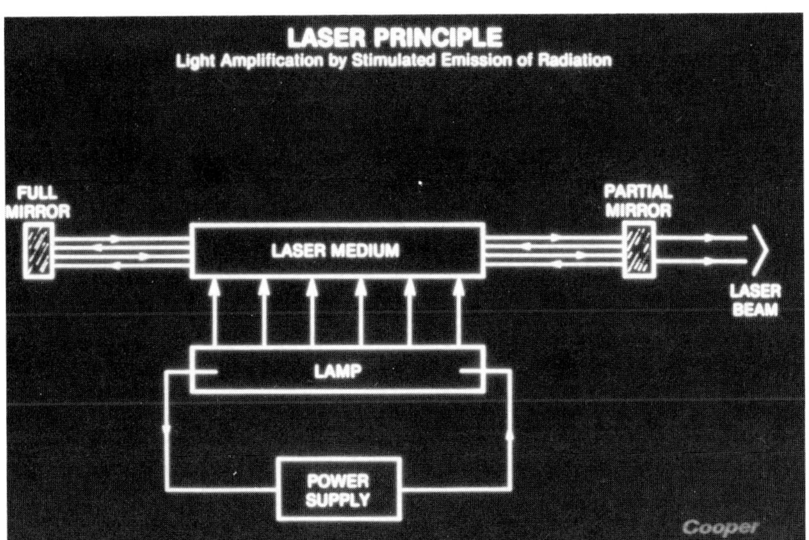

FIG 10–13.
Schematic demonstrating the principle of laser light.

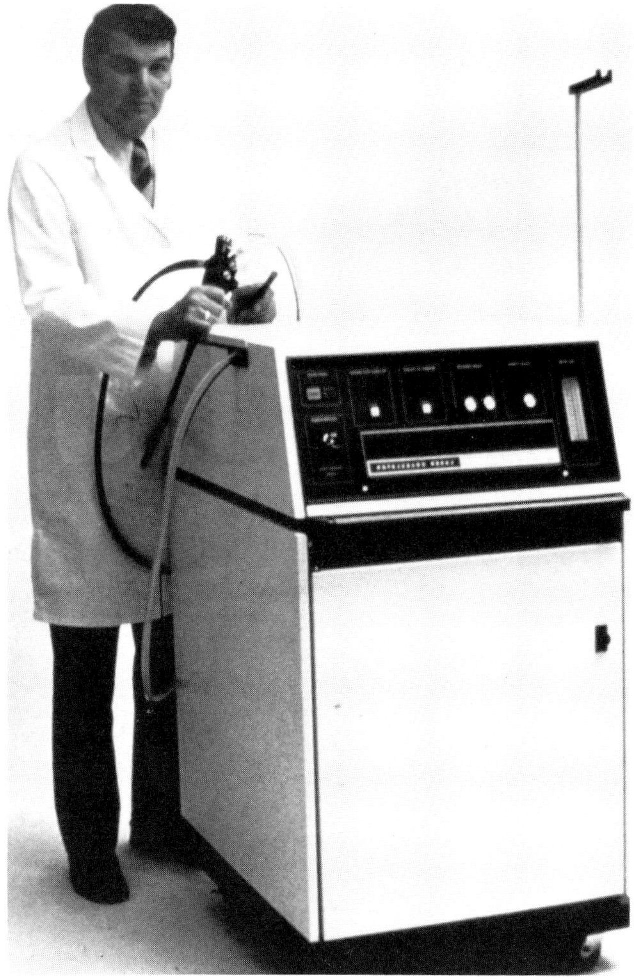

FIG 10–14.
Commercially available Nd:YAG laser.

Many different lasers have been created, and some have been experimented with in therapeutic endoscopy. However, only the Nd:YAG laser is commonly used. Due to its frequency, Nd-YAG is only partially absorbed by blood and not significantly by water; hence, the energy can be carried to a tissue depth of 1 to 4 mm, which is suitable for most applications in gastroenterologic endoscopy.

The laser light is absorbed by the tissue and creates thermal contraction at the site of treatment and the vicinity. The amount of heat generated is inversely related to the square of distance from the end of the fiber and the lesion. With more energy delivered, total destruction of the lesion occurs with a combination of instant vaporization, necrosis, as well as inflammatory changes.[22] As a general rule, protein coagulates at 60°C, and tissue vaporizes at 100°C.[23]

The laser unit itself consists of the laser generator, the cooling system, the gas circulator, and the electrical unit (Fig 10–14). The laser beam is transmitted in a quartz fiber housed within a plastic sheath that encloses free space so that CO_2 or nitrogen gas can coaxially circulate to clean the fiber and help blow away the debris at the surface of the treatment site. This whole plastic sheath is advanced to the lesion via the biopsy channel of the endoscope (see Fig 10–4).

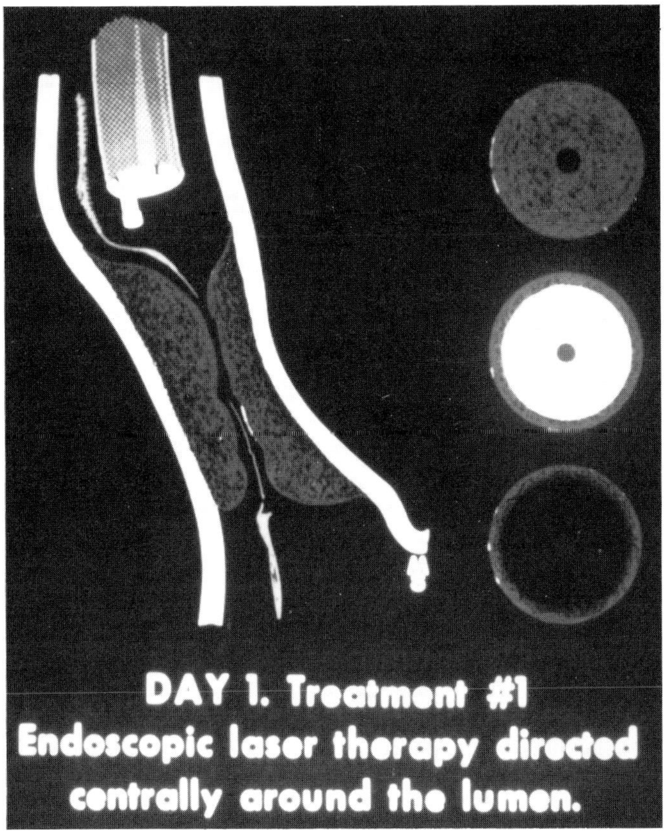

FIG 10–15.
One laser technique to treat esophageal cancer is the antegrade technique. The endoscope is advanced to the proximal tumor margin, and treatment is begun there.

It should be mentioned that laser can cause considerable damage to human eyes if special safety glasses are not used. However, with video endoscopy, since only the television image is observed, such precaution is not necessary.

The laser treatment session is begun in the same fashion as in a regular EGD, with the endoscope's biopsy channel accommodating the laser fiber. The endoscope is then advanced proximal to the esophageal lesion. The laser beam can be utilized in one of several ways:

1. Anterograde method. The laser beam can be focused on the target tissue in anterograde fashion, with the endoscope proximal to the lesion and the endoscopist viewing the obstructed lumen from above.[24] One disadvantage of this approach is that the treated area may swell and prevent the endoscope from passing to the area below (Fig 10–15).
2. Retrograde method. One alternative to circumvent the access difficulty is to begin the treatment at the distal margin and move cephalad. This method requires the endoscope to advance through or beyond the tumor, and therefore, esophageal dilatation may be necessary.[25]
3. Contact method. In both of the above methods, there is no contact between the laser fiber and the target tissue. If the laser beam can be in contact with the tissue, then the energy requirement can be reduced drastically, and potentially less expensive, more portable laser units can be used. The laser beam can be put in contact with the target lesion by one of two ways: placing a tip on the conventional fiber or placing the fiber directly into the tissue—the interstitial method.[26] The tip can be made of metal or aluminum oxide (Al_2O_3) (artificial sap-

phire). The metal tip works solely as a soldering iron and can get up to 1,200° C.[27] It holds some promise as a hemostatic technique. On the other hand, the sapphire tip can be made in different configurations to create different irradiation patterns. The sapphire tip can focus or defocus the laser beam and can chisel, vaporize, and coagulate.[28]

The duration of treatment depends on the tumor and patient's tolerance. Patients may be brought back for repeat treatment in 7 to 10 days, and immediate relief of dysphagia is achieved in 80% to 90% of cases. Quality of life is therefore significantly improved for these patients because they can now consume a normal diet.[24, 29, 30]

Placement of Esophageal Prostheses

Made of plastic compounds, esophageal prostheses are widely available in many sizes and forms. Their basic construction is a hollow tube with flanges on both ends to help anchor in the tumor (Fig 10–16). Some also come with a self-inflated cuff on the outside that serves the same purpose of anchoring, and they are used in patients with large fistulas. Most prostheses are about 14 to 16 mm in diameter and 5 to 20 cm in length. They also have radiopaque markings for verification.

Insertion of esophageal stents requires meticulous advanced planning. The stricture and the extent of the tumor must be predefined with endoscopy and radiology and the exact location reconfirmed prior to stent insertion. Most of the times, dilation with a bougie as previously described is necessary. A stabilizing tube is then placed in position over the guidewire. The appropriate stent is then placed on the pusher tube, and the whole apparatus is advanced over the stabilizing tube under fluoroscopic visualization. Once the stent is at the appropriate location, the stabilizer, pusher tube, and guidewire are withdrawn. A small endoscope is then used to confirm proper placement, and the patient will be kept without anything by mouth for 24 hours and a barium swallow performed the next day to ensure that contrast flows freely and the fistulas, if any, have been sealed.

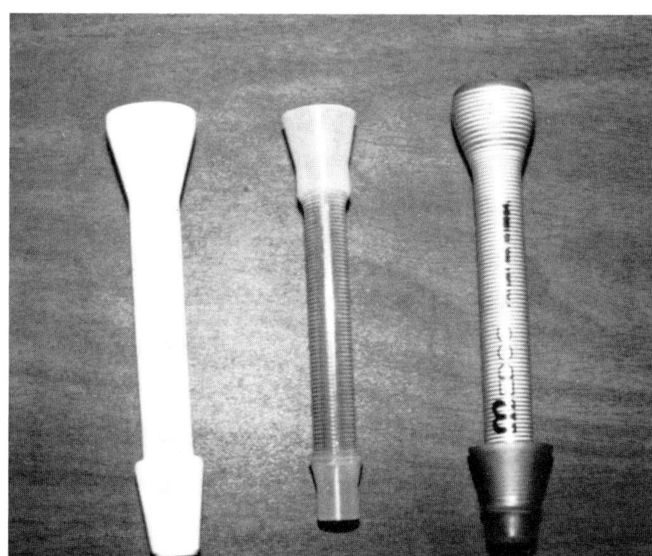

FIG 10–16.
Examples of three commercially available esophageal stents.

Good quality of life with the ability to take a normal diet and immediately improvement of dysphagia occurs in the majority of patients. The results here are comparable to laser ablation but are less costly.[31]

Placement of Percutaneous Endoscopic Gastrostomy Tubes

An alternative to the traditional surgical gastrostomy, percutaneous endoscopic gastrostomy (PEG) was first described in 1980[32] and has since been widely accepted as a means to provide long-term nutrition for a number of patients. Generally, any patient with an intact GI tract but who cannot consume adequate calories may benefit from this procedure. Typical examples are patients with impaired swallowing due to neurologic conditions such as stroke, Guillain-Barre syndrome, or amyotrophic lateral sclerosis (ALS). The other common indication is malignancy from the head, neck, and esophagus.[33]

This procedure can be safely performed in 15 to 30 minutes with minimal sedation. PEG is successfully performed in up to 98% of patients with minimal morbidity and cost as compared with the surgical approach.[34, 35]

A number of modifications of the original approach have been described, but the basic technique involves performing a regular upper endoscopy to rule out any obstructing esophageal lesion, gastric mucosal diseases, or gastric outlet obstruction. With the endoscope in the midstomach, air is then insufflated to bring the anterior gastric wall close to the abdominal skin. The area on the abdominal wall that is best transilluminated with the endoscopc is pushed inward with the finger by the endoscopist's assistant. An indentation of the anterior gastric wall must be seen endoscopically, and the point of maximal ballottement compression on the abdominal wall is then anesthetized locally. A small needle is advanced into the stom-

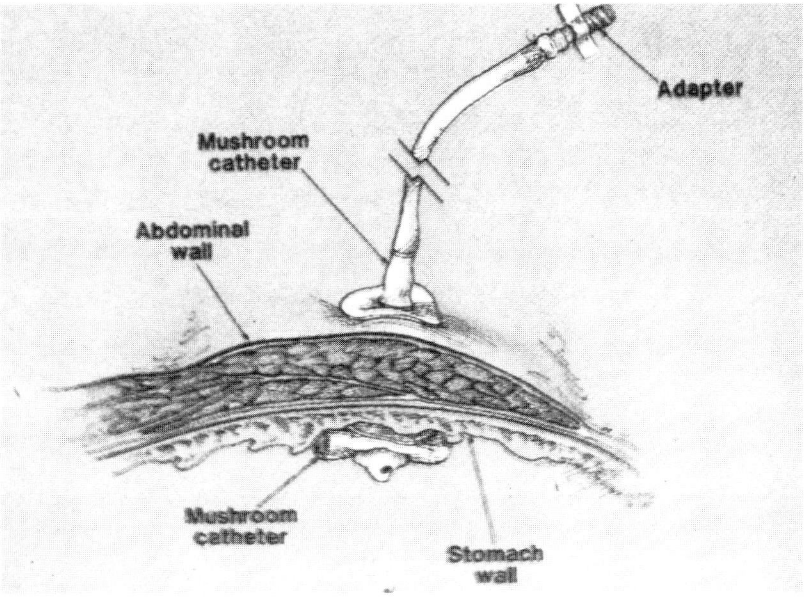

FIG 10–17.
Schematic showing an endoscopically placed gastrostomy tube in position.

ach until air is aspirated. At that juncture, a stylet needle is inserted for passage of a guide wire, which is then snared and brought proximally by the endoscope. Over this guidewire, the gastrostomy tube is advanced distally into the stomach and out the abdominal wall. The gastrostomy tube is prevented from migrating by a mushroom or balloon on the gastric side (Fig 10–17). The patient then undergoes repeat endoscopy to verify the position of the tube, and most often, feeding is possible by the next day.

UPPER GASTROINTESTINAL TRACT HEMORRHAGE

GI hemorrhage is the major indication for emergency endoscopy, and is now universally accepted as the procedure of choice to define the source of bleeding. Additionally, lesions that are at risk for continued bleeding or rebleeding can be identified and therefore can help tailor the management of each individual case. Most importantly, many endoscopic hemostatic interventions are now available and can provide the definitive treatment that can either obviate the need for emergency surgery or allow surgery to be performed electively and hence improve the outcome.[36]

Combined data from four recent studies totaling 3,247 patients indicate that the majority of upper GI hemorrhages are most commonly caused by acute gastric mucosal lesions (32%), peptic ulcer (30%), varices (13%), and Mallory-Weiss tears (7%).[36–39] Endoscopic therapy for gastric mucosal lesions, peptic ulcer, and Mallory-Weiss tears share many common features and will be discussed as a group, separate from the treatment of variceal bleeding.

Treatment of Nonvariceal Upper Gastrointestinal Tract Bleeding

The numerous hemostatic modalities available can be classified into four categories: (1) topical, (2) mechanical, (3) injectable, and (4) thermal. Each of these modalities will be described, with emphasis on the latter two.

Topical and Mechanical Therapy

Topical therapy includes agents that stop bleeding by either physically sealing off the lesion or promoting clot formation at the site of bleeding. Tissue adhesives, clotting factors, collagen, and thrombin-containing ferromagnetic mixtures have been used. However, none of these is currently in clinical use due to a number of reasons, including a lack of efficacy in clinical studies and ineffective delivery systems. For the same reasons, none of the mechanical modalities, which include suturing devices, balloon tamponade, and hemoclips, has found any widespread clinical application.[40] Nevertheless, some of the newer suturing devices and clip delivery systems hold promise.

Injection Therapy

Injection therapy is a simple and inexpensive hemostatic modality since the only necessary accessory is an injection needle. The most common type of injection needle is a plastic probe 1.6 to 2.3 mm in diameter with a 25- or 26-gauge retractable needle that is usually less than 7 mm in length to prevent perforation (Fig 10–18). Common injection agents are absolute alcohol (98% dehydrated), epinephrine (1:10,000), polidocanol (1%), hypertonic saline (15%

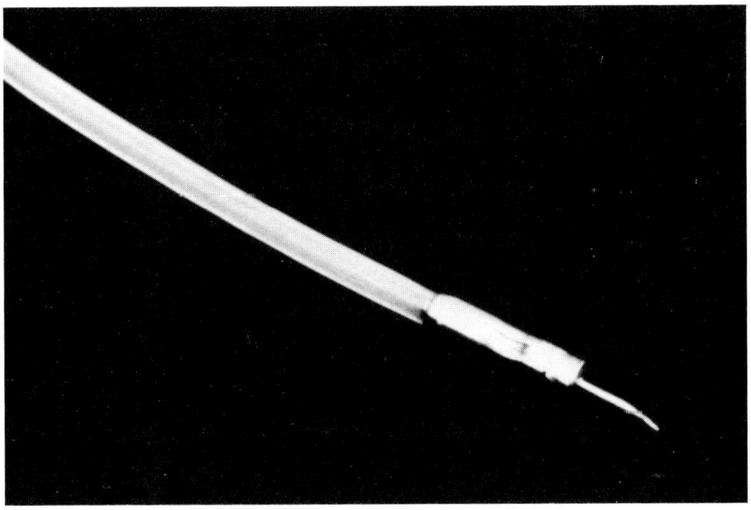

FIG 10–18.
Injection needles used in therapy for GI bleeding.

to 20%), and thrombin (100 IU/3 cc normal saline). Not well defined as yet, the mechanism of hemostasis varies with each agent but is thought to be a combination of compression of the submucosal vessels by the infiltrated solution, local vasoconstriction, fixation of the exposed blood vessel and surrounding tissue, and vascular thrombosis.[41–43]

Most of the times these agents are injected singly; however, some groups have had success with a combination technique with epinephrine injections followed by polidocanol or hypertonic saline.[44] The actual technique involves circumferential injection around the bleeding point with the needle inserted to a depth of 2 to 3 mm. Blanching, swelling, and immediate hemostasis occur after several injections. The least amount of injection is used to avoid extension of the ulceration or perforation. Usual recommendations are not to exceed 2.0 mL of 1:10,000 epinephrine, 1.2 cc of ethanol, or 10 cc of 1:10,000 epinephrine when used with 5 cc of 1% polidocanol.

Six randomized, controlled trials have been carried out, and all have proved that injection therapy is safe and effective. Definitive hemostasis can be achieved in up to 85% of patients with actively oozing or spurting ulcers at the time of endoscopy. Recurrence is usually in the range of 10% to 30%, but repeat injections may be successful.[45]

Thermal Therapy

The most established and promising, thermal therapy includes four different modalities: (1) monopolar electrocoagulation, (2) bipolar electrocoagulation, (3) heater probes, and (4) lasers. Monopolar electrocoagulation and lasers have the largest literature and experience, but bipolar coagulation and heater probes are currently more popular. These devices are pictured in Figure 10–19.

Mechanism of Thermal Hemostasis.—The basic principle underlying thermal therapy is that the heat delivered by various devices would cause protein denaturation and collagen contraction and result in welding of the blood vessel and swelling of the adjacent tissue, which in turn compresses the blood vessel and facilitates its closure. Since protein denatures at 60°C,

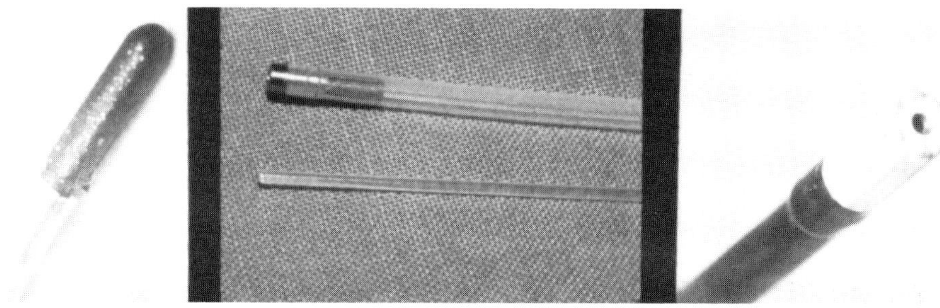

FIG 10–19.
The most commonly employed instruments for endoscopic therapy for bleeding are the heater probe *(left),* laser *(center),* and multipolar coagulation probe *(right).*

collagen contracts at 80°C, and tissue desiccates at 100°C, the goal of thermal hemostasis would be to deliver heat in the range of 60 and 100°C and avoid heat in excess of 250°C, where immediate tissue destruction occurs. This form of coagulation is known as obliterative closure and is effective only with arteries of less than 1 mm. With larger vessels, the continuous flow of blood will carry away heat (heat sink effect) and not allow protein binding of the opposing endothelial surface. However, arteries up to 4 mm can be sealed if the vessels are first occluded by physical apposition followed by delivery of heat.[46] This type of coagulation is referred to as coaptive closure and is the hemostatic mechanism for heater probes and bipolar and monopolar electrocoagulation, whereas traditional lasers, by virtue of noncontact, are presumed to work by the obliterative closure effects.

Monopolar Electrocoagulation.—First used in 1970 to cauterize a bleeding malignant gastric ulcer,[47] monopolar coagulation has become the most widely used clinically among the four thermal modalities. Three controlled trials have shown a significant reduction in the incidence of rebleeding and emergency surgery in patients with nonbleeding visible vessels or bleeding gastric and duodenal ulcers.[48–52] However, since monopolar coagulation is the least predictable and most difficult technique to learn, it has taken second seat to bipolar coagulation and heater probe therapy.

Bipolar/Multipolar Electrocoagulation.—Electrocoagulation here is made possible from the current that flows between a pair of electrodes on the probe tip, thereby bypassing the need for the ground plate on the patient's skin and avoiding the dangerous risk of sparking. The commercial Bicap is a multipolar probe with three pairs of electrodes on its side and tip (Fig 10–19). When any pair of electrodes are in contact with the tissue, the electrical circuit is complete, and heat will be delivered. The distinct advantage of this arrangement is that the probe can be applied to lesions that are hard to reach and allow only tangential contact.

The multipolar coagulation probe can produce temperature only up to 100°C and therefore causes minimal tissue injury[53] as compared with other methods such as monopolar coagulation or lasers, where there is no upper limit of heat delivered.

Currently there are two different sizes of multipolar electrocoagulation probes available. The larger size (3.2 mm) provides much better hemostasis in both experimental models and in clinical use when compared with the smaller (2.3 mm) probe.[54] The probe is connected to a power unit that is typically set between 15 and 25 W. A higher energy level may actually be counterproductive because the tissue may desiccate before the bleeding lesion is sealed off. The most crucial factors in the bipolar technique are the appositional pressure from forceful application of the probe on the lesion[55] and the duration of coagulation.[56] Either multiple short pulses or long pulses lasting a total of 10 to 14 seconds are usually optimal.

The most recent prospective trials on bipolar electrocoagulation have shown that it is a safe and effective modality that can provide immediate hemostasis and prevent rebleeding in actively bleeding patients and patients with visible vessels.[57, 58]

Heater Probe.—Heater probes consist of a hollow metallic cylinder with high thermal conductivity that is coated with a nonstick material on the outside and contains a silicon diode heating element inside. The heater probe is connected to a power unit that controls the amount of thermal energy delivered to the tissue. Typically, the diode can heat the probe up to 250°C, remains on until the preset amount of thermal energy has been transferred to the tissue, and then turns itself off until the next thermal pulse. Usually, about 100 to 120 J is applied at each station before the probe is moved. Just like the bipolar coagulation, the heater probe technique is more effective when a large (3.2 mm) probe is used with firm tamponade pressure on the bleeding lesion.

Numerous studies have been performed to compare heater probes with other hemostatic modalities. Most of the evidence now seems to suggest that for active ulcer bleeding and nonbleeding visible vessels, the heater probe can achieve immediate hemostasis and reduce the incidence of rebleeding and emergency surgery.[59–61]

Laser Coagulation.—Among all the thermal modalities, laser coagulation has been employed for the largest number of patients and publications. Tens of thousands of patients have been treated with Nd:YAG lasers and reported in the literature. Randomized controlled trials have shown that Nd:YAG lasers can control the bleeding and reduce the rate of rebleeding, with a trend toward lower mortality and less emergency surgery.[62–64]

The technique is relatively simple. It involves using an upper endoscope, preferably the therapeutic type, to visualize the bleeding lesions and then treating from afar. A common power setting is 50 W with 0.3- to 0.5-second pulses, depending on the particular circumstance and other variables as described in the section on laser ablation of tumors.

While the Nd:YAG laser has the largest body of evidence in support of its efficacy, laser coagulation does have some limitations. First and perhaps foremost is the cost of setting up a laser unit, which can easily run up to the $100,000 range as compared with $50 to $100 for an injection needle. Other limitations include an inability to produce coaptive compression for the larger vessels, the lack of mobility of the laser unit, and difficulty in mastering the technique. Due to these reasons, laser coagulation is not the treatment of choice for most acute GI bleeding.

Treatment of Esophageal Variceal Bleeding

To date, only three endoscopic modalities are available to treat variceal bleeding. First is laser therapy, which may be of interim benefit but does not represent definitive treatment.[65] Second is sclerotherapy, which is accepted for both acute and long-term treatment, and third is endoscopic variceal ligation.

Sclerotherapy

Sclerotherapy was first reported in 1939,[66] but it did not achieve universal acceptance until recently.[67–71] This method involves visualization of the varix during endoscopy and injection of a sclerosant directly into the varix (the American method) (Fig 10–20) or adjacent to it (the European approach). The injections are begun just proximal to the gastroesophageal junction and repeated at 3- to 5-cm intervals in the cephalad direction. Each injection is 1 to 2 cc of sclerosant, with the total in the range of 20 to 30 cc per each session. Patients are commonly brought back every 1 or 2 weeks until the varices are obliterated.[72]

The sclerosants currently available in the United States are sodium morrhuate (5%), sodium tetradecyl sulphate (1% to 1.5%), and ethanolamine (5%).[73] These agents, when administered intravenously, cause intimal inflammation and thrombosis. Subsequent formation of fibrous tissue will result in obliteration of the varices.[74]

Multiple controlled trials have shown that sclerotherapy is better than medical therapy in controlling the acute bleeding episode, reducing the risk of rebleeding, and once the varices are obliterated, possibly prolonging survival.[75,76] It should be noted that there is no role for sclerotherapy in prophylactic treatment of esophageal varices,[77–79] and neither should it be used for gastric varices, except in the setting of a controlled trial.

It is estimated that from 10% to 15% of patients may have complications from esophageal variceal injections.[80] Esophageal ulcerations, chest pain, and fever occur most frequently. Major complications are stenosis or strictures (1% to 7%), perforation (1% to 5%), and medias-

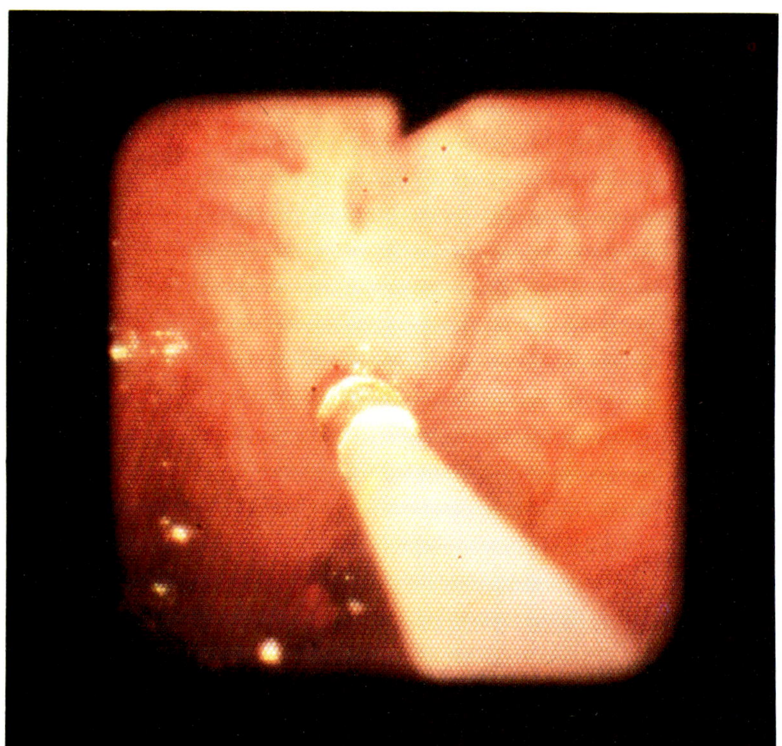

FIG 10–20.
Endoscopic view of an intravariceal injection.

tinitis (1% to 2%). Pericarditis, pleural effusion, pulmonary and systemic hemodynamic perturbations, and minor changes in pulmonary gas exchange can occur transiently without much clinical significance.[81,82]

Esophageal Variceal Ligation

Esophageal variceal ligation is performed with the endoscopic ligating device (ELD), a new instrument that was first described in 1986.[83] This device consists of a housing cylinder, a banding cylinder, a loading device, an O ring, and a trip wire.

About an inch long, the metallic housing cylinder is attached to the distal end of the endoscope. The banding cylinder fits snugly inside the housing cylinder and connects distally to the loading device. The loading device is a cone-shaped piece of metal onto which a plastic O ring is loaded. A trip wire connected to the loading device through the biopsy forceps allows the endoscopist to fire and unload the O ring.

If actively bleeding varices are present, they are treated first; otherwise, ligations can begin with the varices in the far distal portion of the esophagus or proximal 1 to 2 cm of the stomach. Up to 12 ligations can be performed each endoscopic session. Repeat treatment is carried out at 7- to 14-day intervals until the distal varices are obliterated or reduced to grade I, which is less than 4 mm in diameter and 4 cm in length.

A trial of 100 consecutive patients treated with ELD has been reported recently, and the results were comparable to injection sclerotherapy. Bleeding was stopped in 86% of patients. Only 3% had any significant nonbleeding complications as compared with the usually quoted 20% for sclerotherapy.[84] If these results are confirmed by ongoing prospective randomized trials, ELD will be a safe and inexpensive alternative to current treatment options for esophageal varices.

SMALL-BOWEL ENDOSCOPY

A relatively infrequent procedure, small-bowel endoscopy is indicated in three clinical settings (Fig 10–21). First and most common is the scenario of recurrent GI bleeding with negative results from routine radiographic and endoscopic evaluations. The second indication is to search for tumors that may not be seen with barium studies, and the third indication is to obtain mucosal information in the workup of malabsorption.

The small bowel is traditionally a relatively inaccessible organ due to its anatomic location. An upper endoscope can reach only the third part of the duodenum, and the colonoscope, the first several centimeters of the ileum, which makes the jejunum and proximal portion of the ileum out of reach for the endoscopist. Two techniques have been recently developed to rectify this frustrating problem, and they seem to hold some promise.

The more common method is the push technique where the endoscope is passed under direct vision. A pediatric colonoscope can be advanced orally to 50 cm beyond the ligament of Treitz.[85] Special enteroscopes 200 cm in length are now available and can reach an additional 20 cm. The enteroscope can be passed via the overtube to minimize coiling, and it is sometimes performed under fluoroscopy to guide the passage and help localize the lesions.

The second method is to use the Sonde-type enteroscopes, which measure 250 cm in length and 5 mm in diameter and have an inflatable balloon at the tip.[86,87] The enteroscope is actively carried into the duodenum by a regular upper endoscope or a pediatric colonoscope[88]

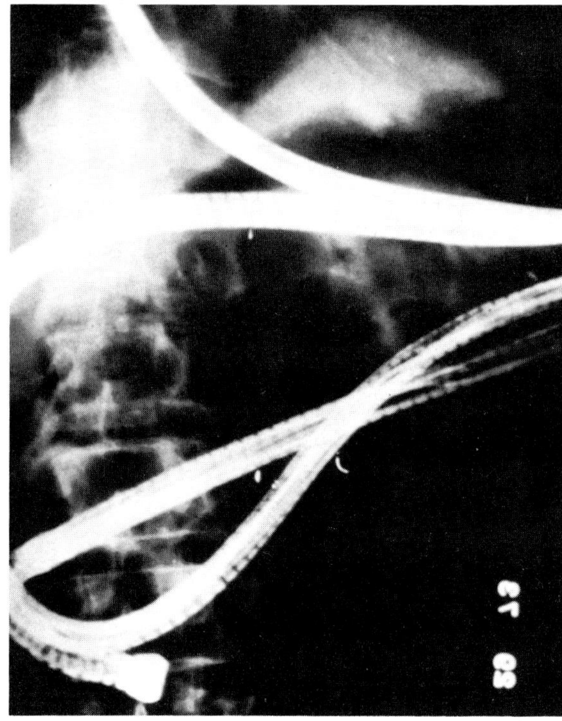

FIG 10–21.
A small-bowel enteroscope enables viewing of a large portion of the small intestine. *(Courtesy of Dr. Blair Lewis.)*

and is propelled distally by the action of peristalsis on the balloon. This method is the only one that allows examination of the entire small bowel. However, several major limitations exist. First of all, the angle of view is limited, and once the enteroscope is pulled back, it can not be readvanced. Second, unlike the push enteroscope, the Sonde-type enteroscope does not have a biopsy channel. And third, since the enteroscope depends entirely on peristalsis for advancement, the procedure may take up to 24 hours before the ileum is reached.

Because of these constraints, further refinements of these two techniques are undoubtedly necessary before they could gain widespread clinical use.

COLONOSCOPY

Conceived of in 1961,[89] the colonoscope has undergone a number of improvements in its design and construction that has enabled its customary use in today's clinical practice. Diagnostically, colonoscopy is indicated in the evaluation of any structural or mucosal defect detected by barium enema, unexplained GI bleeding, chronic inflammatory bowel disease, and surveillance of colonic neoplasia.[5,90]

The day before the procedure, patients are asked to undergo oral lavages at home. Most of the times, the standard regimen is 1 gal of polyethylene glycol/electrolyte mixture or its equivalent. The solution is consumed at the rate of 1.5 L/hr, and bowel action usually starts within several hours.

Just like in upper endoscopy, informed consent, conscious sedation with a combination of midazolam and meperidine, and cardiopulmonary monitoring are also employed in colonoscopy. With the patient in the left lateral decubitus position, a digital examination is carried out to evaluate the anus, rectum, and prostate. Lubricant jelly is also applied to the anal canal during this process. The colonoscope with a well-lubricated tip is then inserted into the rectum and is advanced proximally under direct vision. The patient may need to change his or her position during the procedure to facilitate the passage of the colonoscope. Since the colon can be tortuous with multiple bends, twisting and torquing of the colonoscope are frequently necessary. The cecum is routinely reached in the majority of cases, with the exception being patients with extensive diverticulosis or adhesions due to previous abdominal or pelvic surgery. Up to 20 cm of the distal portion of the ileum can also be accessible with the colonoscope. Once the cecum or distal part of the ileum is examined, the colonoscope is gradually withdrawn with careful, 360-degree inspection of every fold of the colon. When the colonoscope is in the rectum, the instrument is bent backward to form a U-shaped loop to inspect the inferior aspect of the rectum. Air is aspirated and the patient observed until he awakens.

Frequently encountered lesions in the colon are polyps, adenocarcinoma, mucosal ulceration or inflammation, arteriovenous (AV) malformations, and strictures (Fig 10–22,A–D).

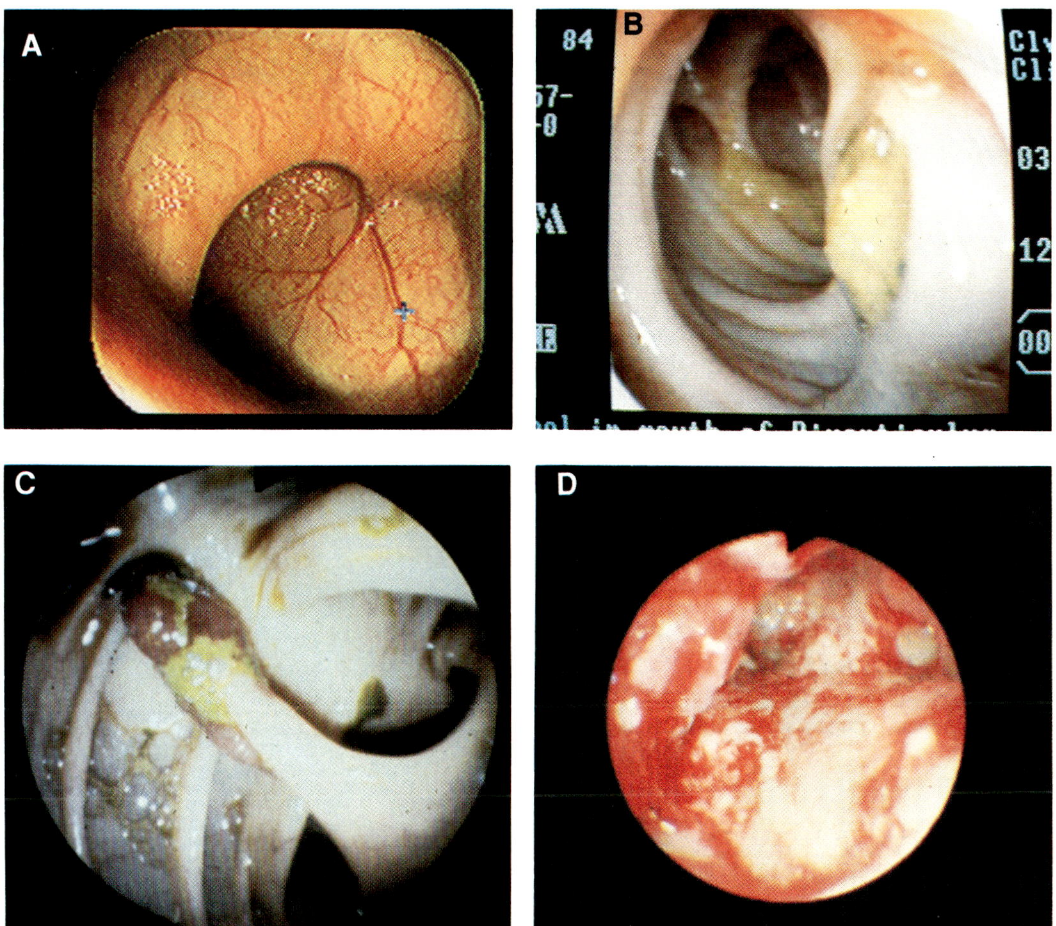

FIG 10–22.
Endoscopic views obtained at colonoscopy reveal normal colon **(A)**, diverticulosis **(B)**, colon polyp **(C)**, and colon cancer **(D)**.

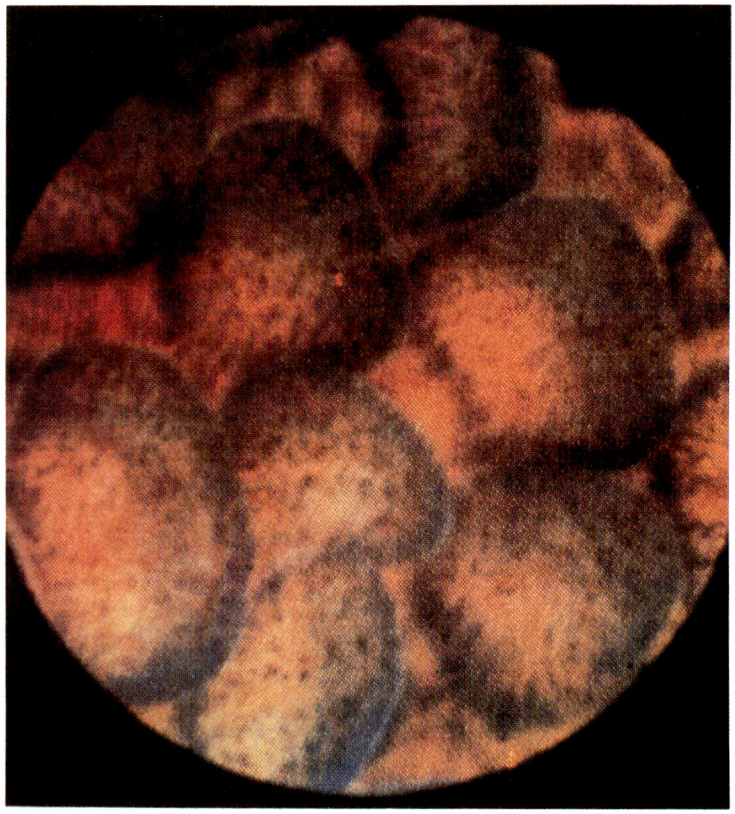

FIG 10–23.
Use of dye to highlight mucosal changes.

Most of the times these lesions are clearly visible with conventional colonoscopy. However, it is also known that some microscopic mucosal abnormalities are not recognized because they are beyond the resolution of the colonoscope. Preliminary work has been done with spraying the mucosa with blue dyes such as methylene blue or indigo carmine (Fig 10–23). Methylene blue is absorbed by the epithelial cells, indigo carmine collects in the mucosal groove and other interstices, and they both enhance the visibility of mucosal irregularities. An example of this technique is in ulcerative colitis, where low levels of disease activity or microscopic erosions or scars of the inactive phase can be identified. Polypoid lesions invisible to conventional colonoscopic observation can also be recognized with this technique.

THERAPEUTIC COLONOSCOPY

Polypectomy

Fiber-optic colonoscopy has revolutionized the management of colonic polyps. Very rarely do patients need open surgery for polyp removal because most polyps can be removed endoscopically with minimal morbidity.

There are many variations of the technique for polypectomy, but basically, a braided wire snare is inserted in the biopsy channel, and the snare loop is placed over the polyp and onto its stalk. Like a noose, the snare loop is closed tightly without transecting the polyp. The colonoscope and the snare are then positioned so that the polyp does not touch the adjacent colonic mucosa. The electrosurgical power unit connected to the snare is activated, with the tension in the snare loop steadily increased. A low power setting with 5- to 20-second application of current is usually necessary to create stalk swelling and desiccation before it can be safely severed. The polyp then falls off and is retrieved for histologic examination.

Larger polyps or polyps with a broad base may require injection of epinephrine to induce local vasoconstriction and edema to reduce the risk of bleeding. Polyps can also be removed in a piecemeal fashion to lessen the chance of injury to the bowel wall. In rare cases, endoscopic removal is not possible, and surgery is the appropriate treatment.

Up to 40% of polyps are less than 6 mm in diameter and hence are classified as diminutive polyps. A large number of these polyps are adenomatous and therefore require removal.[91] They can be removed with either a small snare or, more frequently, a hot biopsy forceps.[92] The hot biopsy forceps differs from a regular forceps in that it is also a monopolar electrocoagulating device. When the diminutive polyp is grasped by the forceps and slightly lifted away from the mucosa, a pseudostalk is formed. When the electrosurgical power unit is turned on, current passes through the pseudostalk and causes thermal damage seen as a small area of whitish coagulum at the base of the polyp. When this area is about 1 or 2 mm wide, current is discontinued, and the polyp is pulled off its base. In 99.8% of cases, the tissue enclosed within the cups of the forceps is not damaged by the electrocoagulating process and can be submitted for histologic study.

With proper precautions, complications are low.[93] Bleeding may occur in 2% of polypectomies and, in some cases, may be treated with local injection. Perforation occurs in the range of 1% and is usually due to entrapment of the serosal surface within the snare loop or to the use of too much heat.

Colonoscopic Decompression of Pseudo-obstruction

Pseudo-obstruction, or Olgivie's syndrome, is a condition characterized by colonic distension without any mechanical cause.[94] The cecum may dilate massively and rupture with mortality in the range of 50%.[95] Decompressive tube cecostomy has been the traditional approach, but the mortality rate for the surgery can approach 20%. An alternative is to decompress the colon with colonoscopy, a procedure first described in 1977.[96] Since that time, multiple reports have documented initial success of 90% for the endoscopic approach, which is now accepted as the standard initial treatment.[97]

Standard colon cleansing is not appropriate in this condition because it may worsen the distension and precipitate perforation. Air insufflation is to be avoided during the procedure for obvious reasons. Frequent irrigation with a small volume of water is necessary to clear the lens and to help visualize the lumen. The procedure can be very tedious, and the endoscopist must be very patient and careful in advancing the instrument. The cecum may not be reached, but adequate decompression can usually be achieved if the colonoscope can pass to only the hepatic flexure.[98] As mentioned above, the success rate is up to 90% with this approach, and the associated morbidity is about 2%.[99]

In about 20% to 30% of cases, cecal dilatation may recur. In these situations, repeat colonoscopy can be performed to deflate the colon. Additionally, at the time of the initial colonoscopy a plastic suction tube can be placed in the cecum or the ascending colon by the "piggyback" method where a loop of thread attached to the leading end of the tube is grasped by the forceps inside the colonoscope. Once it has reached its destination, the thread is released from the forceps and the colonoscope removed.[100]

Colonoscopic Decompression of Colonic Volvulus

An attempt to decompress sigmoid volvulus with flexible sigmoidoscopy[101] is indicated unless perforation or necrosis is suspected (Fig 10–24). Similarly, transverse, right, and cecal volvulus can also be reduced colonoscopically.[102] When the colonoscope is not able to advance past the site of obstruction, a technique has been described where a flexibly tipped wire is used to guide placement of a drainage tube proximal to the lesion.[103]

It should be recognized that due to its high recurrence rate decompression by the colonoscope is only a temporizing measure. If patients are a good surgical risk, elective surgery should be considered.[104]

Palliative Therapy for Malignant Colorectal Cancer

Endoscopic laser therapy is an important alternative for nonoperative candidates with noncurable malignant colorectal neoplasms who suffer from bleeding or obstruction.

At setting of 70 to 80 W, 0.5-second pulse, noncontact laser therapy can coagulate the exophytic tumor, reduce its size, and stop the hemorrhage in one or two sessions. However, pe-

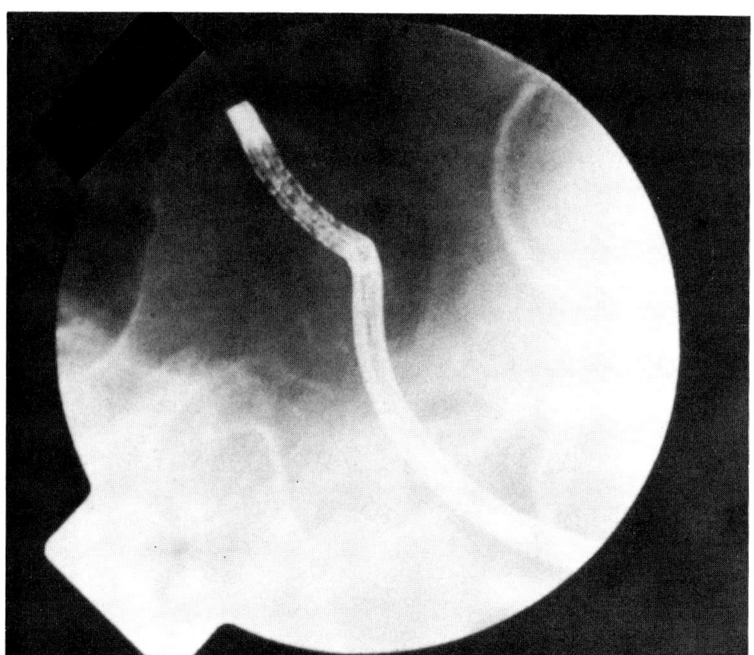

FIG 10–24.
Endoscope advanced via the rectum under fluoroscopic guidance to decompress sigmoid volvulus.

riodic retreatment may be necessary as the tumor sloughs and new surface with new vascularization is formed.

To palliate the obstruction, a higher and longer power setting is necessary. Typically, the noncontact laser can be set at 80 to 90 W for 2-second or longer pulses. The treatment is usually started at the proximal border of the tumor and moved distally. Sometimes, if the stricture is too tight, dilation with a tapered polyvinyl rubber or balloon dilator may be necessary to allow passage of the colonoscope (Fig 10–25). Alternatively, smaller instruments such as an upper GI gastroscope or pediatric colonoscope can be used.

Lumen recanalization and cessation of bleeding and diarrhea have been successful in 70% to 90% of reported cases.[105] Complications are rare, but perforations have been reported in 8 of 179 cases in two large series. Among these 8 patients, 4 died.[106, 107]

Thermal Therapy for Colonic Angiodysplastic Lesions

The most commonly encountered vascular abnormality in the GI tract, angiodysplasia of the right portion of the colon and cecum is an important cause of colonic bleeding.[108] Most of the thermal modalities described for upper GI bleeding can also be applied in the colon in the same manner and will not be repeated[109] (Fig 10–26).

Colonic Tattooing

At times, it is necessary to create a visible marker for the area of interest in the colon. Such a marker is very helpful for both repeat endoscopic examinations and surgical intervention

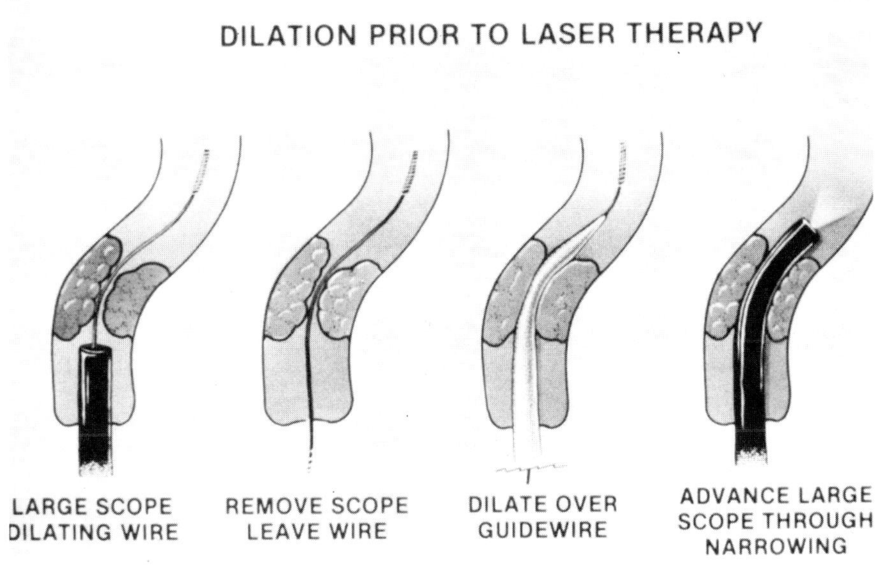

FIG 10–25.
Schematic showing dilation over a guidewire, which may be necessary to define a colorectal neoplasm prior to therapy.

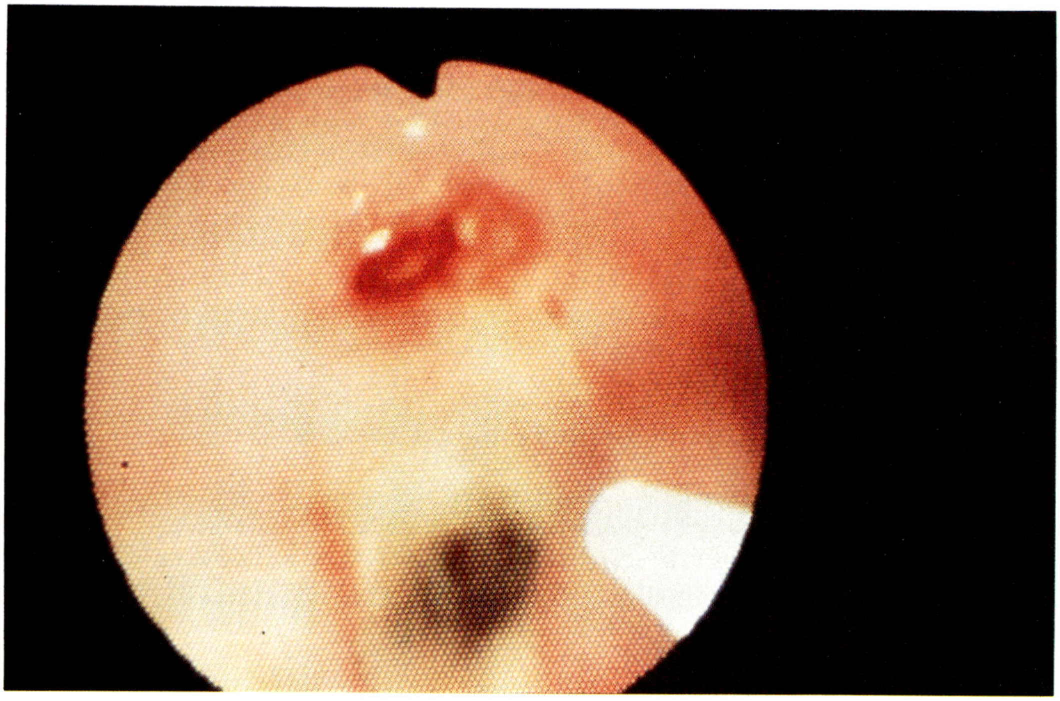

FIG 10–26.
Two cecal angiodysplastic lesions. The *top* one has not been treated. The *lower* has just undergone laser therapy.

because it provides prompt identification for the endoscopist and the surgeon. A common technique for marking the mucosa is to submucosally inject 1 to 2 cc of sterile India ink, which produces a permanent blue-black hue on the mucosal and serosal surfaces of the colon.

REFERENCES

1. Killian G: Geschichte der Oesophago- und Gastroskopie. *Dtsch Z Chir* 1901; 58:499–512.
2. Epstein M: Fiber optics in medicine. *CRC Crit Rev Bio Engr* 1982; 7:79–120.
3. Hirschowitz BI, Curtis LE, Peters CW, et al: Demonstration of a new gastroscope, the "fiberscope." *Gastroenterology* 1958; 35:50–53.
4. Schapiro M, Auslander MO, Schapiro MB: The electronic videoendoscope: Clinical experience with 1200 diagnostic and therapeutic cases in the community hospital. *Gastrointest Endosc* 1987; 33:63–68.
5. *Appropriate Use of Gastrointestinal Endoscopy.* Baltimore, American Society for Gastrointestinal Endoscopy, 1989.
6. Martin TR, Vennes JA, Silvis SE, et al: A comparison of upper gastrointestinal endoscopy and radiology. *J Clin Gastroenterol* 1980; 2:21–25.
7. Habr-Gama A, Waye JD: Complications and hazards of gastrointestinal endoscopy. *World J Surg* 1989; 13:193–201.
8. Fleischer D: Monitoring for conscious sedation: Perspective of the gastrointestinal endoscopist. *Gastrointest Endosc* 1990; 36(suppl):19–22.
9. Mandelstam P, Sugawa C, Silvis SE, et al: Complications associated with esophagogastroduodenoscopy and with esophageal dilatation. *Gastrointest Endosc* 1976; 23:16–19.

10. Nandi P, Ong GB: Foreign bodies in the oesophagus: Review of 2,394 cases. *Br J Surg* 1978; 65:5–9.
11. Vizcarrondo FJ, Brady PG, Nord HJ: Foreign bodies in the upper gastrointestinal tract. *Gastrointest Endosc* 1983; 29:208–210.
12. Davidoff E, Towne JB: Ingested foreign bodies. *N Y State J Med* 1975; 75:103–107.
13. Selivano VV, Sheldon GF, Cello JF: Management of foreign body ingestion. *Ann Surg* 1984; 199:187–191.
14. Witzel L, Scheurer J, Muhlemann A, et al: Removal of razor blades from the stomach with fiberoptic endoscope. *Br Med J* 1974; 2:539.
15. Spurling TJ, Zaloga GP, Richter JE: Fiberendoscopic removal of a gastric foreign body with an overtube technique. *Gastrointest Endosc* 1983; 29:226–227.
16. Patterson DJ, Graham DY, Lacy Smith J, et al: Natural history of benign esophageal strictures treated by dilatation. *Gastroenterology* 1983; 85:346–350.
17. Celestin LR, Campbell WB: A new and safe system for esophageal dilatation. *Lancet* 1981; 1:65–75.
18. Cox JG, Winter RK, Maslin SC, et al: Balloon or bougie for dilatation of benign esophageal strictures? An interim report of a randomized controlled trial. *Gut* 1988; 29:1741–1747.
19. Maiman T: Stimulated optical radiation of ruby. *Nature* 1966; 187:493–494.
20. Fleischer D: Lasers and gastrointestinal diseases, in Sivak MV (ed): *Gastroenterologic Endoscopy.* Philadelphia, WB Saunders Co, 1987, pp 158–180.
21. Riemann JE, Ell C: *Lasers in Gastroenterology. International Experiences and Trends.* New York, Thieme Medical Publishers, Inc, 1989.
22. McKenzie AL: Physics of thermal processes in laser-tissue interaction. *Phys Med Biol* 1990; 35:1175–1209.
23. Cummins L: Laser-tissue interaction, in Fleischer D, Jensen D, Brirght-Asare P (eds): *Therapeutic Laser Endoscopy in Gastrointestinal Disease.* Boston, Martinus Nijhoff Publishers, 1983.
24. Fleischer D, Kessler F, Haye O: Endoscopic Nd:YAG laser therapy for carcinoma of the esophagus: A new palliative approach. *Am J Surg* 1982; 143:280–283.
25. Rienman JF, Ell C, Lux G, et al: Combined therapy of malignant stenosis of the upper gastrointestinal tract by means of laser beam and bougienage. *Endoscopy* 1985; 17:43–48.
26. Sabben G, Lambert R, Lenz P: Laser therapy with fibers in tissue contact. *Gastrointest Endosc* 1983; 29:183.
27. Gourgouliatos Z, Wilcox B, Tores J, et al: Application of new laser probes in the treatment of gastrointestinal bleeding. Presented at the Seventh Congress of the International Society for Laser Surgery and Medicine, Munich, 1987.
28. Daikuzono N, Joffe S: Artificial sapphire probe for contact photocoagulation and tissue vaporization with the Nd:YAG laser. *Med Instrum* 1985; 19:173–178.
29. Bown SG, Hawes R, Matthewson K, et al: Endoscopic laser palliation for advanced malignant dysphagia. *Gut* 1987; 28:799–807.
30. Fleischer D, Sivak MV: Endoscopic Nd:YAG laser therapy as palliation for esophagogastric carcinoma: Parameters affecting initial outcome. *Gastroenterology* 1985; 89:827–831.
31. Bown SG: Endoscopic laser therapy for oesophageal cancer. *Endoscopy* 1986; 18:26–31.
32. Gauderer MW, Ponsky JL, Izant RJ: Gastrostomy without laparotomy: A percutaneous endoscopic technique. *J Pediatr Surg* 1980; 15:872–875.
33. Flock MH: Indications for percutaneous gastrostomy. *Am J Gastroenterol* 1990; 85:1074–1075.
34. Foutch P, Gregory H, Williams C: P.E.G.: A new procedure comes of age. *J Clin Gastroenterol* 1984; 8:10–15.
35. Stiegmann GV, Goff JS, Silas D, et al: Endoscopic versus operative gastrostomy: Final results of a prospective randomized trial. *Gastrointest Endosc* 1990; 36:1–5.
36. Sugawa C: Upper GI bleed in an urban hospital. *Ann Surg* 1990; 212:521–526.
37. Dagradi AE, Ruiz RA, Weingarten ZG: Influence of emergency endoscopy on the management and

outcome of patients with upper gastrointestinal hemorrhage. *Am J Gastroenterol* 1979; 72:403–415.

38. Gilbert DA, Silverstein FE, Tedesco FJ, et al: The national ASGE survey on upper gastrointestinal bleeding. (III) Endoscopy in upper gastrointestinal bleeding. *Gastrointest Endosc* 1981; 27:94–102.
39. Larson G, Schmidt T, Gott J, et al: Upper gastrointestinal bleeding. Predictors of outcome. *Surgery* 1986; 100:765–772.
40. Fleischer D: Endoscopic therapy of upper gastrointestinal bleeding in humans. *Gastroenterology* 1986; 90:217–234.
41. Asaki S: Tissue solidification in coping with digestive tract bleeding. Hemostatic effect of local injection of 99.5% alcohol. *Tohoku J Exp Med* 1981; 134:223–227.
42. Sugawa C, Ikeda J, Fujita Y, et al: Endoscopic hemostasis of gastrointestinal hemorrhage by local application of 98% ethanol: An experimental study. *Gastrointest Endosc* 1984; 30:155.
43. Hirao M, Kobayashi T, Masuda K, et al: Endoscopic local injection of hypertonic saline-epinephrine solution to arrest hemorrhage from the upper gastrointestinal tract. *Gastrointest Endosc* 1985; 31:313–317.
44. Soehendra N, Grimm H, Kempeneers I: Sclerosing therapy in gastrointestinal hemorrhages. *Acta Endosc* 1986; 16:47–53.
45. Sugawa C: Injection therapy for the control of bleeding ulcers. *Gastrointest Endosc* 1990; 36(suppl):50–52.
46. Siegel B, Dunn M: The mechanism of blood vessel closure by high frequency electrocoagulation. *Surg Gynecol Obstet* 1965; 121:823–831.
47. Youmans CR: Cystoscopic control of gastric hemorrhage. *Arch Surg* 1970; 100:721–723.
48. Papp JP: Endoscopic electrocoagulation in upper gastrointestinal hemorrhage. *JAMA* 1976; 236:2076–2079.
49. Matek W, Fruhmorgan P, Kaduk B, et al: Modified electrocoagulation and its possibilities in the control of gastrointestinal bleeding. *Endoscopy* 1979; 11:253–258.
50. Papp JP: Endoscopic electrocoagulation in the management of upper gastrointestinal bleeding. *Surg Clin North Am* 1982; 62:797–806.
51. Freitas D, Donato A, Monteiro JG: Controlled trial of liquid monopolar electrocoagulation in bleeding peptic ulcers. *Am J Gastroenterol* 1985; 80:853–857.
52. Moreto M, Zaballa M, Ibanez S, et al: Efficacy of monopolar electrocoagulation in the treatment of bleeding gastric ulcer: A controlled trial. *Endoscopy* 1987; 19:54–56.
53. Johnston JH, Jensen DM, Auth D: Experimental comparison of endoscopic yttrium-aluminum-garnet laser, electrosurgery, and heater probe for canine gut arterial coagulation: Importance of compression and avoidance of erosion. *Gastroenterology* 1987; 92:1101–1108.
54. Morris DI, Brearley S, Thompson H, et al: A comparison of the efficacy and depth of gastric wall injury with 3.2 and 2.3 mm bipolar probes in canine arterial hemorrhage. *Gastrointest Endosc* 1985; 31:361–363.
55. Siegel B, Hatke FL: Physical factors in electrocoaptation of blood vessels. *Arch Surg* 1967; 95:54–58.
56. Harrison JD, Morris DL: Does bipolar coagulation time affect vessel wall strength (abstract)? *Gastroenterology* 1989; 96:199.
57. Laine L: Multipolar electrocoagulation in the treatment of active upper gastrointestinal hemorrhage: A prospective controlled trial. *N Engl J Med* 1987; 316:1613–1617.
58. Laine L: Multipolar electrocoagulation in the treatment of ulcers with nonbleeding vessels: A prospective, controlled trial. *Ann Intern Med* 1989; 110:510–514.
59. Lin HJ, Tsai VT, Lee DS, et al: A prospectively randomized trial of heater probe thermocoagulation versus pure alcohol injection in nonvariceal peptic ulcer hemorrhage. *Am J Gastroenterol* 1988; 83:283–286.
60. Chung S, Leung J: Heater probe or epinephrine injection for actively bleeding ulcers: A randomized comparison. *Gastrointest Endosc* 1989; 35:152.

61. Jensen DM, Machicado GA, Kovacs TO, et al: Controlled randomized study of heater probe and BICAP for hemostasis of severe ulcer bleeding (abstract). *Gastroenterology* 1989; 94:208.
62. Swain CP, Bown SG, Salmon PR, et al: Controlled trial of Nd:YAG laser photocoagulation for bleeding pectic ulcer. *Lancet* 1986; 1:1113–1116.
63. MacLeod IA, Mills PR, MacKenzie JF, et al: Neodymium yttrium aluminum garnet laser photocoagulation for major hemorrhage from peptic ulcers and single vessels: A single blind controlled study. *Br Med J* 1989; 286:345–348.
64. Rutgeerts P, Vantrappen G, Broeckaert L, et al: Controlled trial of YAG laser treatment of upper digestive hemorrhage. *Gastroenterology* 1982; 83:410–416.
65. Fleischer D: Endoscopic Nd:YAG laser therapy for active esophageal variceal bleed. *Gastrointest Endosc* 1985; 31:4–9.
66. Crafoord C, Frenckner P: New surgical treatment of varicose veins of the esophagus. *Acta Otolaryngol* 1939; 27:422–429.
67. Johnston GW, Rogers HW: A review of 15 years' experience in the use of sclerotherapy in the control of acute hemorrhage from esophageal varices. *Br J Surg* 1973; 60:797–800.
68. Westaby D, Macdougall BR, Williams R: Improved survival following injection sclerotherapy for esophageal varices: Final analysis of controlled trial. *Hepatology* 1985; 5:827–830.
69. Schubert T, Smith O, Kirkpatrick S, et al: Improved survival in variceal hemorrhage with emergent sclerotherapy. *Am J Gastroenterol* 1987; 82:1134–1137.
70. Jackson FC, Perrin ED, Felix R, et al: A clinical investigation of the porta-caval shunt: Survival analysis of the therapeutic option. *Ann Surg* 1971; 174:672–701.
71. Reynolds TB, Donnovan AJ, Mikkelsen WP, et al: Results of a 12 year randomized trial of portacaval shunt in patients with alcoholic liver disease and bleeding varices. *Gastroenterology* 1981; 80:1005–1111.
72. Terblanche J, Burroughs AK, Hobbs KF: Controversies in the management of bleeding esophageal varices. *N Engl J Med* 1989; 320:1469–1475.
73. Conn HO: Endoscopic sclerotherapy: An analysis of variants. *Hepatology* 1983; 3:769–771.
74. Korula J, Kage M, Haranda A, et al: The effects of endoscopic variceal sclerotherapy on the esophagus. A prospective clinical and histological study. *J Clin Gastroenterol* 1987; 9:639–643.
75. Copenhagen Esophageal Varices Sclerotherapy Project: Sclerotherapy after first variceal hemorrhage in cirrhosis. *N Engl J Med* 1984; 311:1594–1600.
76. Korula J, Balart LA, Radvan G, et al: A prospective randomized controlled trial of chronic esophageal variceal bleeding. *Hepatology* 1985; 5:584–589.
77. Santagelo WC, Dueno MI, Estes BL, et al: Prophylactic sclerotherapy of large esophageal varices. *N Engl J Med* 1988; 313:814–818.
78. Gregory P, Hartigan P, Amodes D, et al: Prophylactic sclerotherapy for esophageal varices in alcoholic disease: Result of a VA cooperation randomized trial. *Gastroenterology* 1987; 92:1414.
79. Larson AW, Cohen H, Zweiban B, et al: Acute esophageal variceal sclerotherapy: Results of a prospective randomized controlled trial. *JAMA* 1986; 255:497–500.
80. American College of Physicians Health and Policy Committee: Endoscopic sclerotherapy for esophageal varices. *Ann Intern Med* 1984; 100:608–610.
81. Schuman BM, Beckman JW, Tedesco FJ, et al: Complications of endoscopic injection sclerotherapy: A review. *Am J Gastroenterol* 1987; 82:823–830.
82. Baydur A, Korula J: Cardiorespiratory effects of endoscopic esophageal variceal sclerotherapy. *Am J Med* 1990; 89:477–482.
83. Stiegmann GV, Cambre T, Sun JH: A new endoscopic elastic band ligating device. *Gastrointest Endosc* 1986; 32:230–233.
84. Stiegman GV, Goff JS, Sun JH, et al: Endoscopic ligation of esophageal varices. *Am J Surg* 1990; 159:21–26.
85. Barkin JS, Schonfeld W, Thomsen S, et al: Enteroscopy and small bowel biopsy—an improved technique for the diagnosis of small bowel disease. *Gastrointest Endosc* 1985; 31:215–219.

86. Tada M, Misaki F, Kawai K: Pediatric enteroscopy with a Sonde-type small intestinal fiberscope. *Gastrointest Endosc* 1983; 29:44.
87. Bowden TA: Endoscopy of the small intestine. *Surg Clin North Am* 1989; 69:1237–1248.
88. Lewis BS, Waye JD: Total small bowel enteroscopy. *Gastrointest Endosc* 1987; 33:435.
89. Haubrich WS: History of endoscopy, in Sivak MV (ed): *Gastroenterologic Endoscopy.* Philadelphia, WB Saunders Co, 1987.
90. Fleischer DE, Goldberg SB, Browning TH, et al: Detection and surveillance of colorectal cancer. *JAMA* 1989; 261:580–585.
91. Waye JD, Lewis BS, Frankel A, et al: Small colon polyps. *Am J Gastroenterol* 1988; 83:120–122.
92. Williams CB: Diathermy-biopsy—a technique for the endoscopic management of small polyps. *Endoscopy* 1973; 5:215.
93. Gilbert DA, Hallstrom JP, Shaneyfelt SL, et al: The national ASGE colonoscopy survey—complications of colonoscopy. *Gastrointest Endosc* 1984; 30:156.
94. Olgivie H: Large intestine colic due to sympathetic deprivation. *Br Med J* 1948; 2:671.
95. Wojitalik RS, Lindenauer SM, Kahn SS: Perforation of the colon associated with adynamic ileus. *Am J Surg* 1973; 125:601–606.
96. Kuhora JS, Dent TL: Colonoscopic decompression of massive nonobstructive cecal dilatation. *Arch Surg* 1977; 112:512–515.
97. Nano D, Prindiville T, Pauly M, et al: Colonoscopic therapy of acute pseudoobstruction of the colon. *Am J Gastroenterol* 1987; 82:145–148.
98. Strodel WE, Nostrant TT, Eckhauser FE, et al: Therapeutic and diagnostic colonoscopy in nonobstructive colonic dilatation. *Ann Surg* 1983; 197:416–421.
99. Vanek VW, Al-Salti M: Acute pseudo-obstruction of the colon (Olgivie's syndrome). An analysis of 400 cases. *Dis Colon Rectum* 1986; 29:203–210.
100. Messmer JM, Wolper JC, Loewe CJ: Endoscopic-assisted tube placement for decompression of acute colonic pseudo-obstruction. *Endoscopy* 1984; 16:135–136.
101. Arnold GJ, Nance FJ: Volvulus of the sigmoid colon. *Ann Surg* 1973; 177:527–537.
102. Anderson MJ, Okike N, Spencer RJ: The colonoscope in cecal volvulus: Report of three cases. *Dis Colon Rectum* 1978; 21:71–74.
103. Janardhanan R, Bowman D, Brodmerkel GJ, et al: Cecal volvulus: Decompression and detorsion with a colonoscopically placed drainage tube. *Am J Gastroenterol* 1987; 82:912–914.
104. Strodel WE, Brothers T: Colonoscopic decompression of pseudo-obstruction and volvulus. *Surg Clin North Am* 1989; 69:1327–1335.
105. Kiefhaber P, Kiefhaber K, Huber F: Preoperative neodymium:YAG laser treatment of obstructive colon cancer. *Endoscopy* 1986; 18:44.
106. Brunetaud JM, Manoury V, Ducrotte P, et al: Palliative treatment of rectosigmoid carcinoma by laser endoscopic photoablation. *Gastroenterology* 1987; 92:663–668.
107. Mathus-Vliegen EM, Tytgat GN: Nd:Yag laser photocoagulation in gastroenterology—its role in the palliation of colorectal cancer. *Lasers Med Sci* 1986; 1:75–80.
108. Skibba RM, Hartong WA, Mantz FA, et al: Angiodysplasia of the cecum: Colonoscopic diagnosis. *Gastrointest Endosc* 1976; 22:177–179.
109. Rutgeerts P, Van Gompel F, Geboes K, et al: Long-term results of treatment of vascular malformations of the gastrointestinal tract by Nd:YAG laser photocoagulation. *Gut* 1985; 26:586–593.

Chapter 11

Gastrointestinal Endoscopy: Evaluation of Hepatobiliary Tree and New Technology

Cuong C. Nguyen, M.D.
David E. Fleischer, M.D.

Whereas the preceding chapter focused on the history of endoscopy, the mechanics of endoscopes, and diagnosis and therapy of the upper digestive tract, small intestines, and colon, this chapter focuses on evaluation and therapy of the hepatobiliary tree. Afterward, new technology, such as endoscopic ultrasound is addressed.

The most sophisticated endoscopic procedure, endoscopic retrograde cholangiopancreatography (ERCP) was first accomplished in 1968.[1] Since then, it has gained increasing popularity and has evolved into many therapeutic applications.

Diagnostic ERCP is indicated in the evaluation of suspected biliary obstruction, pancreatic malignancy, unexplained pancreatitis, and preoperative evaluation of chronic pancreatitis. In addition to simply obtaining a radiographic view of the pancreatic and biliary systems, manometric evaluation of the sphincter of Oddi can be performed.[2]

ERCP is a very complex procedure that involves a team of an endoscopist, a radiologist, and specially trained assistants. On the fluoroscopic table, the patient lies with his arm behind the back and then is consciously sedated in the controlled fashion. When the side-viewing endoscope is passed through the pylorus and duodenal bulb, the patient is turned to the prone position. The major papilla is then visualized, and a catheter, through the biopsy channel, is inserted via the ampulla of Vater. Depending on the orientation of the catheter, the pancreatic duct or the biliary tract can be visualized using fluoroscopy and contrast materials. With appropriate maneuvers, the entire pancreatic and biliary ductal system can be seen radiographically. A manometric catheter can be used to study contractions of the sphincter of Oddi. Tissue diagnoses can also be established with endoscopic brushing cytology or forceps biopsy.[3]

Common pathologic conditions that can be diagnosed with ERCP are stone disease, biliary tract or pancreatic stricture, pancreatic neoplasm, and sphincter of Oddi dysfunction (Fig 11–1). Many of these conditions are amenable to endoscopic therapy.

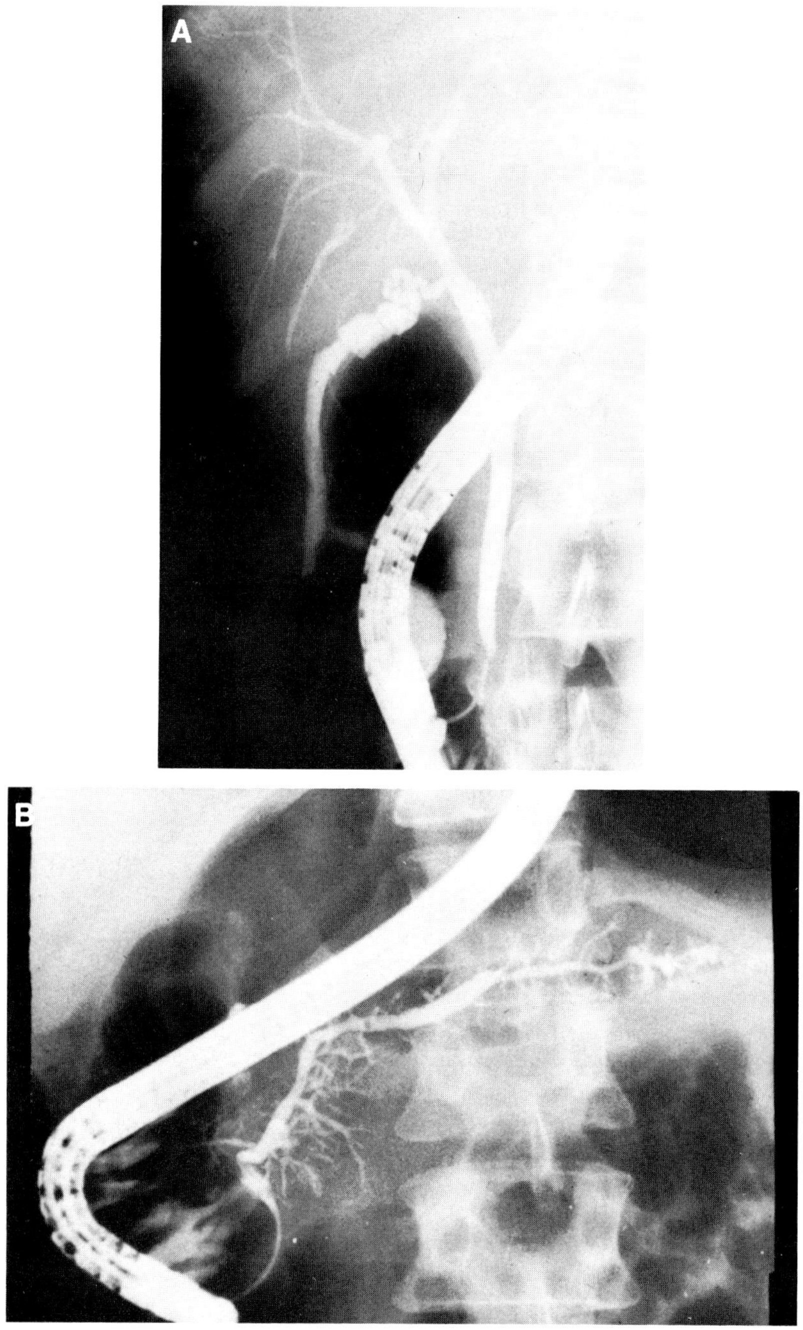

FIG 11–1.
ERCP demonstrating a normal common bile duct **(A)** and, moderate chronic pancreatitis **(B)**. *(Continued.)*

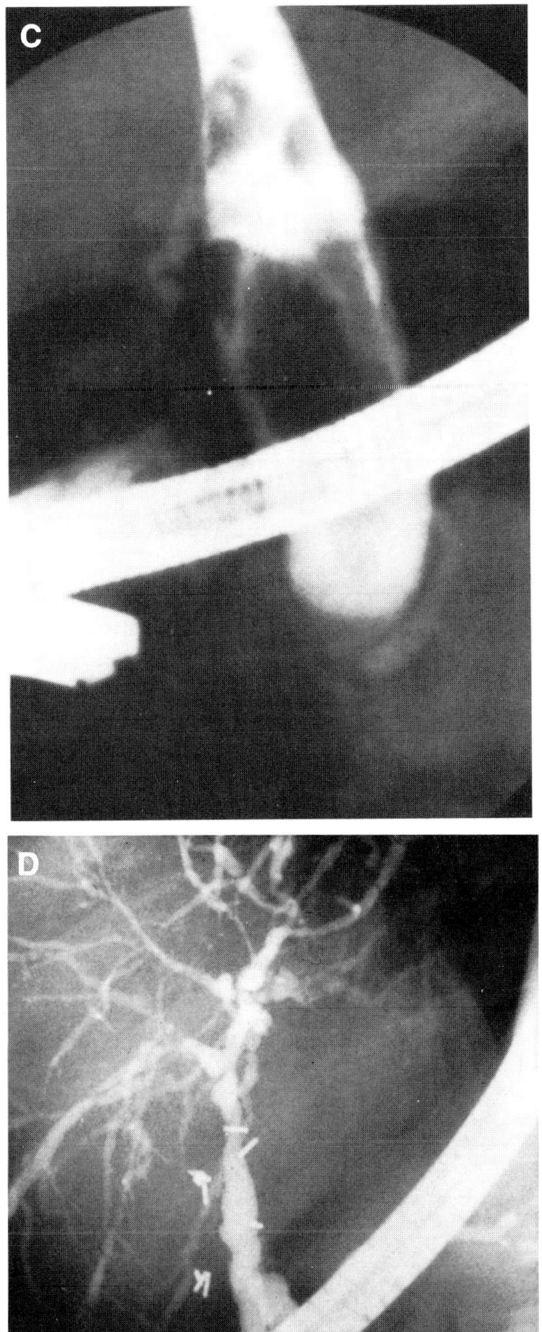

FIG 11–1 (cont.).
ERCP demonstrating multiple common bile duct stones **(C)** and sclerosing cholangitis **(D)**.

ENDOSCOPIC SPHINCTEROTOMY AND STONE REMOVAL

Because common bile duct stones can be missed by ultrasound in up to 20% of patients,[4] ERCP is an important diagnostic tool for this entity. More importantly, the endoscopist now can extract these stones and offer a safe alternative to a celiotomy.

First described in 1974,[5,6] endoscopic stone removal now is a commonplace procedure. It is indicated for patients who are high-risk candidates for surgery or who have septic cholangitis or acute biliary pancreatitis.[2]

This procedure employs a special device called a sphincterotome, which is basically a catheter with a thin steel wire inside (Fig 11–2). The wire exits the catheter at or near the tip and re-enters the catheter several centimeters proximally. Tension can be applied to the wire to produce a bowing effect in the catheter, with the wire forming the bowstring. The wire is connected with the electrosurgical power unit, and when current is applied, a sequential incision of the tissue in contact with the wire occurs. Some sphincterotomes have only a sharp metal tip that can act like a knife to cut through the roof of the papilla.

In addition to the sphincterotomes, a family of stone extraction devices have also been developed. The basic design here is a catheter that houses a wire mechanism that can hold the stones or even crush them for easier passage. An array of baskets, balloons, and crushing devices exists.

To prepare for the procedure, routine preoperative blood studies such as coagulation are performed. Prophylactic antibiotics with standard regimens such as ampicillin and gentamicin are administered. ERCP is then performed to identify the stone(s). Two variations of technique exist: (1) a guidewire is passed through the catheter and is advanced proximal to the stone. The catheter is removed with the guidewire in place. The sphincterotome is then inserted into the papilla via the guidewire. (2) Alternatively, the sphincterotome can be inserted without a guidewire.

After the position of the sphincterotome is verified endoscopically and radiographically, a

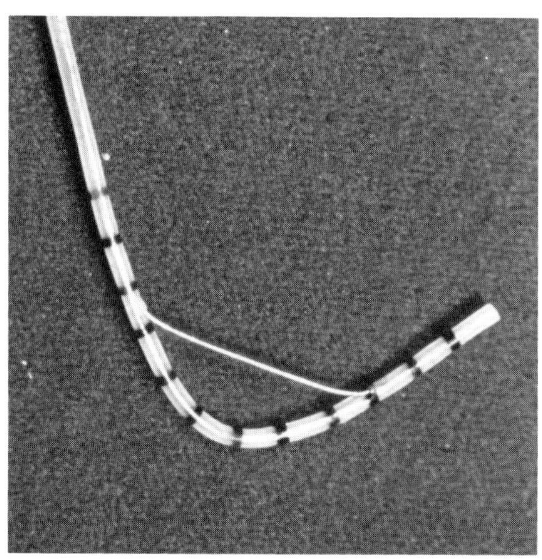

FIG 11–2.
Commercially available sphincterotome.

small incision, usually 10 to 15 mm, is made along the roof of the papilla (Fig 11–3). The sphincterotome is then exchanged for the stone extraction device, which removes the stone from the common bile duct.

For small bile duct stones, it is sometimes possible to remove them without performing sphincterotomy. In these cases, the papilla may be dilated with a balloon or by using glyceryl trinitrate.[7]

In experienced hands, endoscopic sphincterotomy (ESP) and stone removal are successful over 90% of the time.[8] If the stones are too large (greater than 2.5 cm in diameter), extracorporeal shockwave lithotripsy can be utilized with good results.[9] Additionally, experimental trials with laser lithotripsy and electrohydraulic shock wave lithotripsy are ongoing; a thin fiber-

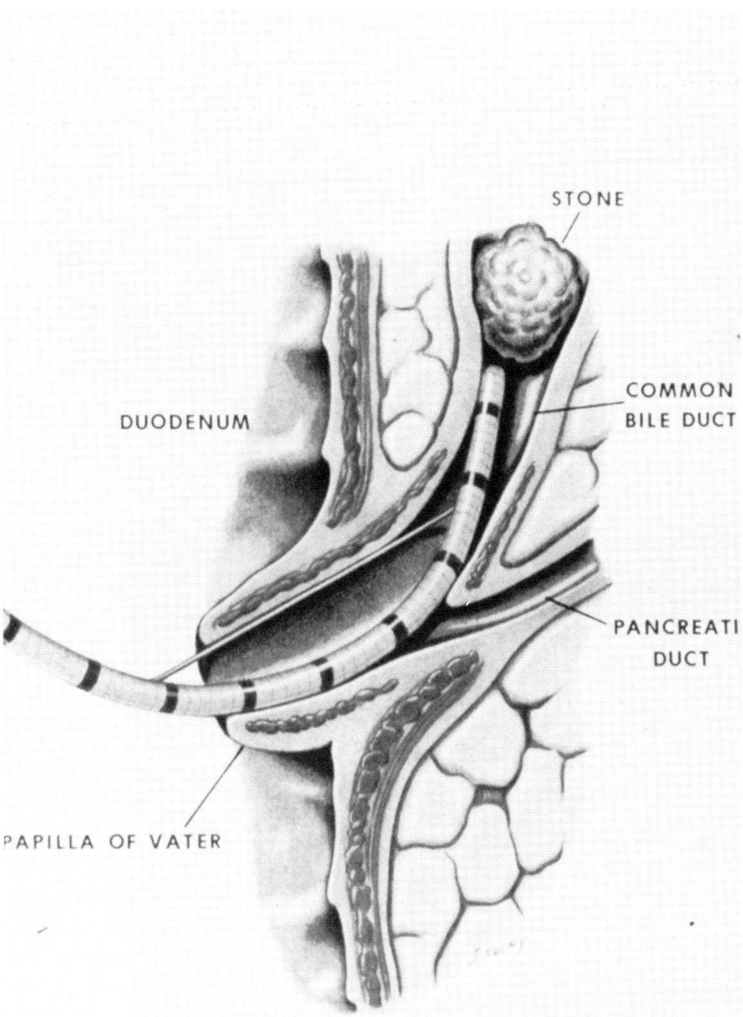

FIG 11–3.
Schematic of a sphincterotome positioned in the common bile duct.

optic endoscope is used in the instrumentation channel of a duodenoscope, the "mother-baby-scope system."[10]

The incidence of complications is about 5% to 10%, with bleeding, perforation, and pancreatitis being the most common.[8] Bleeding can sometimes be treated with a submucosal injection of epinephrine. Retroperitoneal perforation is usually managed conservatively with antibiotics and nasogastric tube. Emergency surgery is necessary in only 1%. Mortality in most published series is about 1%.[11]

ENDOSCOPIC STENTING OF MALIGNANT BILIARY STRICTURES

Malignant biliary stricture is rarely curable, and palliative resection or bypass surgery carries a mortality of 20% to 40%.[12] Percutaneous drainage or a transhepatic internal stent may be associated with high morbidity due to hepatic puncture. An endoscopically placed stent is now considered a safe alternative.[13]

Two kinds of biliary stents are available. They are both made of polyvinyl and are available in different sizes and lengths. The internal type can be up to 15 to 20 cm in length, and the external type is up 150 to 200 cm long, extending out the nostril. In order for the stent to stay in place, pigtails or flaps are incorporated at either end of the stent.

The technique for endoscopic stenting was first reported in 1980. It involves performing the ERCP to define the location of the stricture. A guidewire is then advanced past the stricture. Guidewires with a hydrophilic coating to promote slipperiness are available to slide past the obstruction.[14] There are also guidewires that can be slightly torqued in different directions for this purpose.

Once the wire is in place, it may be necessary to dilate the stricture with stiff tapered dila-

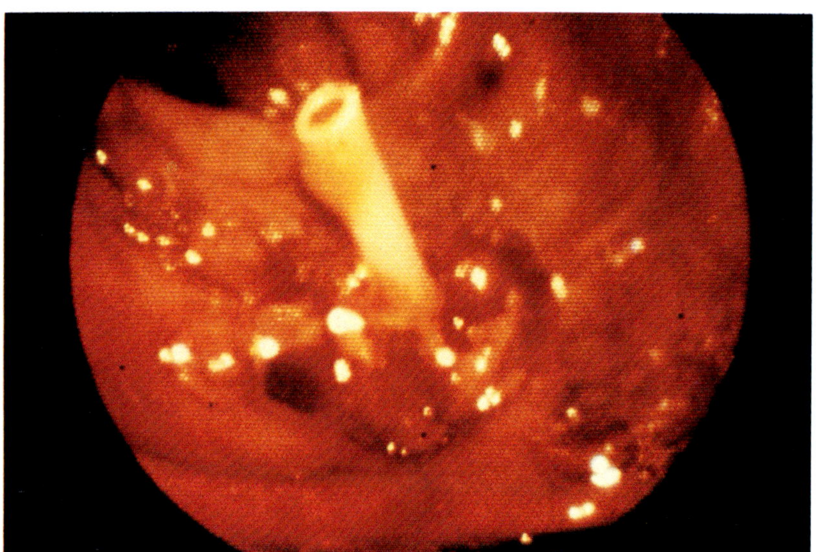

FIG 11–4.
Stent protruding from the distal bile duct into the duodenum.

tors. Over the guidewire, the stent is then pushed past the stricture. For the internal type, the other end of the stent is protruding from the papilla into the duodenum (Fig 11–4). The external stent, on the other hand, is brought back into the mouth and then rerouted out the nostril.[15] This is referred to as a nasobiliary drain.

At large centers, this procedure can succeed in 90% of patients.[16] The overall 30-day mortality is 10% for pancreatic carcinoma and 20% for malignant hilar obstruction.[17] The main immediate complication of placing biliary stents is the 10% risk for cholangitis, which can be minimized with antibiotic prophylaxis and maintaining sterility during the procedure. On the other hand, the main long-term complication is stent blockage, which occurs in 20% to 30% of cases.

The average stent's useful life is about 4 months, but the interval the stent can remain patent is a function of its size as the volume of bile passing through the stent obeys Poiseuille's law. This law states that flow is proportional to the fourth power of the radius. In other words, the flow through a 10 F stent would be 16 times that of a 5 F stent. The slower the flow, the more likely bile stasis and blockage will occur.

Electron microscopic examination of the occluding materials has suggested that stents are colonized with bacteria whose enzymes are responsible for the formation and deposition of insoluble calcium bilirubinate and palmate within the stent. To slow this process, work is underway to impregnate stents with biocides, antibiotics, and metals.[18] A self-expanding stent is also under investigation.[19]

ENDOSCOPIC STENTING OF BENIGN STRICTURES

Postoperative strictures or extrahepatic strictures from primary sclerosing cholangitis can be successfully managed with balloon dilatation and temporary stenting.[20] Good short-term results have also been achieved with temporary stenting for biliary fistulas or bile leakage from surgical intervention.[21]

ENDOSCOPIC ULTRASONOGRAPHY

A perfect marriage between endoscopy and ultrasound, endoscopic ultrasonography (EUS) is a recent major innovation in gastroenterologic endoscopy. This new technology was first described in 1976[22] and is a powerful diagnostic tool capable of producing high-resolution ultrasonic images of lesions that are either inaccessible or poorly visualized by conventional extracorporeal imaging techniques.

Central to EUS is a transducer mounted at the distal tip of the endoscope. The transducer contains crystals that can (1) generate a voltage when placed under compressive stress or (2) change shape when subjected to an electrical voltage, properties referred to as piezoelectricity.[23] When electrically stimulated, the crystals contract and expand to create small pressure waves or ultrasound wavefronts. The transducer is mechanically rotated to produce a real-time image that is a radial sector scan of 360 degrees perpendicular to the long axis of the endoscope.

Since ultrasound waves are not efficiently conducted through air, a cylindrical balloon inflatable with de-aerated water is used to encase the transducer to provide a sufficiently conducive interface between the target and the transducer. Alternatively, sometimes water can be used to fill organs such as the stomach to facilitate the ultrasonic transmission.

As mentioned above, the transducer is housed at the distal tip of the endoscope. This portion of the endoscope is rather rigid and can be up to 4 to 5 cm in length. The fiber-optic component of the endoscope is located proximal to the transducer and to the side of the instrument; this provides an oblique field of view that is rather limited when compared with standard endoscopes. The latest generation of EUS instruments also has an accessory channel for biopsy forceps. The physical characteristics of a common ultrasound fiber-optic endoscope are listed in Table 11–1.

Most current ultrasound endoscopes can generate two different frequencies: 7.5 and 12 MHz, as compared with 2 to 5 MHz in extracorporeal ultrasound transducers. The 7.5-MHz frequency permits a depth penetration of approximately 10 cm with an axial resolution of 0.2 mm. Higher frequencies improve resolution at the expense of penetration, for example, the depth penetration of 12-MHz frequency is only 5 cm.[24]

The reflected ultrasound signals are received by the transducer and are transferred to a digital scan converter connected to a display unit (Fig 11–5). The unit can be set to display ranges of 6, 9, 12, and 15 cm. The 6-cm range is most suitable for examination of the gastric or rectal wall, and the 9 and 12 cm ranges are used for retroperitoneal structures. Images from the display unit can also be captured on video floppy disks or videotapes.

Images seen on the display unit are echoes produced when the ultrasound beam encounters an interface between two adjacent structures that have different acoustic impedances. When scanned at frequencies between 7.5 and 10 MHz, five sonographic layers of the gastrointestinal (GI) tract are recognized: (1) an innermost hyperechoic layer, (2) an inner hypoechoic layer, (3) a middle hyperechoic layer, (4) an outer hypoechoic layer, and (5) an outermost hyperechoic layer.[25] It is not clear whether this sonographic division corresponds to the actual histologic differences within the GI wall or whether it is just reverberated ultrasonic energy.

EUS is most useful in five clinical settings: (1) staging GI cancer, (2) defining mucosal infiltrative diseases, (3) evaluating submucosal lesions, (4) identifying vascular structures, and (5) studying abdominal, retroperitoneal, and pelvic structures adjacent to the hollow-organ GI tract.

The technique for upper GI EUS is similar to standard esophagogastroduodenoscopy (EGD). However, due to the limited endoscopic view of the EUS instrument, patients are typically examined first with the standard upper GI endoscope to identify the area of interest. The standard upper GI endoscope is then replaced by the EUS upper endoscope, which is intubated with digital guidance. The EUS upper endoscope is advanced to the area of interest,

TABLE 11–1.

Specifications of an Ultrasound Fiber-Optic Endoscope

Parameter	Value
Diameter	13 mm (distal tip)
Length of distal rigid tip	45 mm
Working length	1,300 mm
Angle of view	80°, oblique
Suction channel	2.8 mm

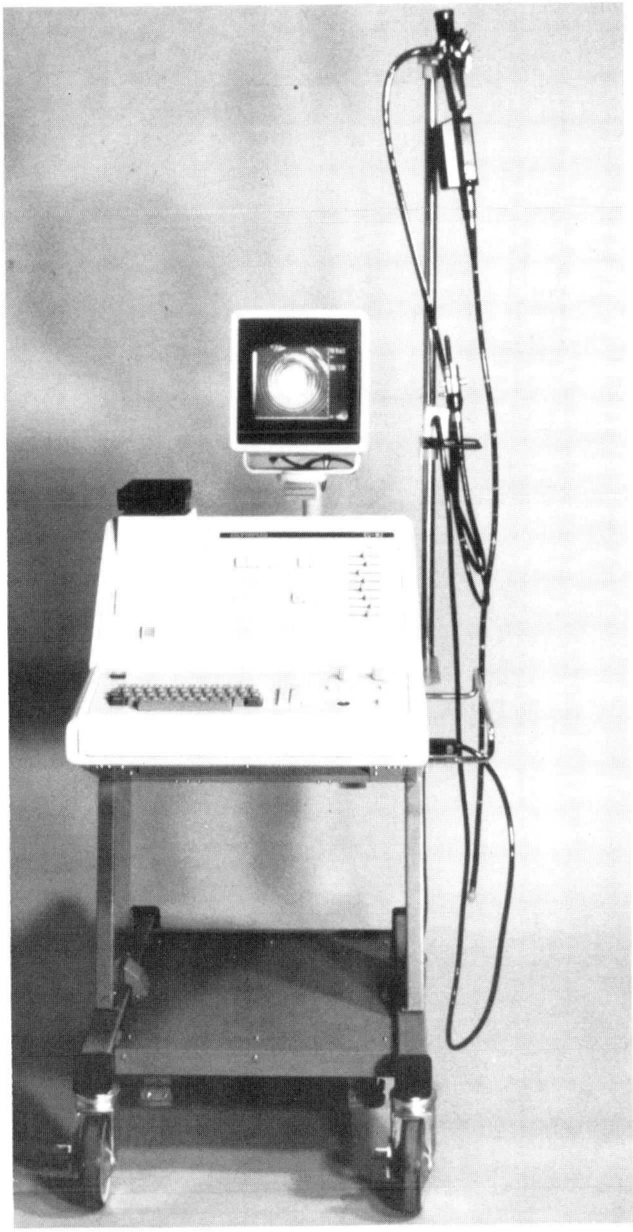

FIG 11–5.
Endoscopic ultrasound equipment consisting of an endoscope with an ultrasound component, display monitor, and keyboard, as well as a processing unit.

and the balloon is inflated with degassed water. As mentioned above, de-aerated water can also be used to examine the stomach.

An example of the usefulness of EUS in staging GI cancer is in the esophagus. Recent studies have shown that preoperative EUS was superior to computed tomographic (CT) studies, with EUS having accuracy of 89% as compared with 59% for CT. Lymph node involvement was also better seen on EUS.[26]

Other examples include the characteristic appearance of diffuse intramural hypoechoic in-

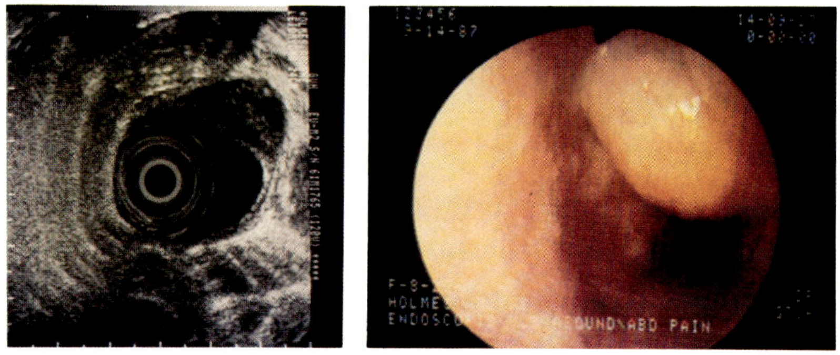

FIG 11–6.
Esophageal leiomyoma: endoscopic view *(right)* and ultrasound view *(left)*.

filtration of non-Hodgkin's lymphoma, the roundish echo-free space of gastric varices, or the homogeneous echo pattern of leiomyoma[24] (Fig 11–6).

Many other structures such as the pancreas, the gallbladder, the biliary tree, the kidneys, the aorta, the heart, etc., have also been studied with EUS. Additionally, there is an extensive literature on EUS of the rectum. These areas are beyond the scope of this chapter and will not be discussed.

To summarize, EUS have several unique features: high frequency, high resolution, and proximity to target lesion. It allows immediate definitions of the mucosa, submucosa, and adjacent organs. Mucosal infiltrative diseases can be diagnosed, vascular structures identified, and carcinoma staging determined. However, because EUS is still in its developmental stage, refinement in the equipment and better familiarity with its images will be necessary to fully utilize this new diagnostic modality.

CONCLUSION

GI endoscopy has come a long way since the first description of the fiber endoscope by Hirschowitz and Hopkins in the late 1950s. It has unequivocally revolutionized the practice of gastroenterology and has become a primary tool for both the diagnosis and treatment of GI diseases. In addition to its remarkable alterations of the practice of diagnostic gastroenterology, it is continuing to emerge as a potent therapy for a large number of GI diseases. In addition to the procedures listed heretofore, several innovations are likely to change the practice of GI endoscopy in the future. The changes in endoscopy can be expected in four areas: (1) mechanical changes, (2) miniaturization, (3) visual images, and (4) new objectives.

Mechanical Changes

Modular endoscopes are being developed in which one viewing head is used with several attachable shafts. It is also conceivable that there may soon be disposable endoscopes. A prototype self-advancing endoscope has been developed. The concept is that the tip of the endoscope would have sensors that could actually seek out the lumen.

Miniaturization

The second major advance that is likely to be realized with endoscopy is in the area of miniaturization. The first fiber-optic endoscopes were between 13 and 16 mm in diameter. Commonly used instruments today are between 8 and 11 mm in diameter. It is probable that endoscopes as small as 1 to 2 mm will be utilized in the future for examination of the biliary and pancreatic ducts. Slightly larger instruments with biopsy channels are also being developed.

Visual Images

As discussed previously, video endoscopy has been another dramatic chapter in the advancement of endoscopy. In addition to the current applications, which have already been enumerated, the most valuable potential for video endoscopy may be to marry it to computers so that its full analytic potential could be realized. Therefore, it may be possible by using computer analysis to find signatures for disease states that can be recognized with the computer without a biopsy specimen being required for a definitive diagnosis.

New Objectives

With the use of high-magnification lenses, images can be magnified. In addition, by using chromoscopy with tissue dye, color enhancement can be accomplished that may alter the image and prove useful for both direct visual assessment as well as computer analysis.

Because with video endoscopy images can be digitalized, three-dimensional reconstruction may be possible. In addition, passing signals such as Doppler through endoscopes (which may give information about blood flow), fluorescent spectroscopy (which may give information based on spectral reflectance), and further utilization of endoscopic ultrasonography may be possible.

In addition, endoscopy may provide for new forms of treatment. Previously mentioned, the endoscopic sewing machine may allow the endoscopist to do through an endoscope what a surgeon does at open surgery. Ulcer healing may be made possible endoscopically either by the performance of vagotomy and pyloroplasty via an endoscope, photostimulation to heal ulcers, or the delivery of medical therapies to the ulcer site. Treatment of neoplastic diseases may be possible by injecting substances into tumors that will elicit an immunologic response. Esophageal reflux may be treated by the injection or delivery of thermal therapies to the lower esophageal sphincter, which may alter its function. Photodynamic therapy already exists and may localize a therapeutic substance to a site that can be activated by light shined upon it endoscopically. Finally, the use of a smart laser system may allow the definition of the pathologic process by one laser wavelength and its therapy by a second wavelength.

The future of GI endoscopy seems limitless with exciting advances to be expected.

REFERENCES

1. McCune WS, Shorb PE, Moscowitz H: Endoscopic cannulation of the ampulla of Vater: A preliminary report. *Ann Surg* 1968; 167:752–756.

2. American Society for Gastrointestinal Endoscopy: *Appropriate Use of Gastrointestinal Endoscopy.* Baltimore, American Society for Gastrointestinal Endoscopy, 1989.
3. Rabinovitz N, Zajko AB, Hassamein T, et al: Diagnostic value of brush cytology in the diagnosis of bile duct carcinoma. *Hepatology* 1990; 12:748–752.
4. Laing FC: Ultrasound diagnosis of choledocholithiasis. *Semin Ultrasound CT MR* 1987; 8:103–113.
5. Classen M, Demling L: Endoskopische Spjinkterotomie der papilla Vateri und Steinentraktion aus dem Ductus Choledochus. *Dtsch Med Wochenschr* 1974; 99:496–497.
6. Kawai K, Akasak Y, Nurakanmi K, et al: Endoscopic sphincterotomy of the ampulla of Vater. *Gastrointest Endosc* 1974; 20:148–150.
7. Staritz M, Poralla T, Dormeyer HH, et al: Endoscopic removal of common bile duct stones through the intact papilla after medical dilatation. *Am J Gastroenterol* 1985; 88:1807–1111.
8. Cotton PB: Critical appraisals of therapeutic endoscopy in biliary tract diseases. *Annu Rev Med* 1990; 41:211–222.
9. Sauerbruch T, Stern M: Fragmentation of bile duct stones by extracorporeal shock waves. *Gastroenterology* 1989; 96:146–152.
10. Classen M, Hagenmuller F: Treatment of stones in the bile duct via duodenoscope. *Endoscopy* 1989; 21:375–377.
11. Cotton PB: Endoscopic management of bile duct stones (apples or oranges). *Gut* 1984; 25:587–597.
12. Saar MG, Cameron JL: Surgical palliation of unresectable carcinoma of the pancreas. *World J Surg* 1984; 8:900–918.
13. Shepherd HA, Royle G, Ross AP, et al: Endoscopic endoprosthesis in the palliation of malignant obstruction of the distal common bile duct—a randomized trial. *Br J Surg* 1988; 75:1166–1168.
14. McCarthy JH, Miller GL, Lawrence BH: Cannulation of the biliary tree, cystic duct, and gall bladder using a hydrophilic polymer-coated steerable guide wire. *Gastrointest Endosc* 1990; 36:386–389.
15. Cotton PB: Endoscopic method for relief of malignant obstructive jaundice. *World J Surg* 1984; 8:854–861.
16. Cotton PB: Nonsurgical palliation of jaundice in pancreatic cancer. *Surg Clin North Am* 1989; 69:613–628.
17. Speer AG, Dineen LP: Endoscopic palliation of malignant hilar structures (abstract). *Gut* 1986; 27:601.
18. Speer AG, Cotton PB, Rode J, et al: Biliary blockage with bacterial biofilm. *Ann Intern Med* 1988; 108:546–553.
19. Huibregtse, Cheng J, Coene PP, et al: Endoscopic placement of expandable metal stents for biliary strictures—a preliminary report with 33 patients. *Endoscopy* 1989; 21:280–282.
20. Berkelhammer C, Kortan P, Haber GB: Endoscopic biliary prostheses as treatment for benign post-operative bile duct strictures. *Gastrointest Endosc* 1989; 35:95–101.
21. Johnson JK, Geenen JE, Venu RP, et al: Endoscopic treatment of biliary duct strictures in sclerosing cholangitis. Follow-up assessment of a new therapeutic approach. *Gastrointest Endosc* 1987; 33:9–12.
22. Lutz H, Rosch W: Transgastroscope ultrasonography. *Endoscopy* 1976; 8:203–205.
23. Kittel C: *Introduction to Solid State Physics,* ed 3. New York, John Wiley & Sons Inc, 1988.
24. Tio TL, Tytgat GN: *Atlas of Transintestinal Ultrasonography.* Aalsmeer, Mur-Kostverloren, 1986.
25. Kimmey MB, Martin RW, Haggitt RC, et al: Histologic correlates of gastrointestinal ultrasound images. *Gastroenterology* 1989; 96:431–433.
26. Tio TL, Cohen P, Coene PP, et al: Endosonography and computed tomography of esophageal carcinoma. *Gastroenterology* 1989; 96:1478–1486.

Chapter 12

Percutaneous Endoscopic Surgery of the Biliary and Renal Tracts

Geoffrey H. White
Richard C. Waugh

The advent of very fine fiber-optic endoscopes and high-resolution sterilizable medical video systems has now made it practical to perform endoscopic examinations and interventions of various body cavities, especially within the lumen of tubular anatomic systems, via percutaneous sheaths down to size 6 F. Percutaneous endoscopy has promising applications in interventional procedures of the biliary tract,[1–4] ureters[5,6] and vascular system.[7–9] Video endoscopy techniques may be used as an adjunct to conventional radiologic interventional procedures in a well-equipped radiology suite or may be performed in the operating room. These are distinct to those generally applied within the peritoneal cavity during laparoscopic surgery, although endoscopic inspection of the bile duct may be made during laparoscopic cholecystectomy after the cystic duct has been cannulated.[10]

This chapter describes recent experience with percutaneous video endoscopy and endoscopic intervention of the biliary and renal systems, with particular reference to the instrumentation, techniques, and specific applications as an adjunct or alternative to conventional surgical procedures.

APPLICATIONS

The major applications in the biliary and renal tracts are for precise diagnosis and less-invasive management of stone disease and tumors (Tables 12–1 and 12–2).

Biliary duct stones and ureteric calculi may be accurately located, the diagnosis confirmed, and treatment instituted by basket removal, ultrasound lithotripsy, laser fragmentation, or other means. Access is made via a newly created percutaneous channel or via the track of a previously placed drain (T-tube, cholecystostomy or nephrostomy tube).

TABLE 12–1.
Applications of Percutaneous Endoscopy and Endoscopic Surgery of the Biliary Tract

Endoscopic diagnosis of obstructing lesions of the biliary tree
Endoscopic biopsy of a lesion of the CBD* and intrahepatic bile ducts
Monitoring percutaneous removal of stones
Monitoring lithotripsy or laser treatment
Monitoring stent placement in bile ducts or the CBD
Follow-up of above treatments or of radiation implants in the CBD

*CBD = common bile duct.

Tumors of the bile duct or ureter may be diagnosed and biopsy specimen samples taken endoscopically. Selected tumors that are not suitable for surgical excision may then be palliated by percutaneous interventions, including placement of stents or radiation implants.

EQUIPMENT AND METHODS

Since these procedures are performed percutaneously, experience and expertise with guidewire techniques and access devices are required. Medical quality video cameras and monitors are coupled to the endoscope systems to provide a magnified, easily accessible image.

Access to the various anatomic systems requires standard guidewires, contrast media, dilatation catheters, and introducing sheaths. Sheaths of diameter 6 F to 15 F are commonly used, depending on the size of endoscope and instruments to be introduced and the luminal diameter of the structure to be examined.

Needles, Guidewires, and Sheaths

Beveled needles of various lengths are used, especially a Chiba-type needle with a hollow structure to allow passage of a guidewire.

TABLE 12–2.
Applications of Percutaneous Endoscopy and Endoscopic Surgery of the Renal Tract

Endoscopic diagnosis of lesions of the renal pelvis or ureter
Endoscopic biopsy of lesions of the renal pelvis or ureter
Monitoring stone removal, stone crushing, or lithotripsy in the ureter
Monitoring laser treatment of the ureter
Monitoring guidewire and stent placement in the ureter

Guidewires should be atraumatic (with a soft, shaped tip) and steerable and have low friction characteristics. Standard vascular guidewires constructed of an inner core wire, outer coiled spring, and bonded coating of Teflon are often used. J-shaped guidewires, floppy-tipped guidewires, and steerable guidewires may all be selected for access.

Percutaneous dilators and access sheaths of various configurations are passed over the guidewire and provide access for subsequent passage of endoscopes and instruments. A hemostatic valve system may be used to prevent egress of fluid used for irrigation.

Endoscopes

The most suitable endoscopes currently available are those that were originally designed for angioscopy or bronchoscopy. The principle requirements are flexibility and a narrow diameter. Three basic designs of fiber-optic endoscopes were used in the procedures reported in this chapter (Table 12–3):

1. Ultrafine optical fiber bundle with an incorporated light source fiber within a catheter body of diameter 2.5 to 5 F (type 1). These endoscopes are less flexible than the other two types and were originally designed for angioscopy within fine arteries such as the tibial or coronary tree. This type is relatively expensive and has no working channel.
2. Midrange-diameter fiber-optic endoscopes of diameter 4.2 to 10 F (type 2). These include an instrumentation channel that is mainly used for passage of guidewires or infusion of an irrigation fluid to clear the lumen of the structure under examination. These endoscopes are nonsteerable; the most commonly used was an angioscope of 2.3-mm external diameter (Baxter Inc, Santa Ana, Calif); this diameter endoscope can be introduced via an 8 F sheath. Relatively inexpensive, disposable angioscopic catheters of this type are available.
3. Larger-diameter endoscopes of size 10 to 15 F with internal mechanisms for deflecting the tip to provide a degree of steerability (type 3). These endoscopes are similar to those used for bronchoscopy or intraoperative choledochoscopy.

TABLE 12–3.
Endovascular Systems Used for Biliary, Renal Tract, and Vascular Endoscopy

System	Features	Manufacturer (Diameter)
Ultrafine angioscopes, 2.5 to 5 F (type 1)	Optical fiber bundle + incorporated light fiber No irrigation/instrument channel Nonsteerable Requires a guiding catheter for many uses	Baxter (0.5 mm) Baxter (1.0 mm) Intramed (2.2 F) Olympus (0.8 mm)
Mid-diameter fiber-optic angioscopes, 4.2 to 9 F (type 2)	Incorporated irrigation/instrument channel Nonsteerable	Baxter (2.3 mm) Intramed (4.2 F) Olympus (2.8 mm) Storz (7 F) Storz (9 F)
Large-diameter endoscopes, 10–15 F diameter with a deflectable tip (type 3)	Incorporated irrigation/instrument channel Steerable	Pentax (10 F) Pentax (15 F) Intramed (10 F)

Light Source and Video Equipment

For type 2 or 3 endoscopes we have used 300-W xenon light sources (Trimedyne, Tustin, Calif, and Olympus Corp, Rye, NY). A light source of this power is required for sufficient illumination via the very fine fiber optics used in the narrow endoscopes. For type 3 endoscopes less power is necessary, and we have used a variable-intensity 200-W quartz light source (Pentax, Japan).

Specific coupling adaptors are available for each brand of endoscope to allow direct attachment to a video camera head that projects the endoscope image via a video camera control unit onto a TV screen. The color monitor image provides magnification by a factor of approximately 200 times. A standard VHS videotape video cassette recorder (VCR) suitable for recording all procedures, and a microphone may be added for live commentary.

TECHNIQUES OF PERCUTANEOUS VIDEO ENDOSCOPY

This section details the techniques that have been used in our practice to date.[8, 9]

Biliary Tract Endoscopy

Most procedures were performed in the radiology suite after the administration of local anesthetic and parenteral sedation. In patients who had undergone recent surgical procedures, access to the biliary tract was made via a T-tube or cholecystostomy tube tract. When these routes were not available, access was made via transhepatic route (Table 12–4). Standard techniques for percutaneous transhepatic cholangiography (PTC) were used,[11] and the tract formed from hepatic ducts to skin was then progressively dilated, at intervals of several days, to a diameter of 12 F.

Choice of endoscope was made according to the diameter of the access track available. Large, steerable endoscopes were preferred because of the relatively large diameter of the

TABLE 12–4.
Access Routes for Endoscopy and Interventions in the Biliary Tree

Status	Route
No previous operation	Percutaneous transhepatic cannulation of the bile duct
Intraoperative	
Laparoscopic	Via cystic duct cannulation
Open surgery	Via choledochotomy incision (intraoperative choledochoscopy)
Postoperative	Via T-tube tract
	Via cholecystostomy tube tract
	Via transhepatic drain tract

common bile duct (CBD) and the desirability of being able to deflect the tip of the endoscope to obtain a thorough inspection. A double-guidewire technique was developed, with the endoscope introduced over one guidewire while a second wire was kept in place to maintain access at all times.

After the endoscope had been introduced to the position of the lesion, the primary guidewire was usually removed to allow irrigation with saline to clear the field of view. This allowed more precise examination of the duodenum, bile duct, and hepatic ducts as the endoscope was retracted. Other instruments such as lithotripter fibers, biopsy brushes, snares, etc., were introduced through the working channel of the endoscope or over the second guidewire.

In several patients endoscopy of the distal portion of CBD was performed during a laparoscopic cholecystectomy operation by introduction of a 4.2 F flexible angioscope (Intramed, San Diego, Calif) through one of the instrumentation ports and then via the cystic duct, which had been cannulated for an intraoperative cholangiogram.[10] In these cases, the image was hampered by lack of steeribility of the endoscopic tip within the ducts.

Renal Tract Endoscopy

Percutaneous access to the ureter or renal pelvis was made by dilatation and sheath insertion over a guidewire. The largest endoscope suitable for the access track was chosen. Again, steerable endoscopes were preferred. The endoscope was initially tracked over a guidewire into the lumen of the ureter. The lumen was then cleared by irrigation of saline solution through the fluid channel, and examinations proceeded as with the biliary inspections.

Percutaneous Vascular Endoscopy

Techniques for vascular endoscopy (angioscopy) were initially developed intraoperatively during vascular surgical operations.[12] Wide exposure, clamping of the arterial inflow vessel and balloon-tipped fine fiber-optic catheters helped overcome the problems of flowing blood obstructing the field of view. Irrigation with heparinized saline was necessary to overcome backbleeding and collateral blood flow.

Percutaneous access was gained by standard Seldinger technique, with an 8 F sheath being inserted over a guidewire. The usual sheath insertion was in an antegrade direction from the puncture site in the common femoral artery, down the lumen of the superficial femoral artery. Experience in the vascular system proved very valuable in developing the related techniques in the biliary and renal tracts.

CASE STUDIES

Case 1.—Endoscopic lithotripsy and removal of gallstones via a cholecystostomy tube track.

A frail 79-year-old woman with severe cardiac disease presented with acute cholecystitis. Operative cholecystostomy was performed via a small incision, and stones were removed from the gallbladder with forceps. Postoperative cholangiography via the cholecystostomy tube showed retained gallstones in the gallbladder and cystic duct (Fig 12–1,A).

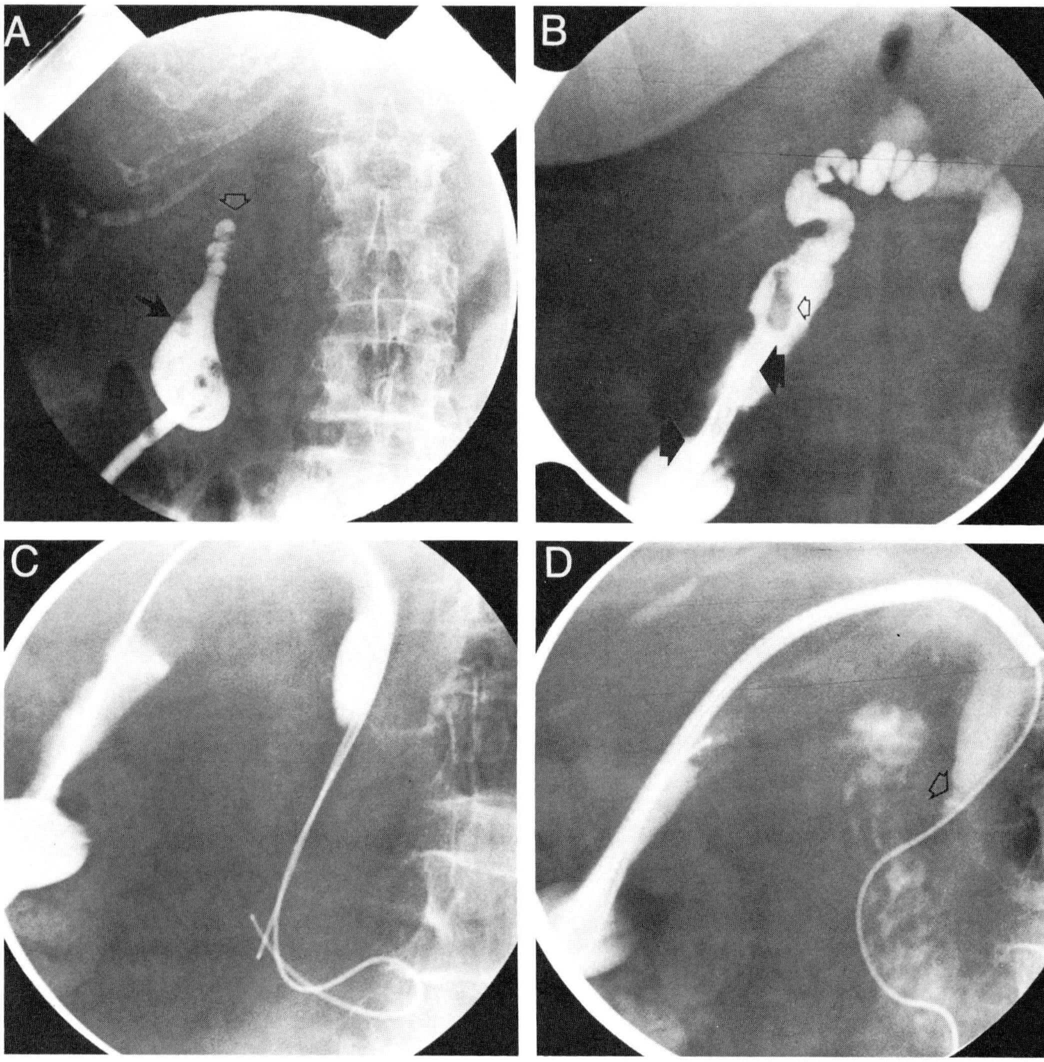

FIG 12–1.

A, postoperative cholangiogram performed via a cholecystostomy tube in an elderly woman who had undergone cholecystostomy 1 week earlier. Stones are in the gallbladder *(arrow)* and the cystic duct are causing duct obstruction *(open arrow)*. **B,** a 10 F diameter endoscope has been introduced percutaneously via the drain track *(large arrows)* for inspection of the gallstones *(small arrow)* and to monitor lithotripsy and stone removal. **C,** two guidewires are manipulated via the gallbladder and cystic duct into the CBD and duodenum. The endoscope is passed over one guidewire, while the second guidewire maintains access for other instruments. **D,** the endoscope is shown as it progresses over the primary guidewire through the cystic duct and into the common bile duct. Several stones identified in the distal portion of the CBD *(arrow)* are causing obstruction of flow into the duodenum. *Facing page:* **E,** after further fragmentation and removal of the CBD stones, the ampulla was dilated with an angioplasty balloon. Contrast now passes freely through the ampulla *(arrow)* into the duodenum. **F,** the endoscope now passes freely along the CBD and through the ampulla into the duodenum. **G,** a final cholangiogram shows free flow of contrast via the biliary tree, with relief of the distal obstruction. One small residual stone in the distal aspect of the gallbladder *(arrow)* was removed with a Dormia basket.

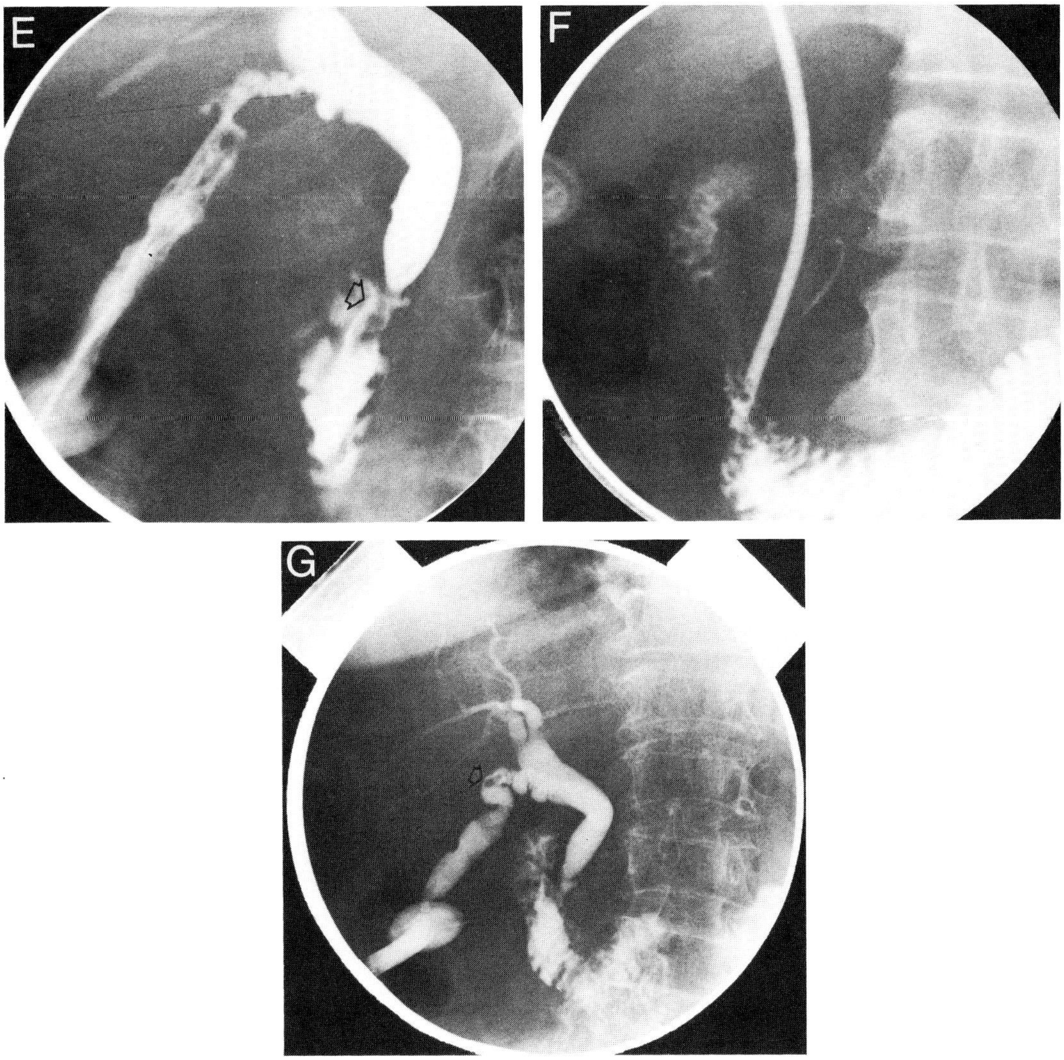

FIG 12–1 (cont.).

Percutaneous endoscopic lithotripsy was subsequently carried out via the cholecystostomy tube tract on two occasions 4 days apart. (Fig 12–1,B and C). Stone fragments were removed with a Dormia basket, and the cystic duct and CBD were dilated with a 6-mm-diameter angioplasty balloon (Fig 12–1,D–G). Final endoscopy and repeat cholangiography showed no residual stones and normal flow of contrast into the duodenum (Fig 12–2).

Case 2.—Endoscopic removal of CBD stones via a T-tube tract.

A 71-year-old woman developed recurrent jaundice 6 weeks after cholecystectomy and exploration of the CBD. (Fig 12–3,A and B) Endoscopic retrograde cholangiopancreatography (ERCP) failed due to previous partial gastrectomy, so sphincterotomy could not be performed. A 10 F steerable endoscope was inserted over a guidewire in the T-tube track, and two stones were imaged in the CBD (Fig 12–3,C). Both stones were extracted with a Dormia basket endoscopically (Fig 12–4), and balloon dilatation of the sphincter of Oddi was performed. A 12 F catheter was left in the biliary tree, and a subsequent cholangiogram was normal.

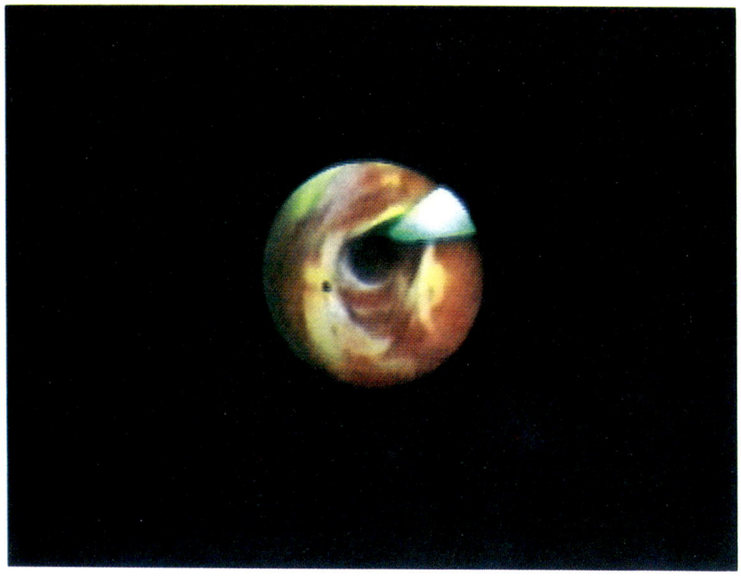

FIG 12–2.
Endoscopic appearance of the distal portion of the CBD after removal of stones and dilatation of the ampulla. The guidewire is seen *(top right)* as it projects from an internal channel of the endoscope. Small amounts of mural blood clot are seen on the duct walls following the manipulations.

Case 3.—Percutaneous transhepatic endoscopic biopsy, dilatation, and stenting of strictured choledochojejunostomy anastomosis.

A 54-year-old woman presented with jaundice 2 years after a Whipple's operation for duodenal carcinoma. Computed tomography (CT) and ultrasound demonstrated dilated intrahepatic bile ducts and a CBD with a mass in the lower end. PTC showed a stricture of the choledochojejunostomy anastomosis (Fig 12–5,A).

A 7 F diameter endoscope was inserted via the PTC tract and used for inspection and guided biopsy of the stricture. The region was then dilated with an 8-mm angioplasty balloon catheter, and a drainage catheter was left in situ (Fig 12–5,B and C).

The biopsy specimen proved to have adenocarcinoma cells. Repeat percutaneous cholangiography and endoscopy via the same access demonstrated that the stricture had not been adequately relieved by the dilatation alone (Fig 12–5,D and E), and since surgical management of this recurrent malignancy was not considered indicated, two expandable 3-cm-long Gianturco-Rösch biliary Z-stents were placed across the stricture (Fig 12–5,F).

Final endoscopy demonstrated an excellent-caliber lumen at the previous stricture site.

Case 4.—Endoscopic crushing and extraction of stones in intrahepatic ducts via a T-tube tract (Oriental cholangiohepatitis).

A 36-year-old Taiwanese woman with features of Oriental cholangiohepatitis underwent operative cholecystectomy and exploration of the CBD. Intraoperative choledochoscopy showed that the left hepatic duct was full of small stones and pus. Following clearance of these ducts, a transhepatic drainage tube was brought out through the skin from the left hepatic duct system, and a T-tube was inserted in the CBD.

Six weeks postoperatively, residual or recurrent stones were identified in the left duct system by a T-tube cholangiogram. A 10 F endoscope was introduced via the percutaneous drain tract to the left ducts, and stones were removed with a Dormia basket. Subsequently, percutaneous transhepatic access was also made to the right hepatic duct, and endoscopic crushing and removal of stones

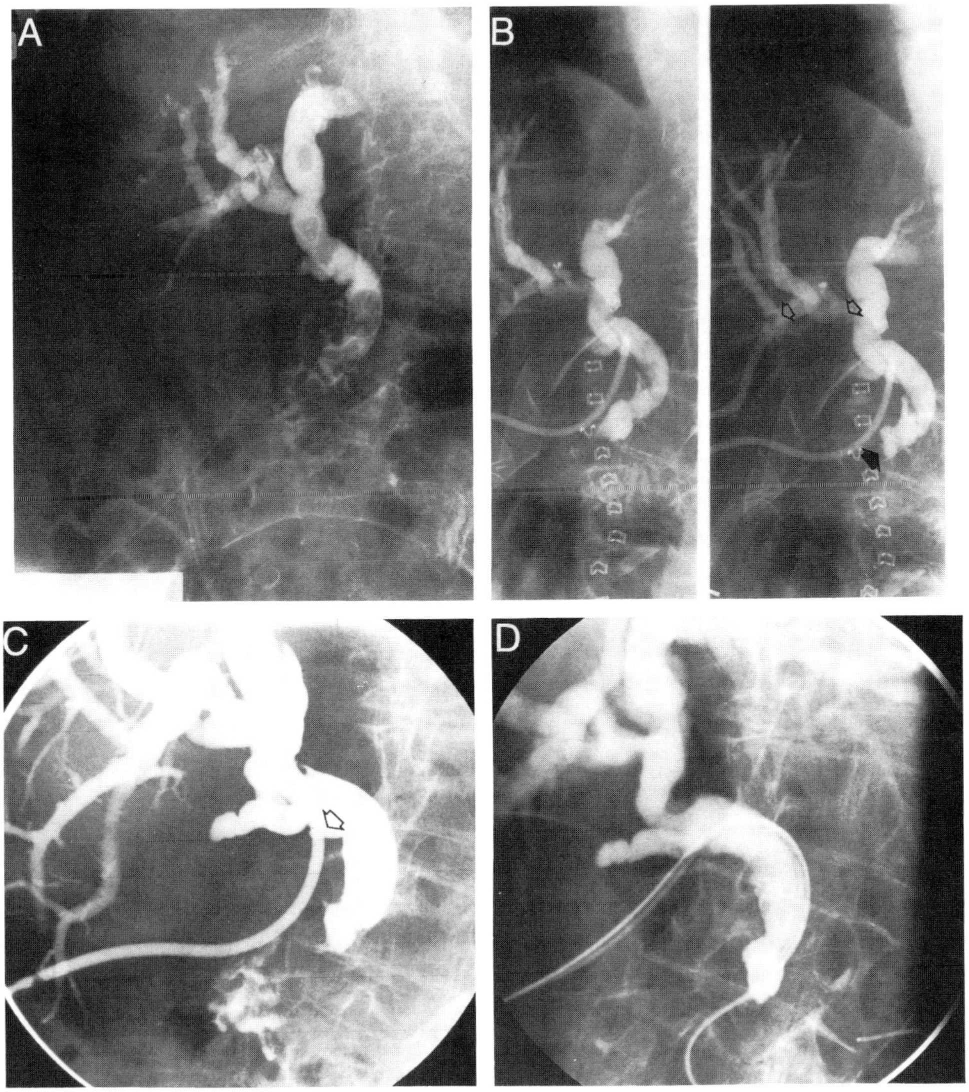

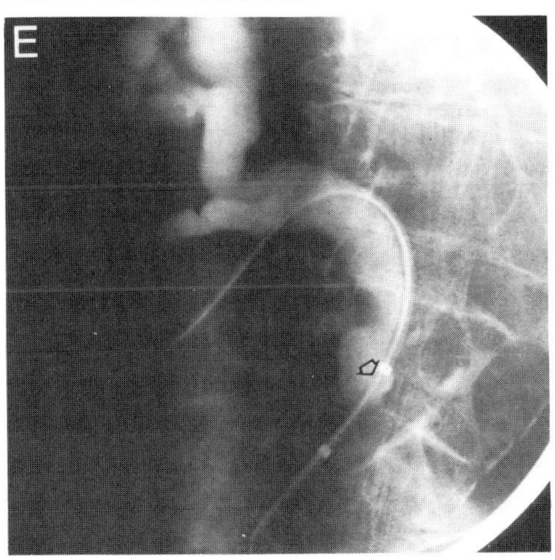

FIG 12–3.
A, an intraoperative cholangiogram (performed via a catheter in the cystic duct) in a 71-year-old woman demonstrates multiple stones in the intrahepatic and extrahepatic bile ducts. Exploration of the CBD and removal of stones was performed. **B,** an early postoperative T-tube cholangiogram demonstrated several retained stones *(open arrows)* and obstruction of the distal portion of the CBD *(large arrow)*. **C,** a 10 F endoscope *(arrow)* is seen as it passes into the proximal aspect of the biliary tree over a guidewire. **D,** a guidewire was passed through the ampulla after extraction of a distal CBD stone. **E,** the sphincter of Oddi was dilated with an angioplasty balloon *(arrow),* and a 12 F drainage catheter was left in the CBD in place of the T-tube. A subsequent repeat cholangiogram several days later was normal.

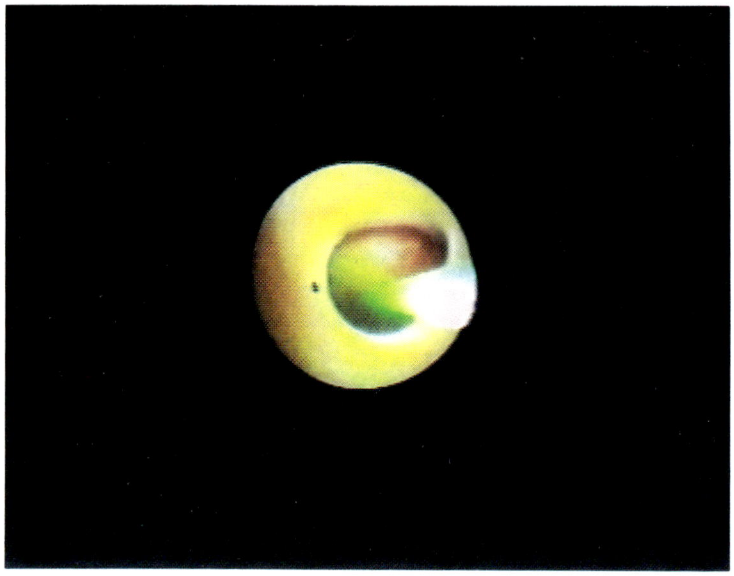

FIG 12–4.
Endoscopic view of the interior of an intrahepatic bile duct radical after Dormia basket removal of a retained stone.

were performed via the right and left hepatic duct tracts and also retrogradely via the T-tube tract. Six days after all systems had been completely cleared of stones, the drainage tubes were removed, and the patient has remained well for the 9 months of follow-up to date.

Case 5.—Percutaneous transhepatic endoscopy for diagnosis and biopsy of cholangiocarcinoma, with endoscopic monitoring of irridium radiation and placement of stents.

A 67-year-old male with obstructive jaundice was shown on CT scanning to have a mass in the bile duct and multiple filling defects in the liver (Fig 12–6,A). PTC demonstrated irregular narrowing of the common hepatic duct system near the porta (Fig 12–6,B). A 10 F drain was left in situ across the strictures into the CBD. Percutaneous endoscopy via the PTC tract showed a polypoid mass in the common hepatic duct that extended for several centimeters into the right and left hepatic ducts (Fig 12–6,C). Biopsy of this lesion was performed, and cholangiocarcinoma was confirmed. Irridium wires were inserted and the position checked endoscopically. Endoscopy was repeated after removal of the irridium. A persistent tumor mass was seen in the distal aspect of the duct. A 10 F stent was placed within the hepatic duct, through into the duodenum. Good palliation was achieved with resolution of his jaundice.

Case 6.—Percutaneous transhepatic endoscopy for diagnosis and placement of stents in an ischemic stricture of the hepatic duct in a transplanted liver.

FIG 12–5.
A, percutaneous transhepatic cholangiogram in a 54-year-old woman who presented with jaundice 2 years after a Whipple's operation. Obstruction of the distal portion of the CBD at the choledochojejunostomy anastomosis is demonstrated *(arrow).* **B,** after endoscopic biopsy of the obstructing lesion, a guidewire and dilatation balloon were passed through the stricture. **C,** an inflated dilatation balloon is seen in position through the stricture. **D,** a 10 F endoscope *(arrow)* is shown passing through the dilated stricture into the anastomosis and jejunal loop. **E,** transhepatic cholangiography now demonstrates the stricture more precisely with a thin stream of contrast into the jejunal loop *(arrow).* **F,** a double length of Gianturco-Rösch biliary Z-stent *(arrow)* was positioned across the dilated stricture to enlarge the lumen and maintain patency.

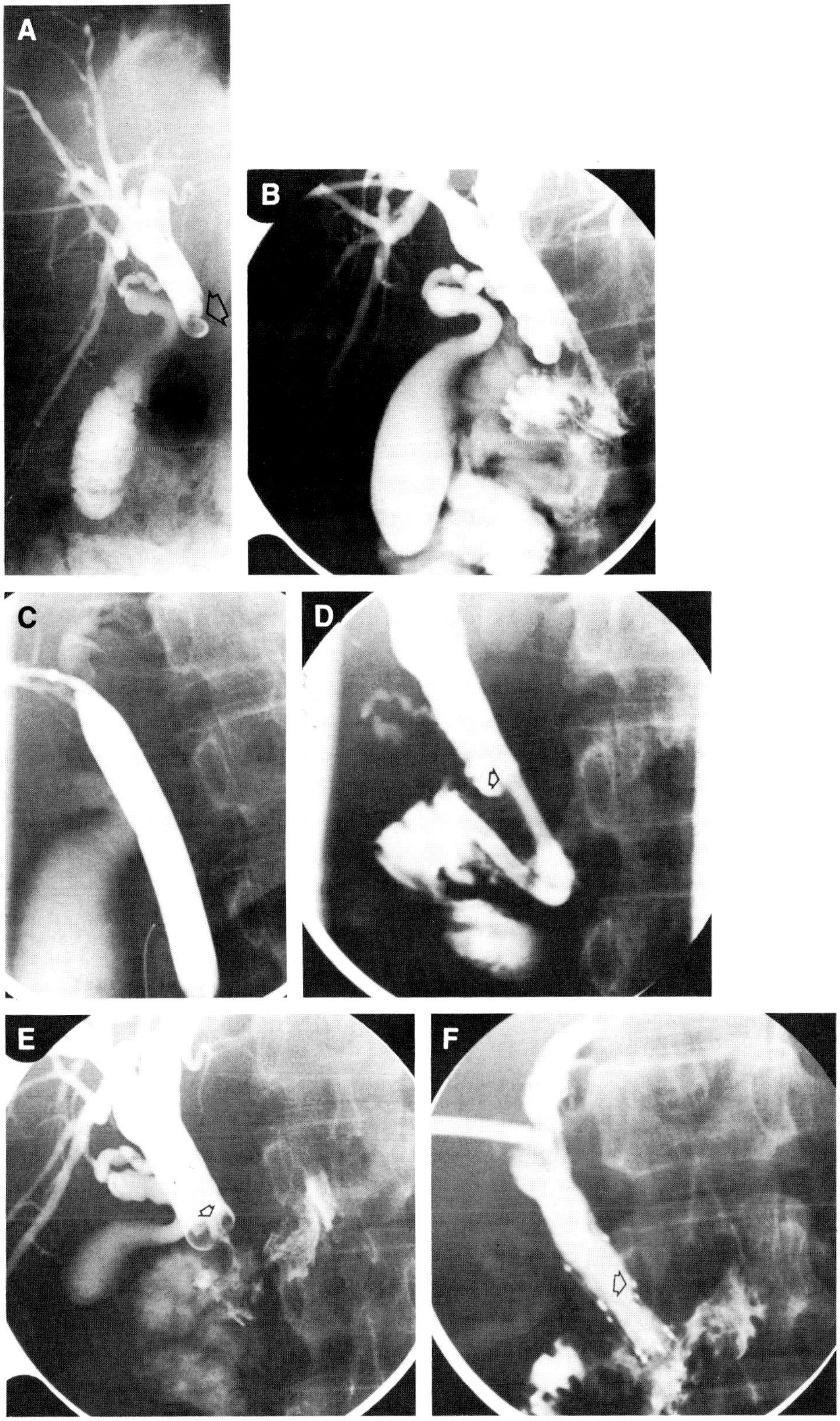
A
B
C
D
E
F

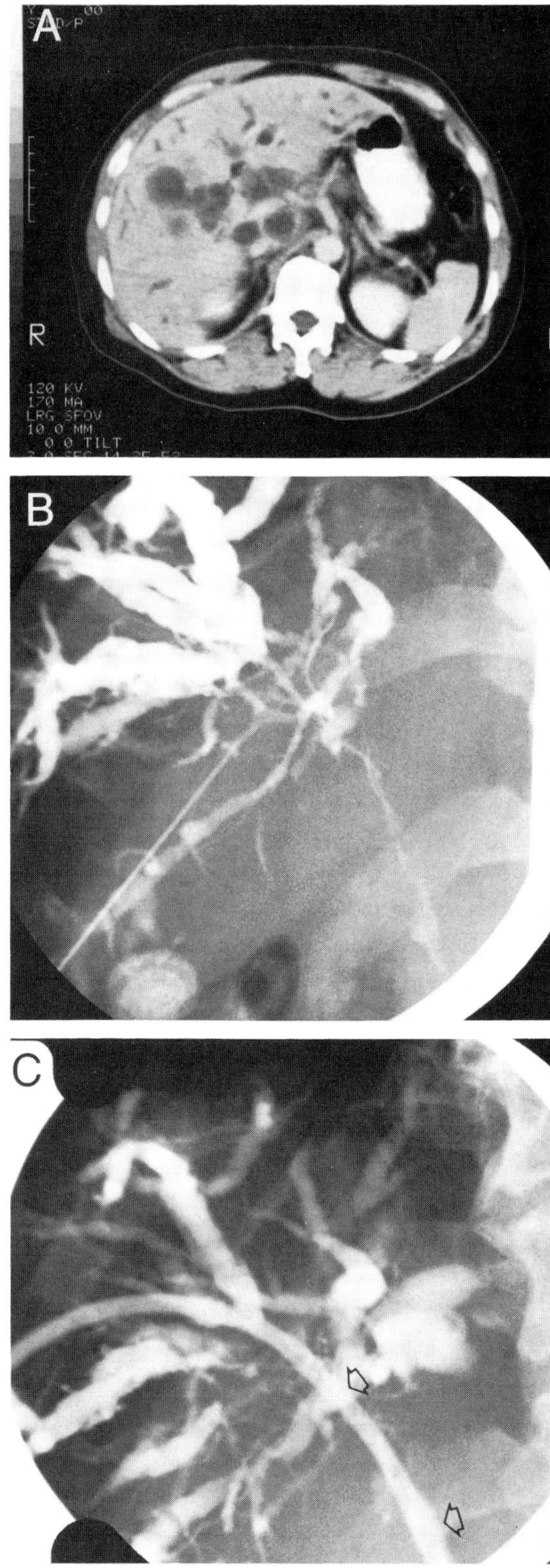

FIG 12–6.
A, a CT scan in a 67-year-old male with obstructive jaundice demonstrates multiple filling defects in the liver due to dilated intrahepatic ducts. A mass in the bile duct was shown on other films. **B,** percutaneous transhepatic cholangiography shows irregular narrowing of the distal hepatic duct system near the porta hepatis. A guidewire was manipulated through this stricture into the CBD. **C,** percutaneous transhepatic insertion of an 8 F diameter endoscope into the biliary tree *(arrows)* allowed inspection and guided biopsy sampling of the obstructing cholangiocarcinoma.

A 46-year-old liver transplant recipient developed a stricture of the right hepatic duct that was associated with fever and raised liver enzyme values. The stricture was diagnosed by PTC, and it was not clear whether the etiology was transplant rejection–related sloughing of the duct endothelium or ischemic stricture. Percutaneous endoscopy showed a segment of ischemic-appearing duct wall without evidence of rejection reaction or filling defects in the lumen. Flexible tantalum stents were placed across the stricture to relieve the obstruction and maintain patency.

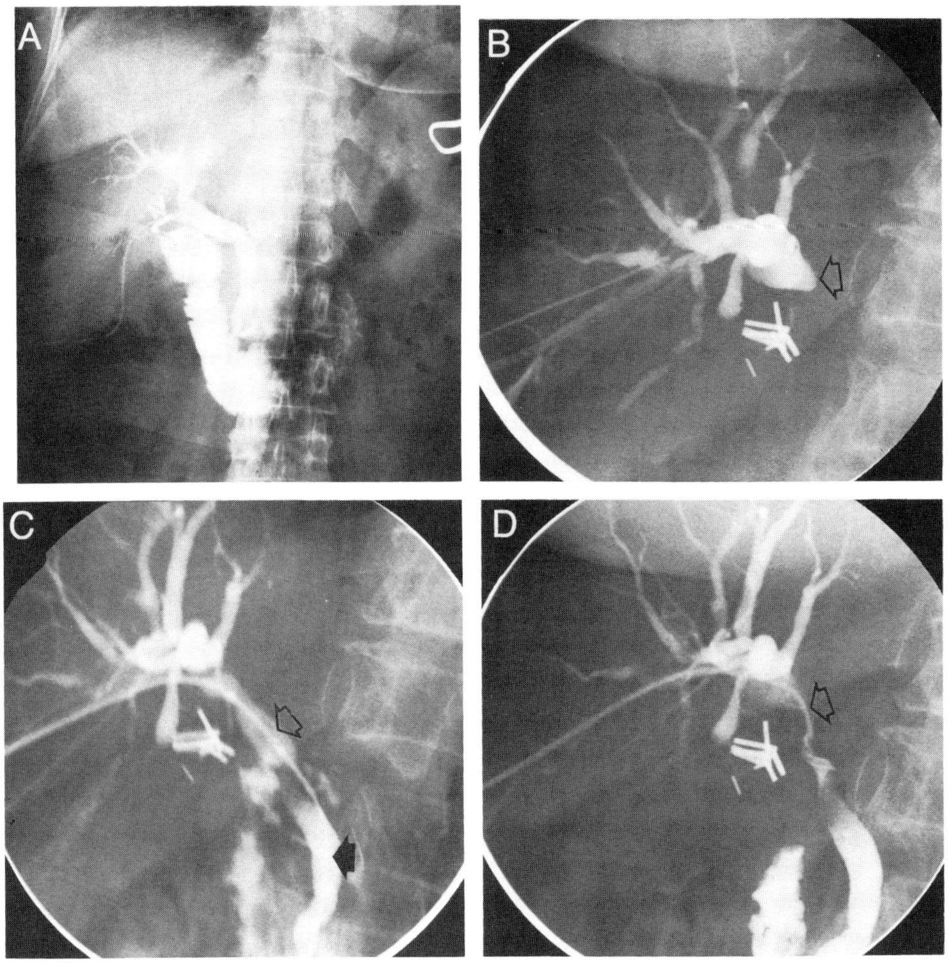

FIG 12–7.
A, intraoperative cholangiography performed via a cannula in the cystic duct at the time of cholecystectomy in a 68-year-old woman. This cholangiogram was considered to be normal, and there were no complications of the surgery. **B,** a percutaneous transhepatic cholangiogram was performed 5 months later to investigate jaundice. This demonstrated total obstruction of the bile duct *(arrow)* near the point of entry of the cystic duct (indicated by the presence of multiple surgical metallic clips). **C,** a guidewire was passed via the same transhepatic access route and was eventually manipulated through the area of obstruction into the distal portion of the CBD *(filled arrow)* A dilatation balloon was passed over the guidewire and is shown to be fully inflated within the stricture *(open arrow).* **D,** an irregular, narrow stricture of the CBD remains after the dilatation procedure *(arrow).* **E** (p. 232), the radiologic appearance of the strictured area *(arrow)* several days later demonstrates a poor lumen and partial obstruction to bile flow. The endoscopic image of the stricture appeared benign (see Fig 12–8). **F** (p. 232), an expansile, metallic stent *(arrows)* was implanted across the stricture to maintain patency with an expanded lumen.

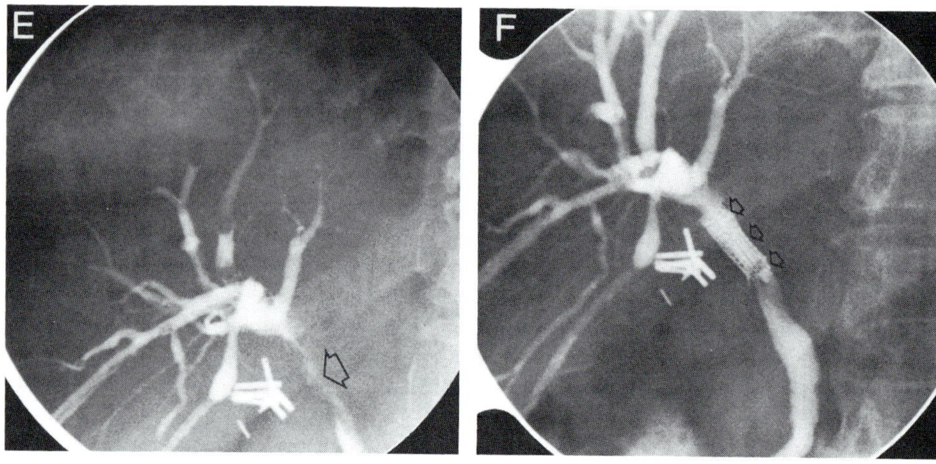

FIG 12–7 (cont.).

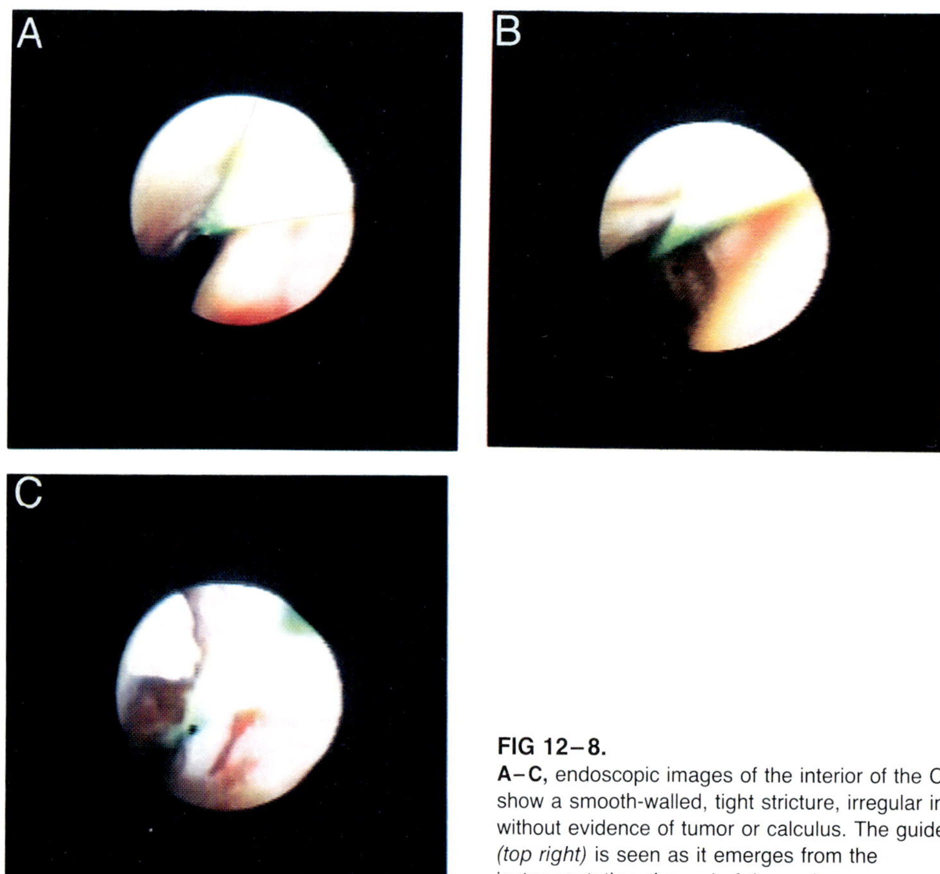

FIG 12–8.
A–C, endoscopic images of the interior of the CBD show a smooth-walled, tight stricture, irregular in parts, without evidence of tumor or calculus. The guidewire *(top right)* is seen as it emerges from the instrumentation channel of the endoscope.

Case 7.—Percutaneous transhepatic endoscopy and stenting of postoperative bile duct stricture.

A 68-year-old woman developed obstructive jaundice 5 months after an uncomplicated cholecystectomy operation. An intraoperative cholangiogram performed via the cystic duct during the cholecystectomy operation had been normal (Fig 12–7, A).

A CT scan showed no evidence of tumor. PTC showed a total occlusion of the extrahepatic bile duct at the approximate site of entry of the cystic duct (Fig 12–7,B). A guidewire was eventually able to be passed through the obstruction into the distal portion of the CBD. The stricture was then dilated with a 5-mm-diameter angioplasty balloon, which resulted in an irregular, stringy stricture (Fig 12–7,C and D).

Two days later, endoscopy via the percutaneous transhepatic tract showed a long, smooth-walled stricture with moderate wall cracking due to the dilatation but no evidence of malignancy (Fig 12–8). Since the endoscopic image confirmed a residual tight stricture, a metallic expansile stent was inserted (Fig 12–7,E and F).

Post stent endoscopy showed that the lumen was now widely patent (Fig 12–9) with the metallic struts of the stent well incorporated into the wall of the CBD.

Case 8.—Percutaneous nephroscopy and placement of ureteric stents.

A 78-year-old man developed bilateral ureteric obstruction due to iliac and para-aortic lymphadenopathy associated with prostatic carcinoma. Bilateral nephrostomy tubes were placed with radiologic monitoring. Three weeks later, J-stents were to be placed in each ureter to relieve the obstruction. However, injection of contrast via the right nephrostomy tube revealed a filling defect in the right ureter that could have been a stone or bloodclot. An 8 F endoscope was introduced over a guidewire to the site of the lesion, but no abnormality was seen. The filling defect was considered to be an artifact, and uneventful placement of internal J-stents was readily accomplished via the guidewires. There were no complications.

Case 9.—Percutaneous endoscopic removal of ureteric calculi.

A 45-year-old woman had a history of incomplete removal of large ureteric calculi via open nephrolithotomy on two occasions. She was transferred from another hospital for management of

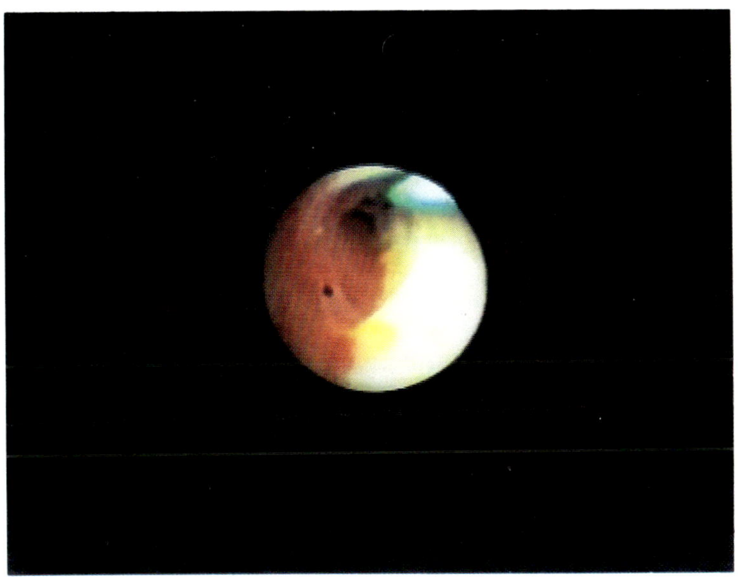

FIG 12–9.
Endoscopic image of the CBD after stenting, with an enlarged lumen including some soft, mural blood clot. The stent has become embedded into the wall and is only partially visible in the distal portion of the duct.

recurrent stones in the renal pelvis and ureter. Initial attempts to remove the ureteric calculus via ureteric cannulation from a cystoscope were unsuccessful. Percutaneous nephrostomy was performed. A 12 F steerable endoscope was used to examine the renal pelvis over a guidewire, and an 8 F nonsteerable endoscope was then substituted for examination of the downstream ureter. Stone fragments were identified in the upper pole and lower pole calyces and in the ureter and were removed endoscopically with Dormia baskets. A stricture of the ureter was also identified, and this prompted insertion of a double-J-stent from the renal pelvis to bladder. The nephrostomy tube was removed after several days, and there were no complications.

DISCUSSION

The techniques presented in this chapter have evolved, in the main, by the combination of video endoscopy systems (using recently developed ultrafine endoscopes) and conventional interventional radiologic procedures.[13] Use of endoscopy in these cases gives an added dimension of precision for diagnosis and less invasive therapy for biliary tract and ureteric lesions.[14]

Percutaneous endoscopy of the ureter and renal pelvis appears to be most valuable in the diagnosis of lesions that are not well elucidated by other imaging techniques and particularly in the monitoring and control of new devices and techniques for management of stone disease.[5, 6] The large volume and easy distensibility of these structures means that a larger, steerable endoscope can usually be accommodated, which makes it easier to inspect impacted stones and other lesions.

The most valuable application of percutaneous cholangioscopy at present would seem to be in the management of recurrent or retained stones after biliary tract surgery (especially if ERCP is unsuccessful or impossible) or in the complex management of multiple small intrahepatic stones as typically seen in Oriental cholangiohepatitis.[1] Occasionally the same techniques are valuable in the diagnosis of strictures or other lesions of the biliary tree that have not been clarified by more conventional diagnostic studies.[14]

Newer therapeutic devices and techniques may be monitored and controlled by endoscopy to allow a more precise evaluation of the lithotripsy techniques, intraduct radiation, dilatation, and stenting procedure to be made.

As laparoscopic cholecystectomy and related procedures become more widely practiced, further applications of percutaneous biliary endoscopy will become apparent. At present, ultrathin endoscopes are being used to inspect the CBD via a laparoscopic port through the cystic duct after cannulation in the routine way.

Complications of biliary tract endoscopy and interventional therapy include hemobilia (due to mucosal trauma), fevers and rigors, ductal perforation, and pain.[1] Antibiotic coverage is used, particularly when there is an element of duct obstruction and biliary stosis. Biliary lithotripsy may be achieved by mechanical fragmentation (with stone-crushing forceps), ultrasonic probes,[15] electrohydraulic shock waves[11] or an Nd:YAG laser contact probe.[16] Basket forceps manipulation and removal of stones may be performed by ERCP or by the percutaneous transhepatic route, but this is limited in some patients with anatomic variations, previous operations, intrahepatic stones, or large impacted duct stones.[1, 4] Lithotripsy may be applied in these more difficult cases.

Electrohydraulic lithotripsy is a recently developed technique by which stones are fragmented by a series of shock waves generated by an electric discharge into a liquid medium. There have been descriptions of its use for biliary stones with fluoroscopic guidance alone or during choledochoscopy via a T-tube tract,[17] by percutaneous transhepatic access,[11, 18] or by ERCP after sphincterotomy.[19]

Use of an Nd:YAG contact laser for endoscopic biliary lithotripsy was described initially by Orii et al., who introduced the endoscope and laser probe via a T-tube tract.[16] With the use of direct vision by choledochoscopy, electrohydraulic probes or laser probes may be kept in direct contact with the stone during lithotripsy procedure, thereby avoiding trauma to the bile duct wall and surrounding structures.[1] Nd:YAG laser probes passed via the cystic duct have potential applications for fragmenting bile duct stones during laparoscopic procedures, but widespread use is currently limited by the expense, difficulty of use, and limitations of access to the segment of CBD distal to the entry of the cystic duct.[10] The Nd:YAG laser only disrupts bilirubin stones and requires the presence of a liquid medium; breaking cholesterol stones is almost impossible.[1]

REFERENCES

1. Chen MF, Jan YY: Percutaneous transhepatic cholangioscopic lithotripsy. *Br J Surg* 1990; 77:530–532.
2. Chen MF, Jan YY: Percutaneous transhepatic removal of common bile duct and intrahepatic duct stones with fiberoptic choledochoscope. *Gastrointest Endosc* 1986; 32:347–349.
3. Chen MF, Jan YY, Lee TY: Percutaneous transhepatic cholangioscopy. *Br J Surg* 1987; 74:728–730.
4. Huang MH, Yang TC, Lee SA: Choledochofiberoscopy in the post-operative management of intrahepatic stone. *Am J Surg* 1980; 139:860–864.
5. Taylor TA, Mander J, Manning K, et al: Criteria audit of percutaneous nephrolithotomies. *Aust N Z J Surg* 1990; 60:849–853.
6. Segura JW, Patterson DE, LeRoy JA: Percutaneous removal of kidney stones: Review of 1000 cases. *J Urol* 1985; 134:1077–1081.
7. White, GH, White RA, Kopchok GE, et al: Endoscopic intravascular surgery removes intraluminal flaps, dissections and thrombus. *J Vasc Surg* 1990; 11:280–286.
8. Rees MR: Percutaneous video endoscopy in peripheral vascular disease. *Clin Radiol* 1989; 40:347–351.
9. White GH, Kopchok GE, White RA: Percutaneous angioscopy as an adjunct to laser angioplasty in peripheral arteries. *Lancet* 1989; 2:99.
10. White GH, Storey D: Percutaneous endoscopy of the common bile duct during laparoscopic cholecystectomy. *Surg Gynecol Obstet,* submitted for publication.
11. Lear JL, Ring EA, Macoviak JA: Percutaneous transhepatic electrohydraulic lithotripsy. *Radiology* 1984; 150:590–598.
12. White GH, White RA, Kopchok GE, et al: Intraoperative video endoscopy compared with angiography during peripheral vascular operations. *J Vasc Surg* 1987; 8:488–495.
13. Waugh RC, Malthouse S, White GH: Percutaneous video endoscopy as an adjunct to interventional radiology. *Radiology,* submitted for publication.
14. White GH, Waugh RC, Malthouse S, et al: Percutaneous endoscopy and endoscopic intervention of the biliary and renal tracts. *Aust N Z J Surg,* submitted for publication.
15. Gacetta DJ, Cohen MJ, Crummy AB: Ultrasonic lithotripsy of gallstones after cholecystectomy. *AJR* 1984; 143:1088–1089.
16. Orii K, Nakahava A, Takase Y: Choledocholithotomy by YAG laser with a choleochofiberscope: Case reports of two patients. *Surgery* 1981; 90:120–122.

17. Burhenne JH: Electrohydrolytic fragmentation of retained common duct stones. *Radiology* 1975; 117:721–722.
18. Tanaka M, Yoshimoto H, Ikeda S: Two approaches for electrohydraulic lithotripsy in the common bile duct. *Surgery* 1985; 98:313–318.
19. Koch H, Stolte M, Walz V: Endoscopic lithotripsy in the common bile duct. *Gastrointest Endosc* 1980; 26:16–18.

Chapter 13

Interventional Radiologic Adjuncts and Alternatives to Biliary Surgery

Lindsay Machan, M.D.

Interventional radiology, i.e., "surgical" radiology, refers to a group of diagnostic or therapeutic procedures requiring the insertion of specialized needles, catheters, or other devices by using imaging guidance. For the most part, the diagnostic procedures consist of aspiration, biopsy, or venous sampling, and the therapeutic procedures involve drainage, dilatation, occlusion, fragmentation, or extraction. The most common guiding modality is fluoroscopy, but ultrasound, computed tomography (CT), or even magnetic resonance imaging may be used alone or in combination with fluoroscopic imaging. Interventional radiologic techniques have been applied to every organ system literally from head to toe, but this chapter will be confined to the discussion of those techniques that can be offered to patients as an alternative to, a combined procedure with, or applied to complications after laparoscopic cholecystectomy.

GALLBLADDER INTERVENTION

Percutaneous Cholecystostomy

Gallbladder puncture can be performed for diagnostic or therapeutic indications (Table 13–1).

Diagnostic cannulation with a fine needle, usually guided by ultrasound, allows aspiration of bile for chemical or bacteriologic examination or cellular material for cytology. Cholangiography can also be performed via gallbladder puncture when the intrahepatic ducts are nondilated (Fig 13–1) or transhepatic cholangiography is incomplete or unsuccessful.

Gallbladder puncture is most frequently performed under ultrasound guidance, although CT or fluoroscopy (after oral contrast administration) can also be used. Theoretically, the safest route of puncture is transhepatically through the gallbladder bed where it is adherent to the liver; however, it is important to enter the gallbladder as close as possible to the fundus if a tract is to be established for therapeutic maneuvers. Some authors[1] prefer the subhepatic route and use an anchoring device if a large tract is formed or if there is sepsis.

Percutaneous cholecystostomy has been proposed as an alternative to surgical cholecystec-

TABLE 13–1.
Indications for Percutaneous Gallbladder Puncture*

- Diagnosis
  - Chemical or bacterial bile analysis
  - Cytology
  - Cholangiography when PTC† unsuccessful
- Therapy
  - Gallbladder drainage
    - Acute cholecystitis
    - Empyema
    - Biliary obstruction
    - Gallbladder perforations
  - Gallstone therapy
    - Mechanical removal
    - Chemical dissolution
    - Electrohydraulic lithotripsy
    - Laser lithotripsy
    - Rotational contact lithotripsy
  - Access to biliary tree via the cystic duct

*Adapted from Cope C: *Percutaneous Biliary Decompression.* New York, Gower Medical Publishing, 189, p 13.3.
†PTC = percutaneous transhepatic cholangiography.

tomy or cholecystostomy in the treatment of patients with acute cholecystitis[2,3] (Fig 13–2). In selected high-risk patient populations, the mortality for emergency open cholecystectomy is as high as 10% to 30%.[4,5] In this high-risk group, percutaneous cholecystostomy can be performed to decompress the acutely inflamed and obstructed gallbladder. McGahan and Lindfors[6] were able to successfully perform 39 or 40 consecutive attempted percutaneous cholecystostomies in patients with acute cholecystitis with no major complications related to the procedure. The catheter became dislodged in 2 patients, and 2 other patients experienced significant abdominal pain that did not require surgery.

Once the patient's clinical condition has stabilized, the gallbladder can be removed electively, or the stones can be dealt with by radiologically guided mechanical removal or lithotripsy. In one series of 11 elderly patients with acute cholecystitis who were poor surgical candidates due to underlying cardiac and/or respiratory disease, all were successfully drained and the gallstones removed.[7] There were two complications; one minor wound infection and one death secondary to bile peritonitis.

An alternative approach is to perform a surgical cholecystostomy emergently and suture the gallbladder to the abdominal wall with subsequent elective radiologic gallstone removal[8] (Fig 13–3). This renders the possibility of losing access to the gallbladder extremely unlikely. The authors were able to allow all patients to defervesce and removed all calculi in 31 of 36 patients, with no deaths or major complications. Three patients had elective cholecystectomy, one had endoscopic sphincterotomy, and one was observed.

Gallstone Therapy

The role of percutaneous gallstone therapy in the nonemergent patient is less well defined, although a number of techniques have been developed including mechanical removal, solvent

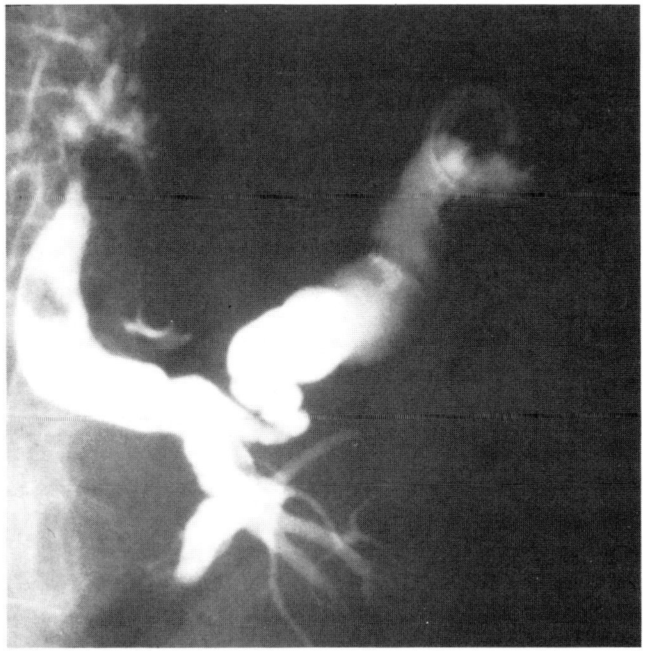

FIG 13–1.
Cholangiography via gallbladder puncture in a patient with nondilated ducts demonstrates a single common bile duct (CBD) stone.

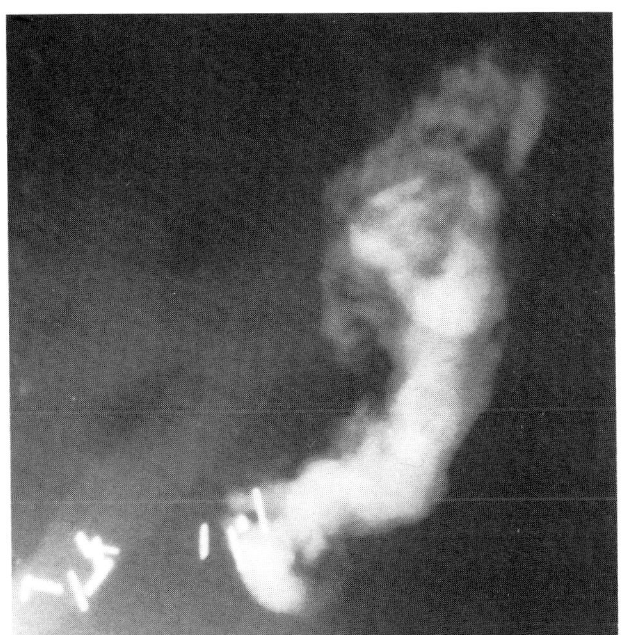

FIG 13–2.
Percutaneous cholecystostomy in a patient with acute cholecystitis. The gallbladder lumen is markedly irregular and reflects the marked inflammatory change.

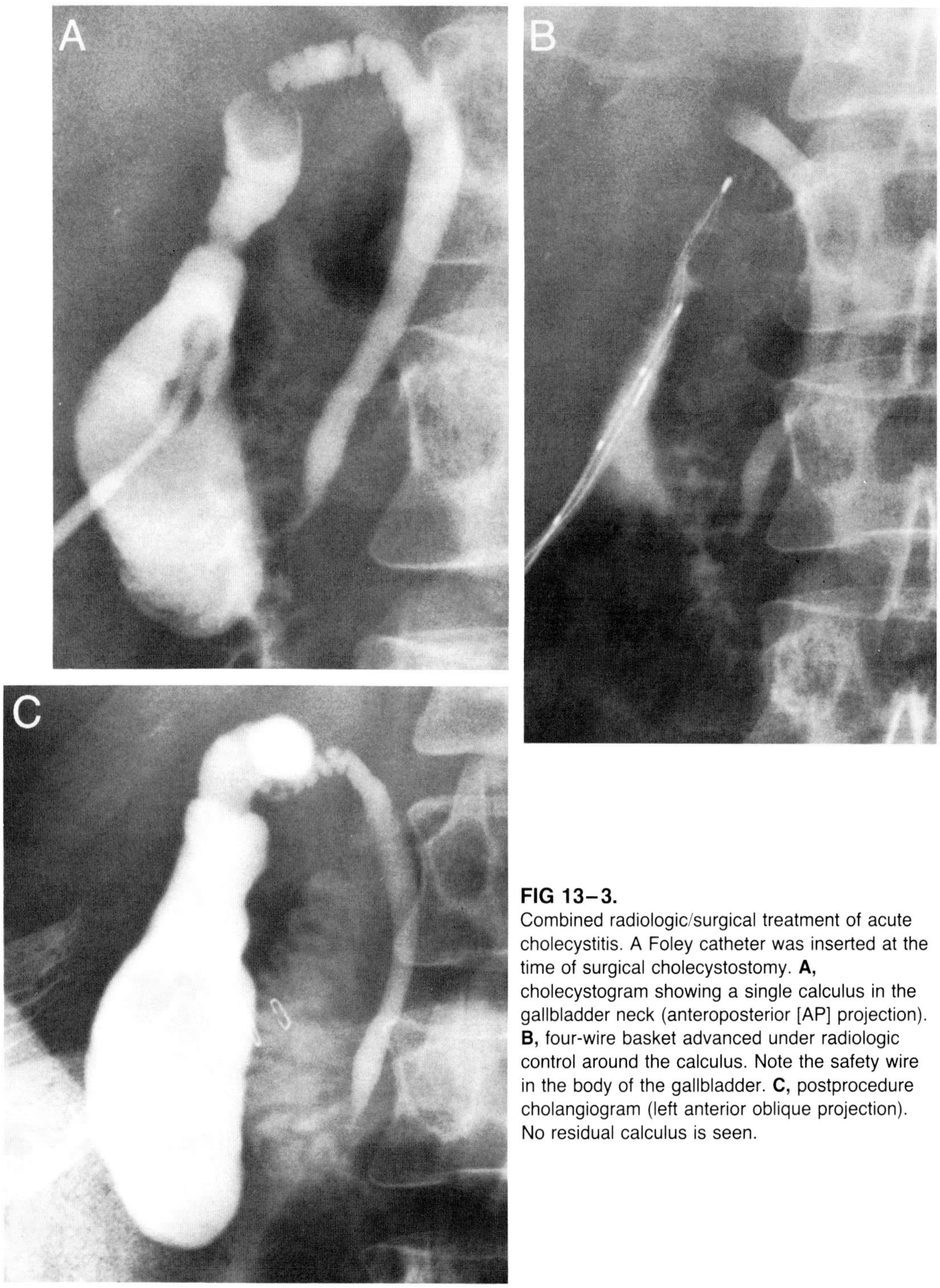

FIG 13–3.
Combined radiologic/surgical treatment of acute cholecystitis. A Foley catheter was inserted at the time of surgical cholecystostomy. **A,** cholecystogram showing a single calculus in the gallbladder neck (anteroposterior [AP] projection). **B,** four-wire basket advanced under radiologic control around the calculus. Note the safety wire in the body of the gallbladder. **C,** postprocedure cholangiogram (left anterior oblique projection). No residual calculus is seen.

dissolution, and intracorporeal or extracorporeal lithotripsy. The method chosen depends upon the size, number, and composition of the gallstones and the experience of the interventionist. The tract to the gallbladder is established in the same manner as in patients with acute cholecystitis.

Mechanical Removal

Mechanical gallstone removal is the easiest to perform, but it requires a large tract (20 to 30 F). Multiple small stones can be removed by irrigation or suction. Medium-sized stones, either solitary or a small number, are easily dealt with by using baskets, forceps, or suction under fluoroscopic or endoscopic guidance. Large stones can be fractured by using forceps or lithotripsy and the fragments dealt with individually.

Gallstone Dissolution

There are two drugs available for gallstone dissolution. Monoctanoin and methyl tert-butyl ether (MTBE). Monoctanoin is the only contact solvent approved by the Food and Drug Administration (FDA) and is successful in only about 30% of common duct calculi.[9] It can be used to potentiate mechanical fragmentation and to clear debris and small particles in both gallbladder and common duct calculi. It requires infusion (usually for days) through a double-lumen catheter with continuous biliary manometry because it is important to avoid a rise in intraluminal pressures during its infusion.

MTBE is investigational in the United States, but it appears to be efficactious in approximately 75% of cholesterol stones[10, 11] (Fig 13–4). It is difficult to use because of its odor and toxicity, and the procedure can still be time-consuming. Frequent fluoroscopic monitoring is required; if the size of the calculus has not changed in 2 to 3 hours, complete dissolution is unlikely.

Lithotripsy

Intracorporeal lithrotripsy most frequently implies fragmentation of calculi by shock waves generated from a catheter tip immediately adjacent to the stone. The most frequent method utilized in the biliary tree is electrohydraulic lithrotripsy (EHL)[12]; a series of high-voltage sparks are produced across an electrode at the catheter tip, and this vaporizes the adjacent fluid and produces a sharp, high-amplitude hydraulic wave. EHL has been reported most frequently in intrahepatic or bile duct stones, but it can also be used to debulk large gallbladder calculi.[13] Biliary calculi can also be fragmented by intracorporeal tunable dye[14] or YAG laser[15] lithrotripsy.

Rotational contact lithotripsy at the time of publication is an experimental technique utilizing a modification of the Kensey-Nash atherectomy catheter. A rotating cam spinning at 40,000 rpm is introduced into the gallbladder via a percutaneous sheath and creates a vortex drawing stones less than 2.5 cm into an impeller that fragments them to particles less than 5,000 μm in size. The resulting slurry is irrigated from the gallbladder.[16]

Extracorporeal shock wave lithotripsy (ESWL) is the fragmentation of calculi by shock waves generated outside the body. The energy, targeted with fluoroscopy or ultrasound, reduces calculi to fragments of 2 mm or smaller to allow their passage from the biliary tract (Fig 13–4). Although its original widespread use was for renal stones, there is now a large experience with gallbladder and bile duct calculi.[17, 18]

Eligibility criteria for treatment of gallstones with ESWL vary between centers, but a typical

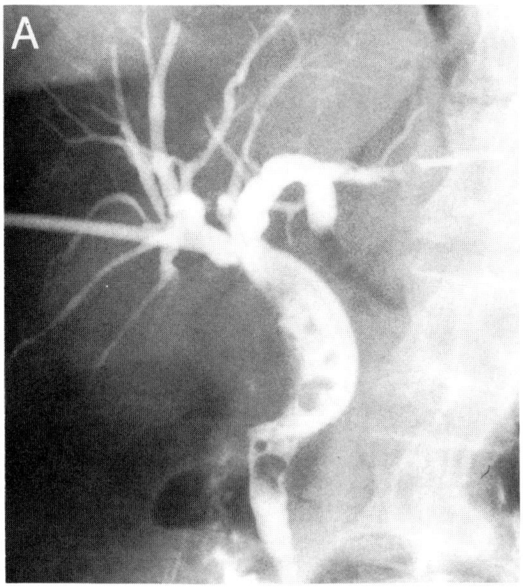

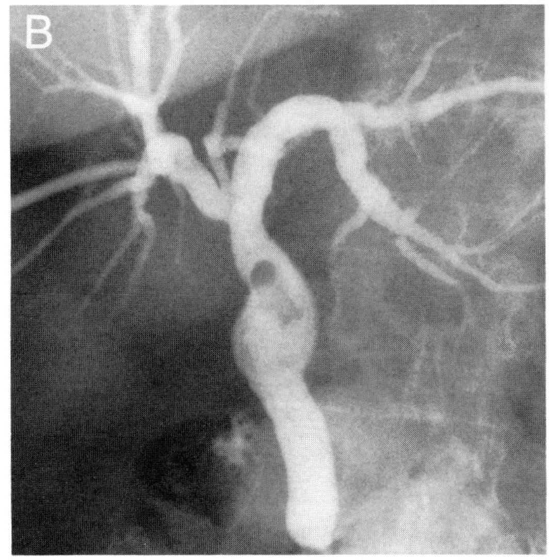

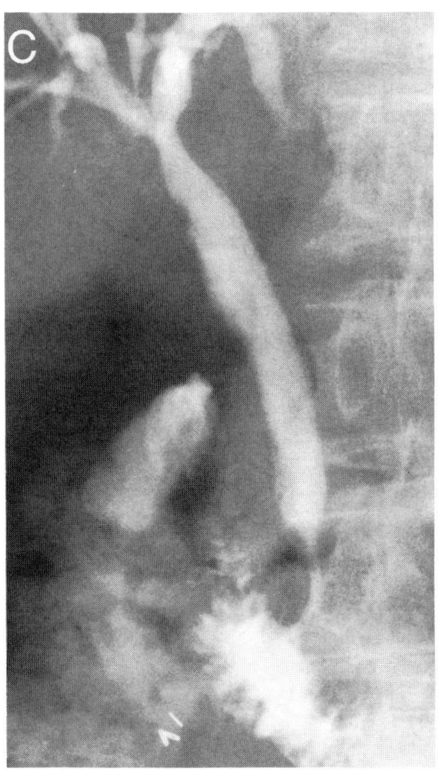

FIG 13–4.
Biliary calculus dissolution and extracorporeal lithotripsy. The patient has had a cholecystectomy. **A,** Cholangiography via a transhepatic tube shows multiple calculi of varying sizes within the common hepatic and common bile ducts. **B,** after 24 hours of MTBE infusion, a single large calculus remains unchanged. The smaller calculi have dissolved. **C,** Cholangiography after extracorporeal lithotripsy demonstrates a small amount of debris within the extrahepatic biliary tree, but the stone has been fragmented. The patient remains well 9 months after removal of the transhepatic tube.

protocol would include a history of pain related to the gallstones, a burden of radiolucent calculi not greater than 9 cm, and fewer than four stones. The gallbladder should be functioning and the stones targetable in the shock wave focus by a path that avoids lungs and bones. The patient should not have acute cholecystitis, cholangitis, or biliary obstruction, peptic ulcer disease, acute pancreatitis, coagulopathy, or vascular aneurysms in the shock wave path. In most protocols, supplemental oral dissolution therapy is given.

In 184 treatments performed on 175 patients by Sackman and colleagues,[17] gallstones disintegrated in all but one patient and completely disappeared in 30% of all patients 2 months after lithotripsy, 48% at 2 to 4 months, 63% at 4 to 8 months, 78% at 8 to 12 months, and 91% at 12 to 18 months. One third of patients experienced biliary colic, and 2 developed pancreatitis. One patient required elective cholecystectomy. Fourteen percent developed percutaneous petechiae, and transient hematuria developed in 3%.

The three major methods of shock wave generation are the spark-gap method, electromagnetic shock wave generation, and the piezoelectric shock wave generator. Efficacy of fragmentation depends upon the type and amount of energy delivered to the target site in addition to the characteristics of the stones. Gallstone size and number are more important factors in outcome than composition.[19]

Calcified gallstones have been excluded from most extracorporeal lithrotripsy protocols. Rawat and Burhenne[20] treated 38 patients with calcified stones. They found that 50% more shock waves were required, fragments cleared more slowly from the gallbladder, and there was an increased incidence of complications as compared with radiolucent stones. The authors concluded that ESWL may be applied occasionally to patients with calcified cholelithiasis if an alternative to surgery is required.

Gallstone recurrence after treatments that do not result in removal of the gallbladder is a major factor limiting the wider application of these techniques. Recurrent gallbladder calculi were found in 27% of patients examined by ultrasound 18 months after cholecystolithotomy.[21] Because of this, numerous methods have been proposed to percutaneously occlude the cystic duct and ablate the gallbladder lumen, mostly unsuccessful.[22, 23] Agents that have been introduced into the gallbladder in an attempt to seal it shut include saline, boiling contrast medium, sodium tetradecylsulfate, tetracycline, ethanol, an ethanol and trifluoracetic acid mixture, and methyl cyanocrylate. In the most recently published series, Becker and coworkers[24] were able to occlude the cystic duct in eight patients by using a radiofrequency electrocoagulation catheter. After occlusion was verified, at a mean of 5 weeks postcoagulation, sclerosis was induced the gallbladder with a mixture of 95% alcohol and 3% sodium tetradecylsulphate in one to four sessions and resulted in near complete obliteration of the gallbladder fossa in all patients.

HEPATOBILIARY INTERVENTION

Bile Duct Puncture and Drainage

The indications for biliary puncture are listed in Table 13–2. The standard approach is via the ninth intercostal space in the right midaxillary line. If the right and left ducts are noncommunicating, if there is severe right-sided atrophy, or if an interventional procedure is more easily done from this approach (see Figs 13–5 and 13–12), a left hepatic duct puncture can also be performed via the epigastric region. Either method is most frequently performed un-

TABLE 13–2.
Indications for Percutaneous Biliary Drainage*

Palliation of unresectable obstructive lesion
Improvement of hepatorenal function before surgery
Gallstone extraction
Dilatation of primary or anastomotic strictures
Cholangitis
Postsurgical or traumatic biliary leak

*Adapted from Cope C: *Percutaneous Biliary Decompression.* New York, Gower Medical Publishing, 1989, p 13.3.

der fluoroscopic guidance, although ultrasound or CT can occasionally be used. If the procedure is for diagnosis only, the needle is withdrawn after introduction of contrast. If a tract is to be established for drainage or intervention, an appropriate point of entry into the biliary tree is chosen and punctured and serial dilatation performed over a guidewire prior to insertion of a catheter at least 10 F in size.

It should be ensured that the patient has normal or correctable coagulation factors. Antibiotic coverage should be given at least 1 hour prior to ductal cannulation and continued for at least 24 hours, longer if there is biliary sepsis.

The most common acute complications are sepsis, biliary leak, and bleeding.[25] Sepsis occurs in 1.6% to 3.1% of patients and can be minimized by administering periprocedure antibiotics, minimizing the manipulation required within the biliary tree, and avoiding overdistension of the biliary radicals with radiopaque contrast. Asymptomatic bile leakage after transhepatic puncture of the bile ducts likely occurs more frequently than is appreciated, but syptomatic leakage, which may result in biliary peritonitis, occurs in 0.8% to 2.6% of cases.[26] Unless the patient is booked for a surgical procedure immediately following, if a partial or complete obstruction is suspected or confirmed at the time of bile duct puncture, a drain must be left in place. If not, a bile leak will almost certainly develop. Bleeding is most frequently venous and usually resolves spontaneously or is tamponaded by the drain. Other, less frequent acute complications include intrahepatic and perihepatic abcess and vasovagal reactions. Inadvertent puncture of the lung and colon have also been reported.

Benign Biliary Strictures

Operative trauma, which may be recognized in only half of patients at open cholecystectomy,[27] is the most frequent cause of benign bile duct stricture and accounted for 58% in one series of 2,665 noncancerous biliary strictures.[28] Stricture formation is due to to focal ischemia and fibrosis and might not manifest itself until years remote from surgery when the patient develops recurrent cholangitis or jaundice. Postoperative strictures can also occur at the site of biliary-enteric anastomosis. Less frequent causes of benign bile duct strictures include chronic pancreatitis, infective or sclerosing cholangitis, perforated duodenal ulcer, adjacent abscesses, blunt trauma, therapeutic embolization or chemotherapeutic infusion of the hepatic artery, and choledocal cysts. Benign strictures of the bile duct prevent adequate biliary drainage and are associated with biliary calculi in one third of patients. Conversely, chronic biliary calculi can cause benign biliary strictures.

Benign strictures are amenable to treatment by dilatation with a balloon angioplasty catheter[29] and should subsequently be stented with an external/internal biliary drain for approxi-

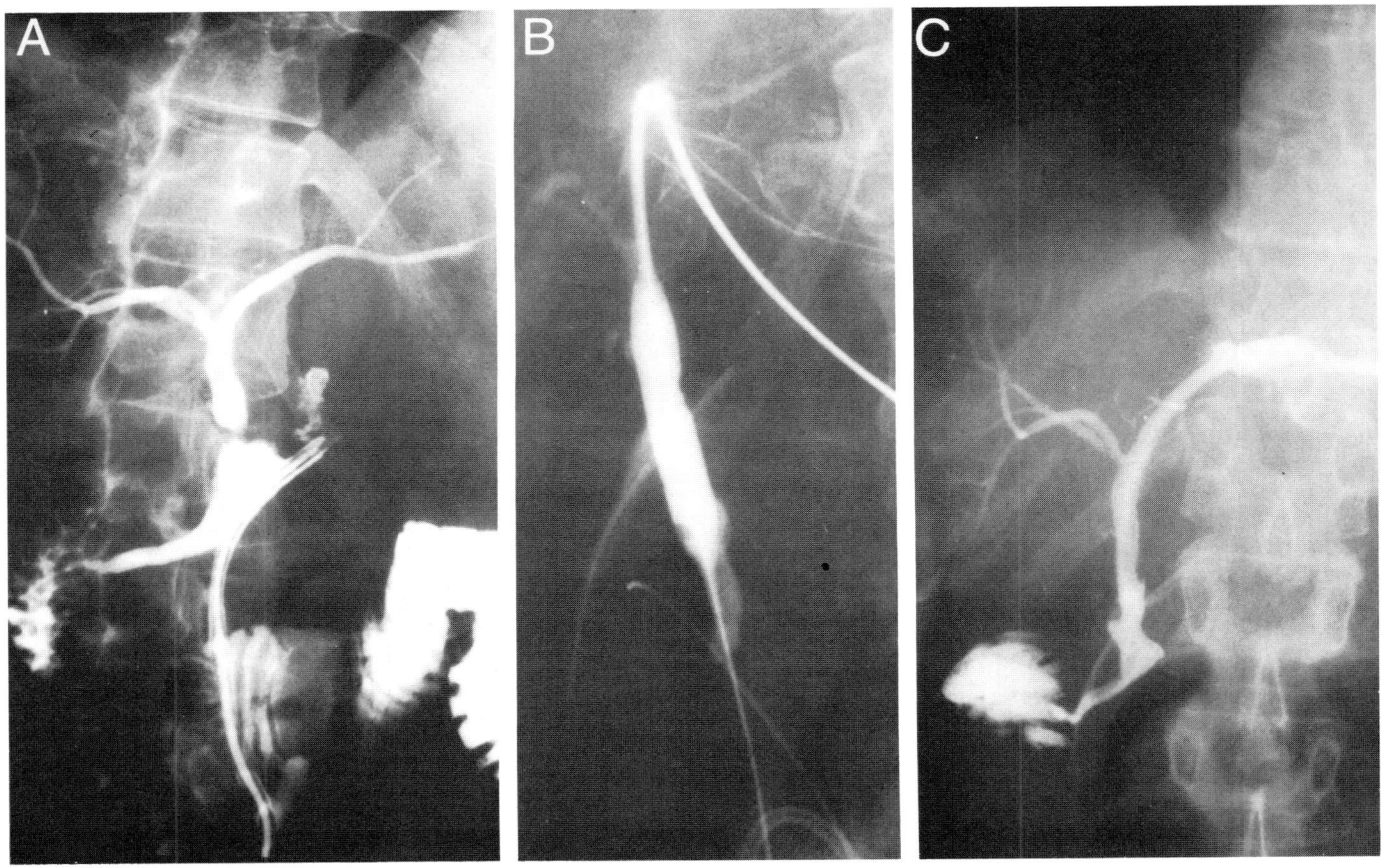

FIG 13–5.
Bile leak associated with a benign biliary stricture at the ductal anastomosis after a hepatic transplant. **A,** injection through a surgical drain reveals a tight anastamotic stricture and contrast pooling outside the bile duct. **B,** after percutaneous stenting via the left hepatic duct to control a bile leak, a balloon dilatation is performed. **C,** 4 weeks postdilatation contrast drains promptly into the duodenum with no extravasation.

mately 6 weeks (see Fig 13–5). Complications of balloon dilatation of biliary strictures occur in fewer than 5% of cases and include perforation of the bile duct, pancreatitis, vasovagal reaction, and sepsis.

The incidence of recurrence after balloon dilatation is greater for postoperative strictures than with those that occur due to other etiologies. Of 74 postoperative strictures dilated by Williams et al.,[30] 73% of 49 biliary-enteric anastamotic strictures and 88% of 25 patients with postinjury strictures were patent (by clinical criteria) at a follow-up of 1 to 58 (mean, 28) months. If the stricture recurs, redilatation via the transhepatic or endoscopic route can be performed, or the patient may be considered for placement of a metallic biliary stent[31, 32] (Fig 13–6). Metallic stents will be discussed in more detail in the section on malignant biliary strictures.

Malignant Biliary Obstruction

Because surgery is often technically difficult and the mean survival for unresectable proximal biliary duct cancer is 13 to 16 months and that for pancreatic or metastatic cancer is 4 to 6 months,[33] percutaneous biliary decompression has become a routine part of the management of malignant biliary obstruction.[34] Patients can be effectively and promptly palliated by catheter drainage without straining their already depleted metabolic reserves. In nearly 100% of cases, resolution of pruritus, fever, and jaundice can be achieved. Occasionally, the patient's

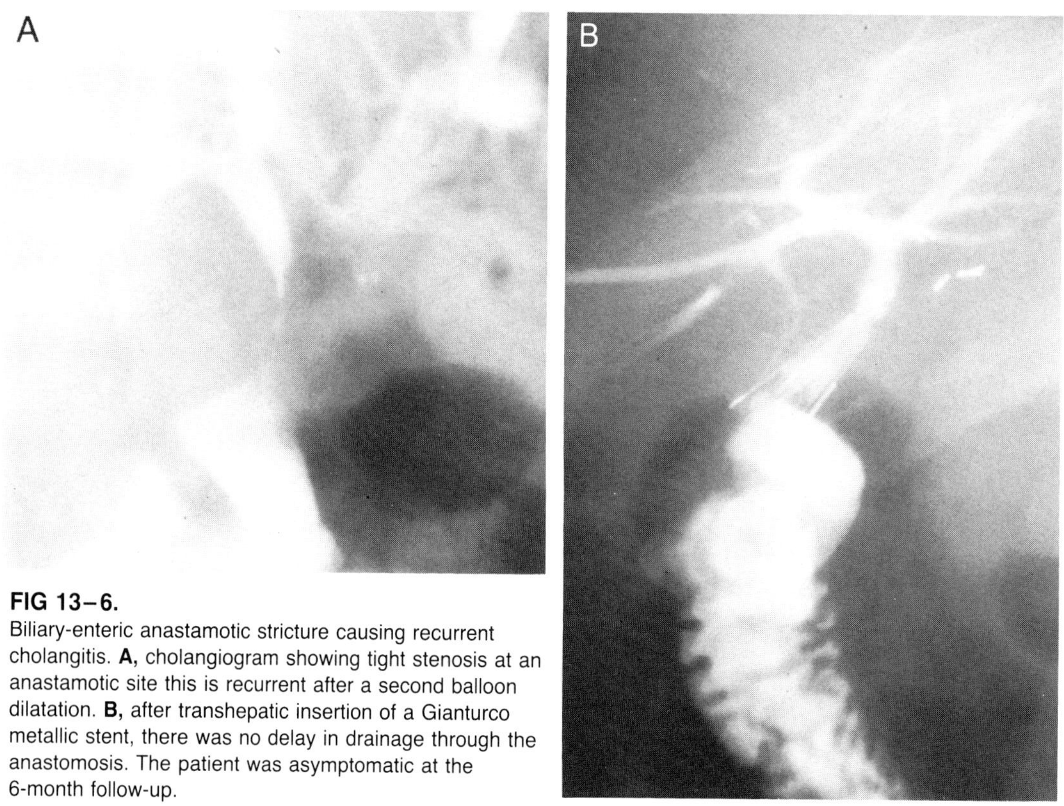

FIG 13–6.
Biliary-enteric anastamotic stricture causing recurrent cholangitis. **A,** cholangiogram showing tight stenosis at an anastamotic site this is recurrent after a second balloon dilatation. **B,** after transhepatic insertion of a Gianturco metallic stent, there was no delay in drainage through the anastomosis. The patient was asymptomatic at the 6-month follow-up.

clinical status will improve so significantly that he may become a candidate for operative bypass treatment.

The choice of method of palliating malignant biliary obstruction in any specific patient is a function of the geometry of the obstructed biliary tree, patient prognosis, patient acceptance, and the bias of the patient's physicians. Neither surgical nor radiologic palliation appears to alter patient survival[35]; therefore the goal is to provide a treatment that will be most functional and least obtrusive to the patient.

The most common method of interventional radiologic treatment is internal/external drainage (Fig 13–7); a plastic stent clamped outside the skin passes through the malignant stricture with sideholes above and below the obstructing lesion. This allows easy access for catheter exchange, which should be performed prophylactically every 12 weeks. However, these drains commonly become clogged by bile encrustations or food particles, or the sideholes can become misaligned by respiratory movements. Internal/external catheters are also prone to skin irritation or infection of the skin around the drain site, and they act as a continuous reminder to the patient of their malignancy.

For these reasons, biliary endoprostheses have been developed. These are completely internalized tubes with sideholes that, when positioned to bridge a bile duct stricture, will conduct the bile passed the stricture (Fig 13–8). These catheters have been made of various types of plastic, the most successful of which appears to polyurethane. The prosthesis should be positioned with its distal end proximal to the papilla of Vater when the location of the obstructing lesion permits. This will maintain bile sterility, and the stent will not be subjected to reflux of duodenal content. Complications include migration in 5%; occlusion by encrustation or tu-

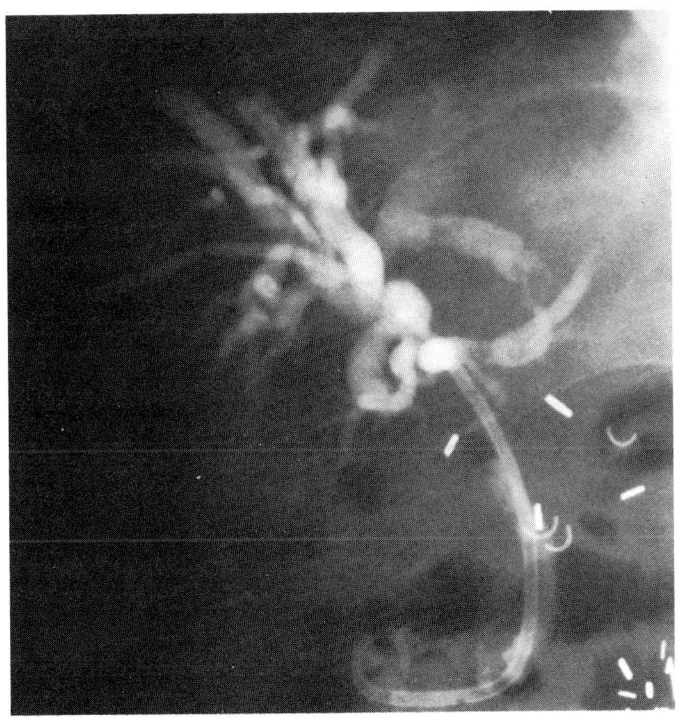

FIG 13–7.
A malignant biliary obstruction due to cholangiocarcinoma was treated with internal/external biliary drainage.

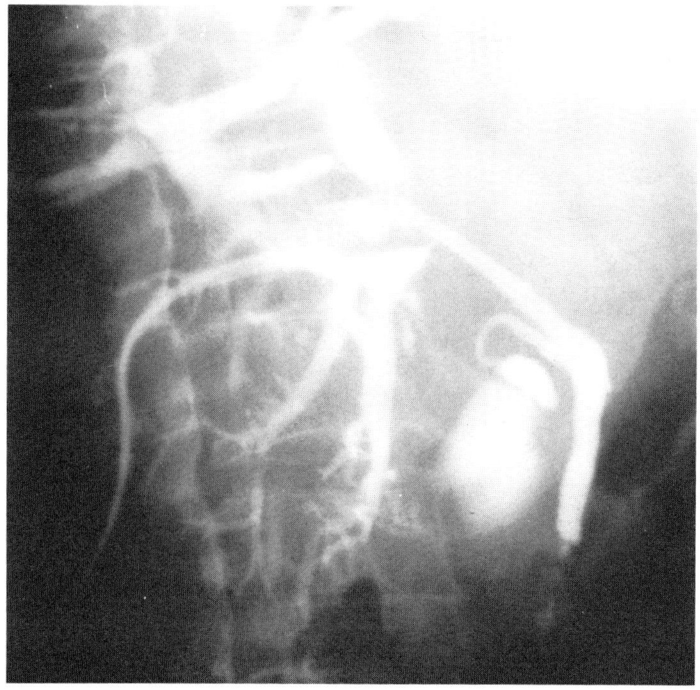

FIG 13–8.
Plastic endoprosthesis relieving a biliary obstruction in a patient with cholangiocarcinoma.

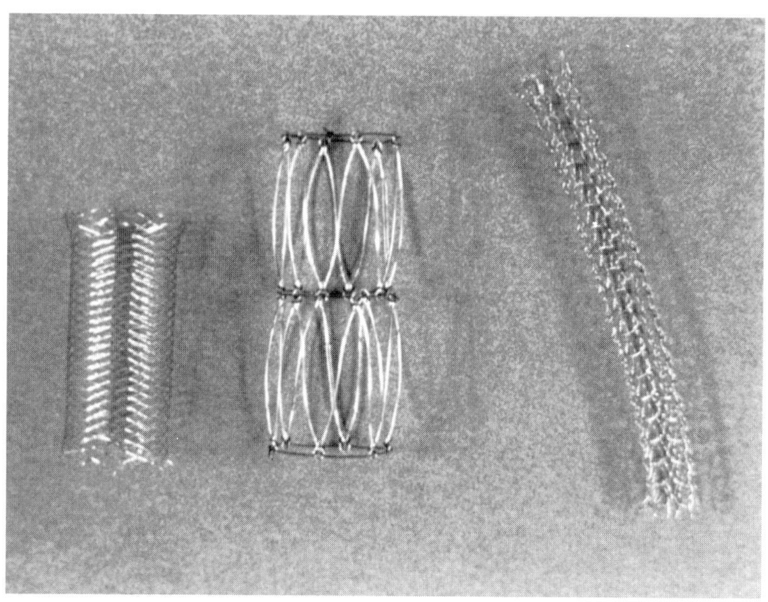

FIG 13–9.
Three types of expandable metallic stent: *Left,* Wallstent (Schneider, Minnetonka, Minn); *middle,* Gianturco Z stent (Cook Inc, Bloomington, Ind); *right,* Strecker stent (Meditech, Watertown, Mass).

mor overgrowth, which occurs in virtually 100% of patients within 1 year of placement[36]; or duodenal perforation. Although once they are occluded these endoprostheses can be removed and replaced endoscopically or radiologically,[37] patients with benign disease or slow-growing tumors whose life expectancy is greater than 1 year should not be considered for plastic endoprostheses.

A recent development, the metallic endoprosthesis ("stent") (Fig 13–9) made of stainless steel or tantalum offers several potential advantages. A large-size stent can be inserted through a relatively small tract because it is expandable. The materials, particularly stainless steel, appear much less prone to encrustation by bile deposits (which appears to be the major factor in the occlusion of plastic stents[38]), and the expanding nature of these devices enable them to hold their position in the biliary tree once deployed.

Coons[31] treated 31 patients with metallic biliary stents: 15 with benign strictures and 16 with malignant obstructions (Fig 13–10). In follow-up to 14 months, occlusions were docu-

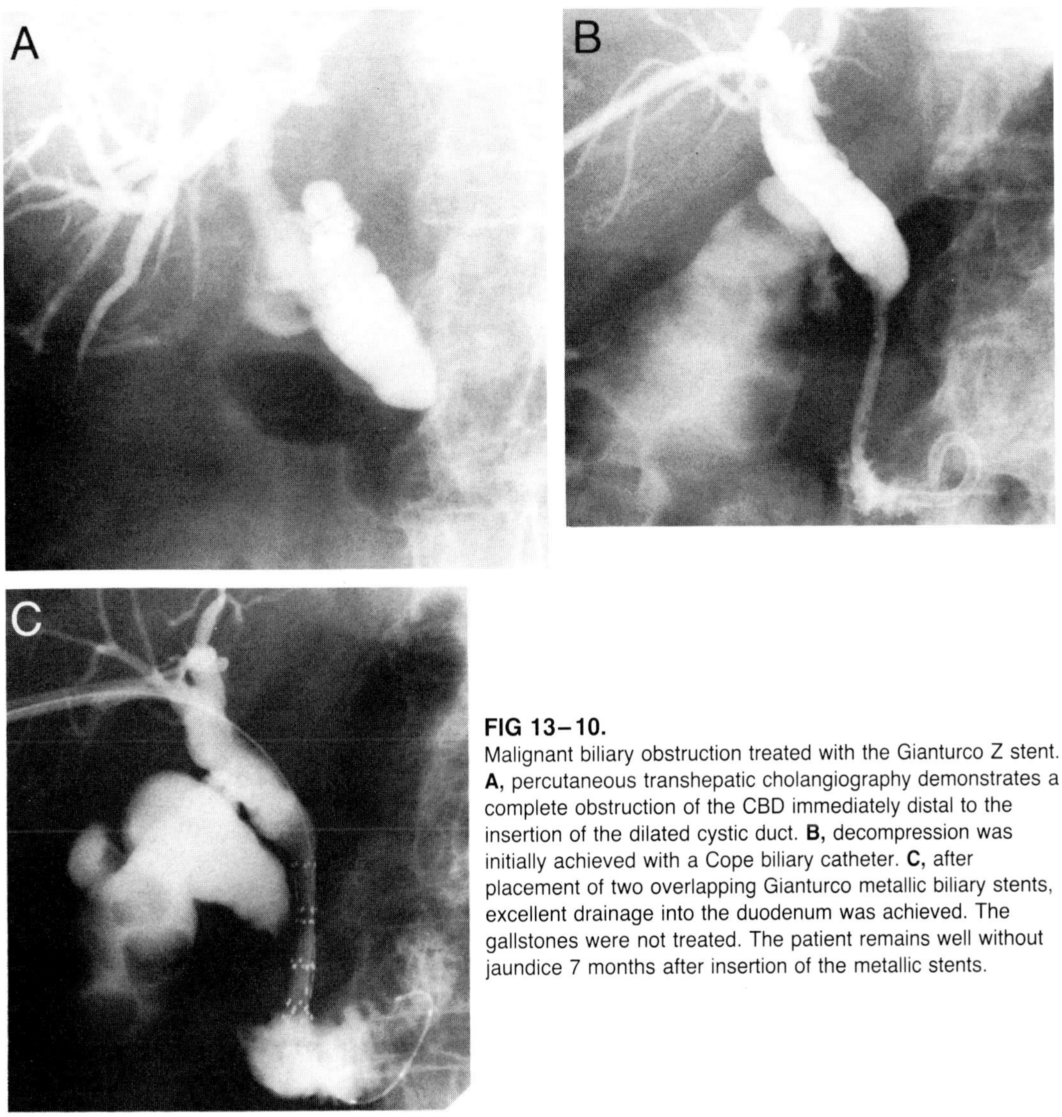

FIG 13–10.
Malignant biliary obstruction treated with the Gianturco Z stent. **A,** percutaneous transhepatic cholangiography demonstrates a complete obstruction of the CBD immediately distal to the insertion of the dilated cystic duct. **B,** decompression was initially achieved with a Cope biliary catheter. **C,** after placement of two overlapping Gianturco metallic biliary stents, excellent drainage into the duodenum was achieved. The gallstones were not treated. The patient remains well without jaundice 7 months after insertion of the metallic stents.

mented in 10% of the patients. No complications directly related to the insertion of the stainless steel stents were encountered. Two patients with malignant obstruction died, 1 at 4 months and 1 at 9 months.

Irving and colleagues[32] treated 11 patients with benign disease and 16 with malignant biliary strictures. All patients with benign disease had failed treatment with surgical reconstruction and transhepatic balloon dilatation. In follow-up to 21 months, 9 of the 11 patients with benign disease were asymptomatic. Of 16 patients with malignant strictures, 4 were alive at follow-up to 13 months without jaundice, and 2 had died without jaundice. The remainder had developed recurrent jaundice except for 1 in whom the stent had migrated within 24 hours and 1 who was lost to follow-up.

It has been suggested that a more tightly woven stent such as the Wallstent (Fig 13–11) might be more resistant to overgrowth by malignancy, although at the present time there is no hard scientific evidence to prove this or to show that metallic biliary endoprostheses justify their extra cost in the palliation of malignant biliary tract obstruction. Metallic stents do appear to be a significant advance in the treatment of benign biliary strictures.

Bile Duct Stones

The incidence of retained stones following cholecystectomy is approximately 3% to 4%. If a T-tube has been inserted at the time of cholecystectomy and the calculi are recognized prior

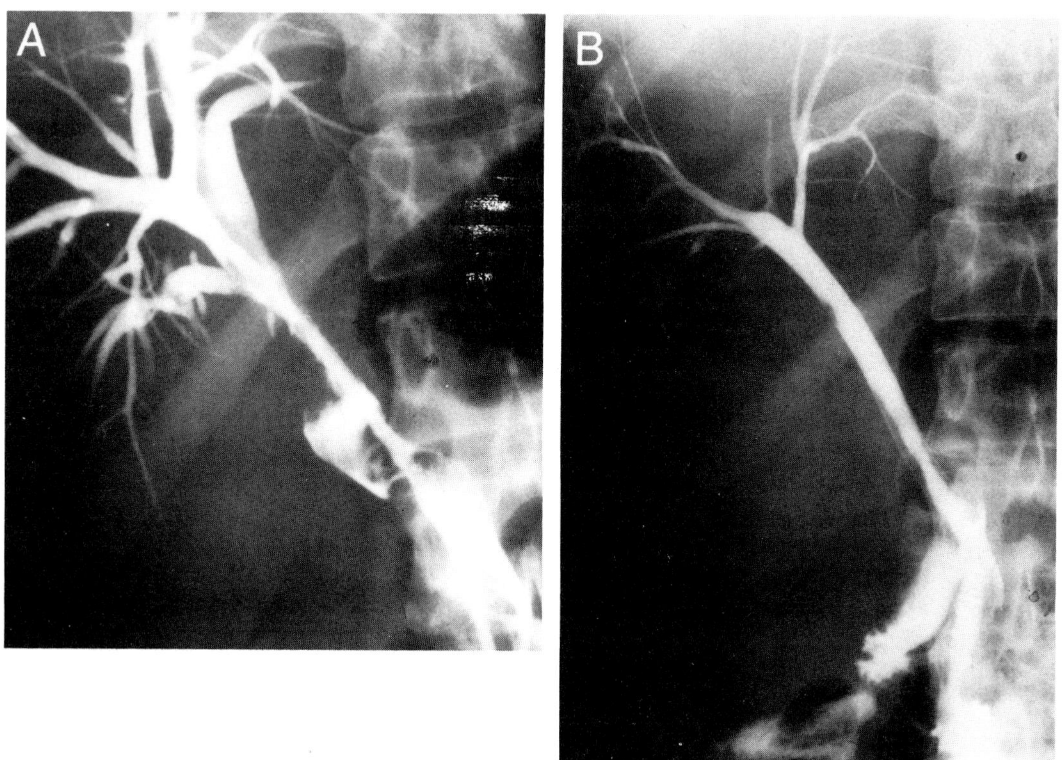

FIG 13–11.
Malignant biliary obstruction treated with the Wallstent. **A,** a long malignant stricture of the common hepatic duct and the CBD is shown. **B,** after placement of two overlapping stents, prompt drainage into the duodenum is seen.

to its removal, the tract should be allowed to mature for 5 to 6 weeks, and the stones can then be extracted via this route.[39] If the patient is not unduly frail and does not have a coagulation disorder or sepsis, the procedure can be performed as an outpatient with a high degree of success. Stones can be removed with a basket or forceps, or if the patient has multiple small stones or stone fragments, they may be pushed through the ampulla into the duodenum with a balloon.

If a CBD stone occurs or is discovered remote from the time of cholecystectomy and the patient is not a candidate for extracorporeal lithotripsy or endoscopic sphincterotomy with stone removal, the stone can be dealt with through a transhepatic tract[40] (Fig 13–12). These patients frequently have nondilated intrahepatic ducts, which makes the bile duct puncture more difficult. In one series of 54 transhepatic CBD stone removals performed on patients who were considered too high risk for surgery and had failed endoscopic procedures, a 93% success rate was achieved.[41] The complication rate was 13%, including gallstone ileus in 1 patient and pancreatitis in 1 patient, and a mortality rate of 4% was documented.

If the stone is large, fragmentation with a basket, intracorporeal lithotripsy, or a combined approach with extracorporeal lithotripsy and endoscopic sphincterotomy is recommended to avoid the creation of an unduly large transhepatic tract. Primary stones are more frequently associated with benign or malignant biliary strictures; therefore these should be looked for on cholangiography at the time of stone removal.

VASCULAR EMBOLIZATION

The deliberate occlusion of arteries, veins, or abnormal vascular spaces by embolic material injected through a selectively positioned catheter can usually be performed through a percutaneous approach under local analgesia, thus making it an attractive alternative to surgery in those patients with appropriate lesions in whom general anesthesia would pose a serious risk.[42] There are also certain lesions amenable to embolization for which no other effective form of medical or surgical therapy exists at present. Many different materials have been used to embolize blood vessels. They range from autologous substances such as fat, blood clot, and chopped muscle fragments to artificial materials such as plastic or glass beads, tantalum powder, radioactive particles, sterile absorbable gelatin sponge, oxidized cellulose, steel coils, alcohol, lyophilized human dura mater, collagen fibrils, polyvinyl alcohol sponge, silicon spheres, detachable balloons, and liquids such as alcohol, acrylates, silicones, or polyurethanes.

Embolization should always be preceded by high-quality angiography to precisely define the vascular territory under consideration, and its anastomotic communications and the catheter should be sited as selectively as possible to avoid the unintentional embolization of adjacent vascular territories.

Embolization has been used extensively in the management of acute gastrointestinal bleeding.[43, 44] Major branches in the celiac territory such as the left gastric, hepatic, gastroduodenal, or gastroepiploic arteries can be individually embolized with very little risk of infarction of normal viscera owing to the rich collateral blood supply in the upper gastrointestinal tract. Ischemic necrosis can occur, however, and the risk of this is increased if previous surgery has compromised the available collateral circulation, if there is pre-existing arterial disease, or if multiple simultaneous embolizations are performed. In the hepatobiliary system, embolization can be used to control acute bleeding from tumors, trauma, aneurysms, vascular malforma-

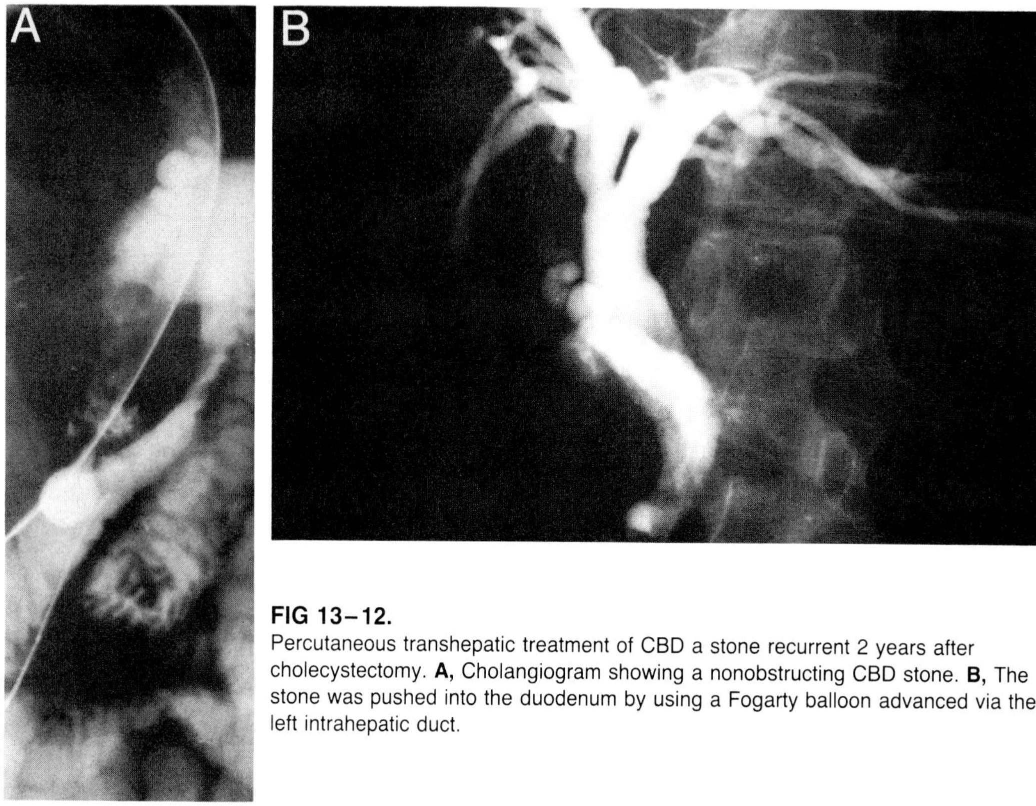

FIG 13–12.
Percutaneous transhepatic treatment of CBD a stone recurrent 2 years after cholecystectomy. **A,** Cholangiogram showing a nonobstructing CBD stone. **B,** The stone was pushed into the duodenum by using a Fogarty balloon advanced via the left intrahepatic duct.

tions, or iatrogenic bleeding due to recent biopsy or surgery.[45] Bleeding from varices can also be controlled by embolization, access to the portal venous system being achieved by a percutaneous transhepatic approach.[46]

Embolization can be used in the nonacute situation in the treatment of hepatobiliary vascular malformations. These can arise spontaneously or can occur secondary to surgical trauma (Fig 13–13). Benign tumors such as hepatic hemangioma can sometimes be successfully treated by embolization alone and can also be used as a primary mode of treatment in inoperable malignancy,[47] and the embolization of metastatic deposits has been shown to extend survival times in patients with advanced disease.[48]

PERCUTANEOUS DRAINAGE OF ABSCESSES AND FLUID COLLECTIONS

Although morbidity and mortality have decreased since the introduction of antibiotics, the overall incidence of postoperative abscess formation has not changed in that time.[49] The ability to localize abscesses precisely and define their position relative to adjacent intra-abdominal viscera has led to the development of radiologically guided percutaneous drainage using angiographic techniques (Fig 13–14). These procedures can be successfully applied to postoperative abdominal abscesses, thereby avoiding the morbidity of repeat surgery, and cure rates

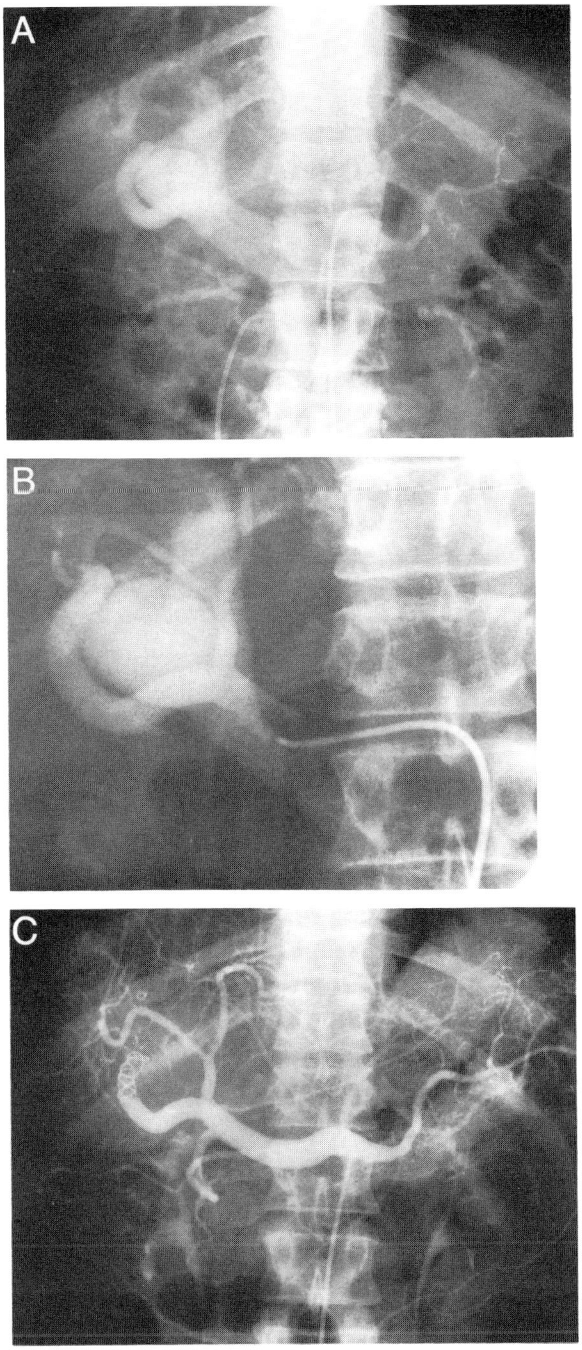

FIG 13–13.

Embolization of the hepatic artery to a portal vein fistula. This patient had unexplained portal hypertension 6 months after cholecystectomy. **A,** celiac artery injection. Simultaneous with filling of the arterial system, there is opacification of the portal vein. Note the faint opacification of the hepatic artery due to the massive flow. **B,** injection of the hepatic artery. There is a large communication between the right hepatic artery and a bulbous dilatation of the right portal vein. **C,** postembolization celiac arteriogram. The celiac axis is now much better opacified, and the shunt has been obliterated.

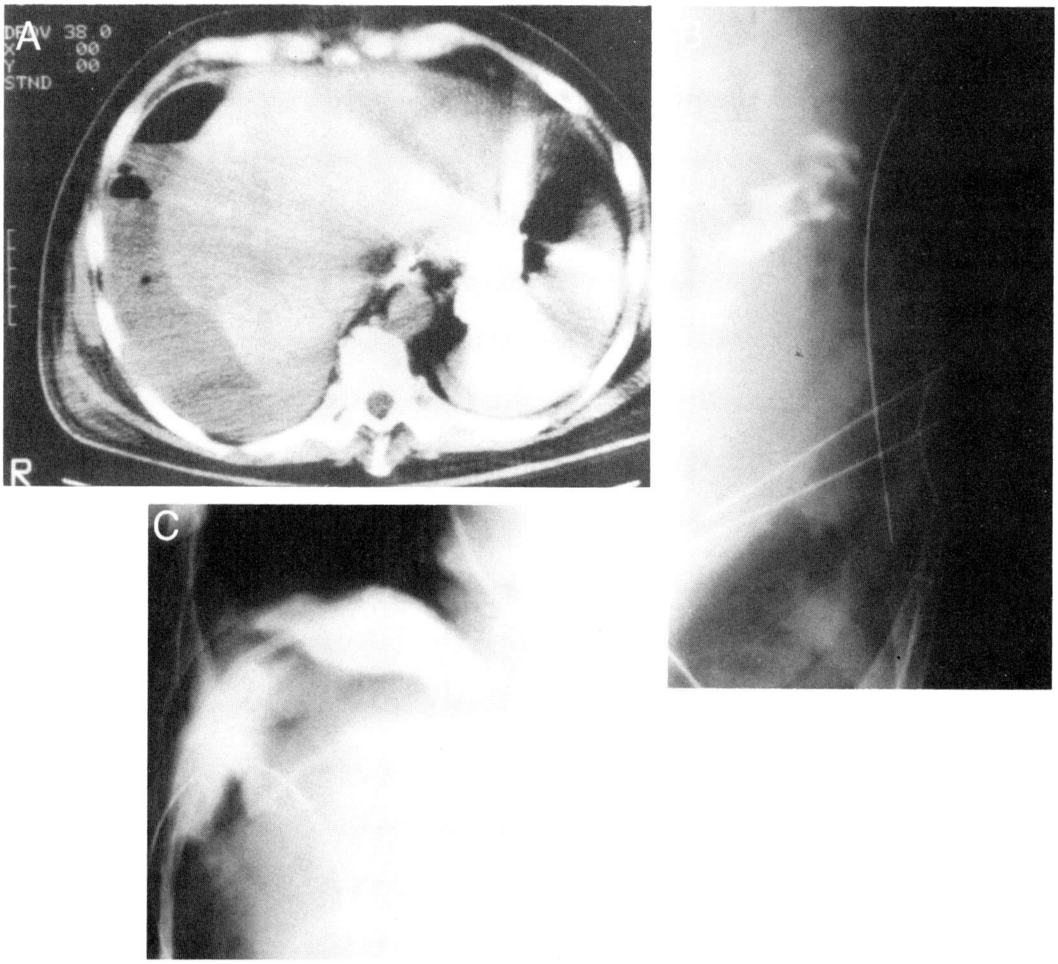

FIG 13–14.
Percutaneous drainage of a hepatic subcapsular abscess. **A,** CT scan showing gas-containing subcapsular fluid collection. **B,** to avoid transgressing the pleural space, a curved needle was angled subcostally. Note the gas in the abscess. **C,** sinogram obtained after one pigtail catheter was placed in each locule of the abscess.

of 80% or better have been reported.[50] However, the prognosis for success in any given patient should be taken on the specifics of that situation rather than from large reported series because each case seems to have some unique features. Factors that can lead to prolongation or failure of percutaneous abscess drainage[51] include multiple abscess cavities or loculations that cannot be drained individually; a drainage route traversing bowel, contaminated peritoneal or pleural spaces, or contaminated organs; a source of continuous contamination; and fungal infections. These are not all absolute contraindications to percutaneous drainage, but if one or more is present, other means of treatment should be considered.

Enteric communications with abdominal abscesses are frequently uncovered after drainage. Most are low-output fistulas and clinically occult. High-output fistulas are extremely difficult to cure with percutaneous techniques and are usually heralded by continuous high output through a percutaneous drain. If a low-output enteric communication to a percutaneously drained abscess is discovered, the success of nonoperative therapy depends upon the absence

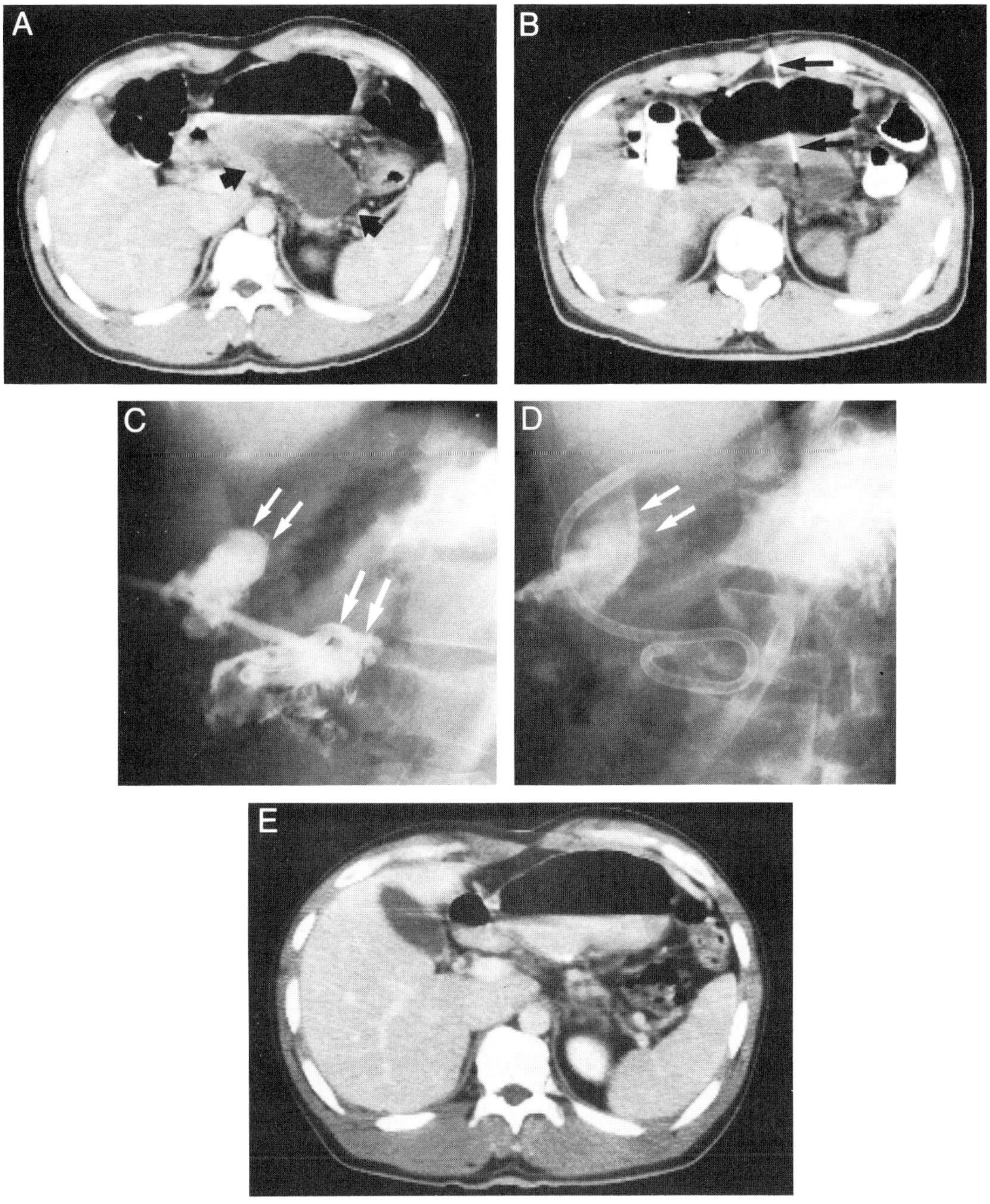

FIG 13–15.

Transgastric drainage of a pseudocyst caused by gallstone-induced acute pancreatitis. **A,** CT of the abdomen demonstrates a pseudocyst *(large arrows)* immediately adjacent to the posterior wall of the stomach. **B,** under CT guidance, a needle *(arrow)* was passed through the anterior abdominal wall and stomach into the pseudocyst. **C,** lateral view after placement of a percutaneous drain through the stomach *(small arrows)* into the pseudocyst *(large arrows).* **D,** 2 weeks later, the tube was internalized by severing at the skin so that the loop remains within the pseudocyst and the stem of the catheter is seen within the stomach *(small arrows).* **E,** CT scan 2 months later. The tube has been spontaneously passed. Resolution of the pseudocyst with only a small amount of residual soft-tissue thickening is seen.

of obstruction in the bowel distal to the site of the fistula, control of the bowel effluent with an adequately sized and positioned catheter, drainage of associated abscesses, nutrional support, and the condition of the involved segment of bowel. More than 80% of patients with a low-output fistula between the bowel and an abdominal abscess cavity can be cured by percutaneous drainage.[52]

Noninfected postoperative fluid collections are common after both operative and laparoscopic cholecystectomy and usually resolve spontaneously. They can be aspirated under ultrasound or CT guidance if fluid is required for bacteriologic analysis or rarely if the patient has local symptoms referable to a loculated collection. Most simple loculated postoperative fluid collections will not recur after aspiration with a skinny needle.

Pseudocyst formation secondary to pancreatitis may occur as a direct result of gallstones or biliary manipulation or surgery, among other causes. Single-step fine-needle aspiration is curative in only 22% of patients[53] and should usually be performed for diagnostic purposes, such as in the differential diagnosis between pseudocyst and cystadenoma or to exclude infection. Percutaneous drainage, either by direct external drainage or preferably via a transgastric route, is more successful. After a percutaneous transgastric tract has been allowed to mature, the drain can be internalized (Fig 13–15), and the catheter will be either digested or passed via the alimentary tract, leaving the cystogastrostomy open and the patient without an operative scar or an external tube. In a large series of percutaneously treated pancreatic pseudocysts reported by Grosso et al.,[54] recurrence was seen in 71% of patients drained with single-step needle aspiration, in 27% of patients treated by direct extragastric percutaneous catheter drainage, and in no patients treated with transgastric external drainage or by percutaneous cystogastrostomy, although there were only seven patients in each of the last two groups.

REFERENCES

1. Cope C: Percutaneous subhepatic cholecystostomy with removable anchor. *AJR* 1988; 151:1129–1132.
2. Teplick SK: Diagnostic and therapeutic interventional gallbladder procedures. *AJR* 1989; 152:9–13.
3. Eggermont AM, Lameris JS, Jeekel J: Ultrasound-guided percutaneous transhepatic cholecystostomy for acute acalculous cholecystitis. *Arch Surg* 1985; 120:1354–1356.
4. Crocker JR: Biliary tract disease in the elderly. *Clin Gastroenterol* 1985; 14:773–809.
5. Glenn F: Surgical management of acute cholecystitis in patients 65 years of age and older. *Ann Surg* 1981; 193:56–59.
6. McGahan JP, Lindfors KK: Percutaneous cholecystostomy: An alternative to surgical cholecystostomy for acute cholecystitis? *Radiology* 1989; 173:481–485.
7. Picus D, Marx MV, Hicks ME, et al: Percutaneous cholecystolithotomy: Preliminary experience and technical considerations. *Radiology* 1989; 173:487–491.
8. Gibney RG, Fache JS, Becker CD, et al: Combined surgical and radiologic intervention for complicated cholelithiasis in high-risk patients. *Radiology* 1987; 165:715–719.
9. Haskin PH, Teplick SK, Sammon JK, et al: Monooctanion infusion and stone removal through the transparenchymal tract: Use in 17 patients. *AJR* 1987; 148:185–188.
10. VanSonnenberg E, Hofmann AF, Neoptolemus J, et al: Gallstone dissolution with methyl tert-butyl ether via percutaneous cholecystostomy: Success and caveats. *AJR* 1986; 146:865–867.
11. Allen MH, Borody TH, Bugliosi TF, et al: Rapid dissolution of gallstones by methyl tert-butyl ether. *N Engl J Med* 1985; 312:217–220.

12. Picus D, Weyman PJ, Marx MV: Role of percutaneous intracorporeal electrohydraulic lithotripsy in the treatment of biliary tract calculi. *Radiology* 1989; 170:989–993.
13. Hruby W, Stackl W, Urban M, et al: Percutaneous endoscopic cholecystolithotripsy: Work in progress. *Radiology* 1989; 173:477–479.
14. Nishioka NS, Levins PC, Murray SC, et al: Fragmentation of biliary calculi with tunable dye lasers. *Gastroenterology* 1987; 93:250–255.
15. Ell CH, Lux G, Hochberger J, et al: Laser lithotripsy of common bile duct stones. *Gut* 1988; 29:746–751.
16. Miller FJ, Kensey K, Nash J: Experimental percutaneous gallstone lithotripsy: Results in swine. *Radiology* 1989; 170:985–987.
17. Sackman M, Delius M, Sauerbruch T, et al: Shock wave lithotripsy of gallbladder stones: The first 175 patients. *N Engl J Med* 1988; 318:393–397.
18. Ferrucci JT: Biliary lithotripsy: 1989. *AJR* 1989; 153:15–22.
19. Schachler R, Sauerbruch T, Wosiewitz U, et al: Fragmentation of gallstones using extracorporeal shock waves: An in vitro study. *Hepatology* 1988; 8:925–929.
20. Rawat B, Burhenne HJ: Extracorporeal shock wave lithotripsy of calcified gallstones: Work in progress. *Radiology* 1990; 175:667–670.
21. Gibney RG, Chow K, So CB, et al: Gallstone recurrence after cholecystolithotomy. *AJR* 1989; 153:287–289.
22. Martin EC, Gertrajdmaj GI: Does the gallbladder have a future? *Radiology* 1989; 170:969–973.
23. Salomonowitz E, Frick MP, Simmons RL, et al: Obliteration of the gallbladder without formal cholecystectomy. *Arch Surg* 1984; 119:725–729.
24. Becker CD, Fache JS, Malone DE, et al: Ablation of the cystic duct and gallbladder: Clinical observations. *Radiology* 1990; 176:687–690.
25. Kadir S (ed): *Diagnostic Radiology.* Philadelphia, WB Saunders Co, 1986, pp 642–678.
26. Juhler GL, Conroy RM, Fuellman RW: Bile leakage following percutaneous transhepatic cholangiography with the Chiba needle. *Arch Surg* 1977; 112:954–958.
27. Way LW, Dunphy JE. Biliary stricture. *Am J Surg* 1972; 124:287–295.
28. Smith R: Obstructions of the bile duct. *Br J Surg* 1979; 66:69–79.
29. Trambert JJ, Bron KM, Zajko AB, et al: Percutaneous transhepatic balloon dilatation of benign biliary strictures. *AJR* 1987; 149:945–948.
30. Williams HJ, Bender CE, May GR: Benign postoperative biliary strictures: Dilatation with fluoroscopic guidance. *Radiology* 1987; 163:629–634.
31. Coons H: Self-expanding stainless steel biliary stents. *Radiology* 1989; 170:979–983.
32. Irving JD, Adam A, Dick R, et al: Gianturco expandable metallic biliary stents: Results of a European clinical trial. *Radiology* 1989; 172:321–326.
33. Ottow RT, August DA, Sugarbaker PH: Treatment of proximal biliary tract carcinoma: An overview of technique and results. *Surgery* 1985; 97:251–266.
34. Ferrucci JT, Mueller PR (eds): *Interventional Radiology of the Abdomen,* ed 2. Baltimore, Williams & Wilkins, 1985, pp 184–249.
35. Bonel D, Ferrucci JT Jr, Mueller PR, et al: Surgical and radiological decompression in malignant biliary obstruction: A retrospective study using multivariate risk factor analysis. *Radiology* 1984; 152:347–351.
36. Lammer J, Neumayer K: Biliary drainage endoprostheses: Experience with 201 placements. *Radiology* 1986; 159:625–629.
37. Lee MJ, Mueller PR, Saini S, et al: Occlusion of biliary endoprostheses: Presentation and management. *Radiology* 1990; 176:531–534.
38. Speer AG, Farrington H, Costerton JW, et al: Bacteria, biofilms and biliary sludge (abstract). *Gut* 1986; 27:601.
39. Burhenne HJ: Percutaneous extraction of retained biliary stones: 661 patients. *AJR* 1980; 134:888–898.

40. Clouse ME, Falchuk KR: Percutaneous transhepatic removal of common duct stones. *Gastroenterology* 1983; 85:815–819.
41. Stokes KR, Falchuk KR, Clouse ME: Biliary duct stones: Update on 54 cases after percutaneous transhepatic removal. *Radiology* 1989; 170:999–1001.
42. Allison DJ: Therapeutic embolization. *Br J Hosp Med* 1978; 20:707–715.
43. Uflacker R: Transcatheter embolization for treatment of acute lower gastrointestinal bleeding. *Acta Radiol* 1987; 28:425–430.
44. Reuter SR, Chuang VP, Bree RI: Selective arterial embolization for control for massive upper gastrointestinal bleeding. *AJR* 1975; 125:119–126.
45. Chang J, Katzen BT, Sullivan KP: Transcatheter gelfoam embolization of posttraumatic bleeding pseudoaneurysms. *AJR* 1978; 131:645–650.
46. L'Hermine C, Chastanet P, Delemazure O, et al: Percutaneous transhepatic embolization of gastroesophageal varices: Results in 400 patients. *AJR* 1989; 152:755–760.
47. Chuang VP, Wallace S: Hepatic artery embolization in the treatment of hepatic neoplasms. *Radiology* 1981; 140:51–58.
48. Blumgart LH, Allison DJ: Resection and embolization in the management of secondary hepatic tumors. *World J Surg* 1982; 6:32–45.
49. Altemeier WA, Culbertson WR, Fullen WD, et al: Intraabdominal abscesses. *Am J Surg* 1973; 125:70–79.
50. Martin EC, Karlson KB, Fankuchen EI, et al: Percutaneous drainage of postoperative intraabdominal abscesses. *AJR* 1982; 138:13–15.
51. Aeder MI, Wellman JL, Haaga JR, et al: Role of surgical and percutaneous drainage in the treatment of abdominal abscesses. *Arch Surg* 1983; 118:273–280.
52. Kerlan RK, Jeffrey RB, Pogany AC, et al: Abdominal abscess with low output fistulae: Successful percutaneous drainage. *Radiology* 1985; 155:73–75.
53. Barkin JS, Smith FR, Pereiras R, et al: Therapeutic percutaneous aspiration of pancreatic pseudocysts. *Dig Dis Sci* 1981; 26:585–586.
54. Grosso M, Gandini G, Cassinis MC, et al: Percutaneous treatment (including pseudocystogastrostomy) of 74 pancreatic pseudocysts. *Radiology* 1989; 173:493–497.

Chapter 14

Intraluminal Ultrasound Imaging

Marwan R. Tabbara, M.D.

Rodney A. White, M.D.

Contrast studies are the oldest available method to image the alimentary tract. Barium sulfate became established as the contrast medium of choice in 1910 and has remained so ever since.[1] Gross obstruction, luminal filling defects, and mucosal irregularities can be diagnosed. The exact nature of the lesions is not always apparent because histologic diagnosis is not possible. The advent of fiber-optic endoscopy in 1956 was a historic event that allowed the physician to actually visualize the mucosal surface of the gastrointestinal (GI) tract and to obtain biopsy specimens.[2] However, submucosal lesions could not be directly visualized, and other imaging modalities like computed tomographic (CT) scanning, magnetic resonance imaging (MRI), or transcutanous ultrasound had to be used. These techniques are all limited by inadequate resolution to clearly define the different layers of the wall of the GI tract and adjacent lymphatic structures or organs.[3–7] The advantage of intraluminal ultrasound (IUS) or endoscopic ultrasound (EUS) is that it can use higher frequencies than transcutanous ultrasound and therefore achieve better resolution.[8, 9] The ultrasound waves are not attenuated by intervening skin and soft tissue.

Intraluminal vascular ultrasound is developing rapidly as a method to define the transmural anatomy of tubular organs. Current devices use various configurations of transducers at the end of an intraluminal catheter to make real-time images. These devices may have diagnostic applications, particularly at the time of endoscopy, angiography, or other diagnostic procedures.[10] The thrust of enthusiasm for current development is as an adjunct to current intraluminal diagnostic and therapeutic procedures. This technology offers a method of three-dimensional diagnostic analysis and is a method of precise guidance of intraluminal instruments to provide concentric recanalizations of stenotic or occluded tubular structures.

Recent advances in the catheter-based technology have led to the current IUS devices. The ultrasound images are generated by using 7.5- to 50-MHz transducers incorporated into the tip of a 3 to 15 F diameter catheter. Although high-frequency ultrasound has limited tissue penetration, it is adequate to produce images when used in an intraluminal position. At 20 MHz, the usable depth of penetration in liquid medium is approximately 2.0 to 4.0 cm.[11] At 50 MHz the resolution of the images is finer but has less penetration. When better tissue penetration is desired, lower frequencies and/or more power from longer aperatures must be

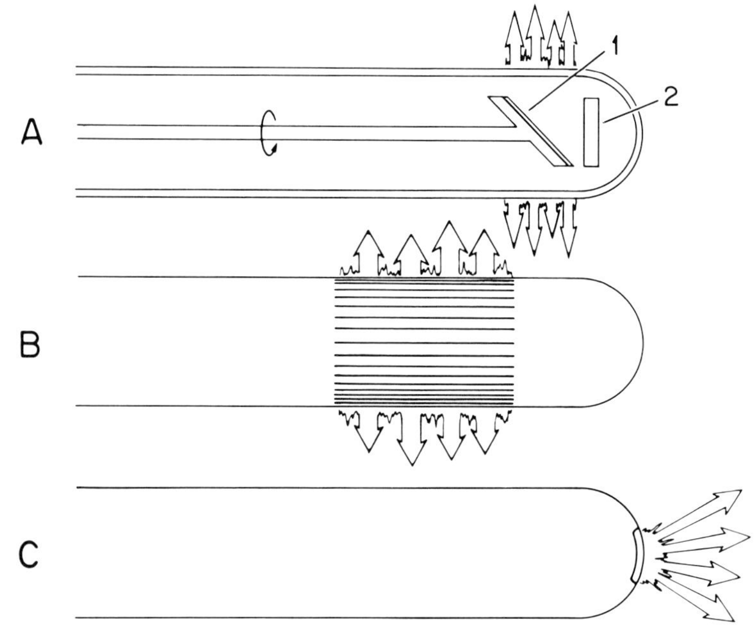

FIG 14–1.
A, schematic of a prototype mechanical ultrasound device with rotating (1) and fixed (2) elements. Either the transducer or the mirror may be fixed with the other element in a rotating position. **B,** schematic of a phased array device with the elements arranged circumferentially around the tip of the catheter. **C,** pizoelectric transducers placed close to each other at the tip of the catheter with a fan-shaped sector scanning pattern.

used. For smaller tubular structures such as blood vessels, higher frequency can provide visualization comparable to lower-frequency devices in larger tubular organs.

Piezoelectric transducers are used to generate the ultrasound images by mechanically rotating either an echotransducer or a mirror on the tip of a catheter and scanning by an array of stationary elements either lateral to or forward from the axis of the catheter (Fig 14–1).

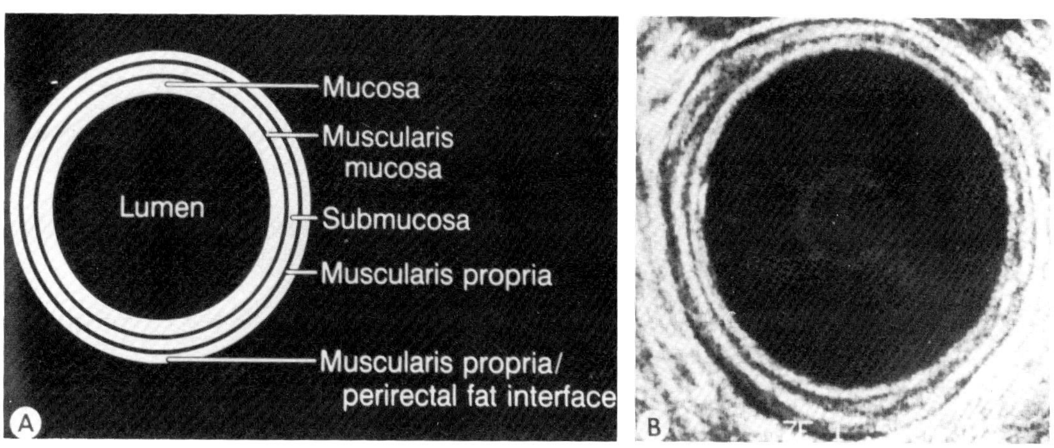

FIG 14–2.
Diagram **(A)** and axial ultrasonogram **(B)** of the five ultrasonagraphically visualized layers of rectal wall. (From Jochem RJ, Reading CC, Dozois RR, et al: *Mayo Clin Proc* 1990; 65:1571–1577. Used by permission.)

Each of these types of device has advantages and limitations that affect the design of functioning catheters, and they require electronics to image-process and display the signals. The rotating intraluminal devices are simpler to manufacture, but the rotating transducer prototypes are more difficult to use in tortuous lumens due to the necessity for rotating transducer connecting wires. This disadvantage is eliminated by the rotating mirror design or the multielement phase array configurations, although the increased electronic connection required in phase-array devices is difficult to miniaturize. Integrated circuits at the catheter tip may permit sequenced transmission while improving flexibility and simplifying manufacturing by reducing the number of wires in the catheter. Phase-array catheters also have a disadvantage

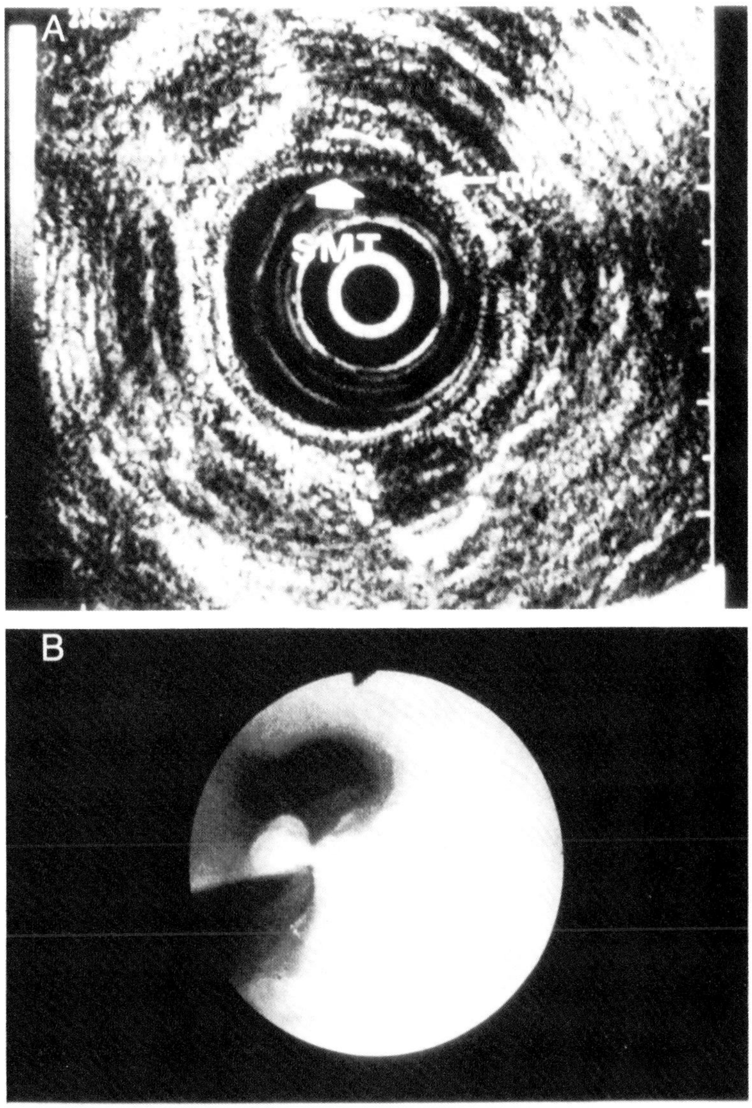

FIG 14–3.
A, leiomyoma *(SMT)* located in the submucosal layer. The fourth layer *(mp)* can be seen under the tumor. **B,** it was removed by endoscopic polypectomy. (From Murata Y, et al: *Surg Endosc* 1988; 2:51–58. Used by permission.)

of image loss close to the perimeter of the device ("dead zone or ring-down artifact"); this can be eliminated in some of the mechanical prototypes. Side-viewing (images being a slice of the vessel perpendicular to the catheter) and forward- and back-viewing images are also possible in certain designs. In general, as catheter size increases, image quality improves. Forward-viewing sector scanning devices produce a fan-shaped viewing field. The drawbacks of these devices are that they have complicated circuits and a narrow viewing field of short distances. It is likely that various systems will be used depending upon the specific application.

ULTRASOUND IMAGING OF THE GASTROINTESTINAL TRACT

In general, the ultrasound image of the wall of the GI tract (mainly the esophagus and rectum) is composed of five layers[12]: (1) fluid/mucosal interface (hyperechoic), (2) deep portion of the mucosa including the muscularis mucosae (hypoechoic), (3) submucosa and submucosa/muscularis propria interface (hyperechoic), (4) muscularis propria (hypoechoic), and (5) serosa and periserosal fat (hyperechoic) (Fig 14–2). This is applicable to most portions of the GI tract that are accessible for ultrasound evaluation including the esophagus, stomach, duodenum, colon, and rectum.

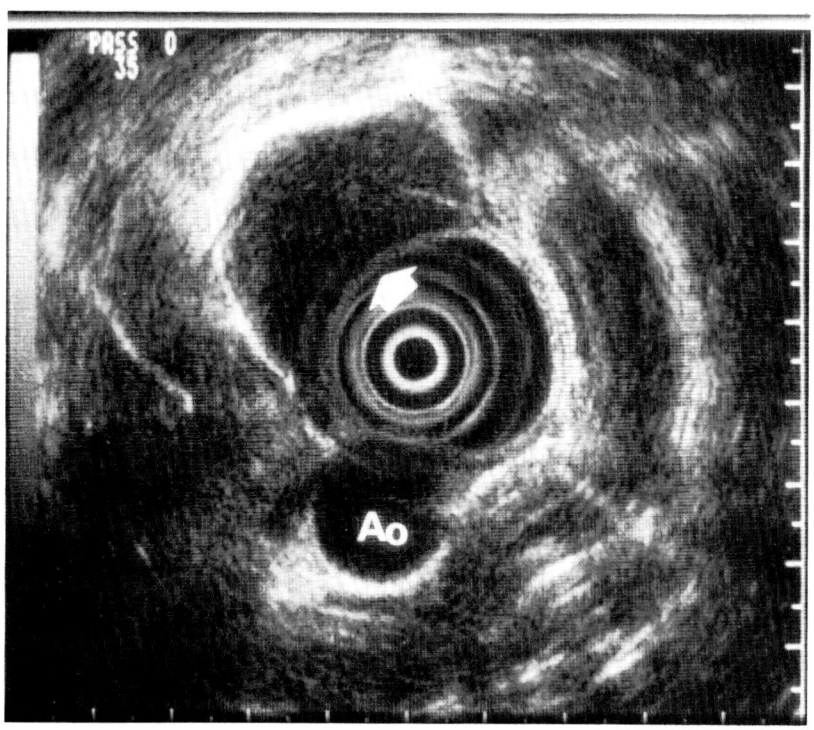

FIG 14–4.
Tracheobronchial cyst *(arrow)* in the esophagus. *Ao* = aorta. (From Murata Y, et al: *Surg Endosc* 1988; 2:51–58. Used by permission.)

BENIGN LESIONS

Diagnosis of benign lesions of the GI tract can be accurately done for the submucosal tumor by demonstrating the tumor tissue, size, and growth direction. A characteristic EUS image has been demonstrated with leiomyoma (Fig 14–3), cysts (Fig 14–4), lipoma, and varices.[13, 14] The ability of EUS to detect malignancy in biopsy proven sessile tubulovillous adenoma by visualization of transmural tumor growth has not been proved in larger series.[15] Peptic ulcer depth can also be determined accurately and the healing process observed. The use of EUS has been reported in patients with perirectal abscesses and fistulas. This technique might have an impact in patients with Crohn's disease and complicated perirectal lesions (Fig 14–5).[16]

MALIGNANT LESIONS

Accurate staging of malignant lesions can be done with EUS. The typical appearance of a malignant tumor is an echo-poor or nonhomogeneous lesion with irregular borders. The in-

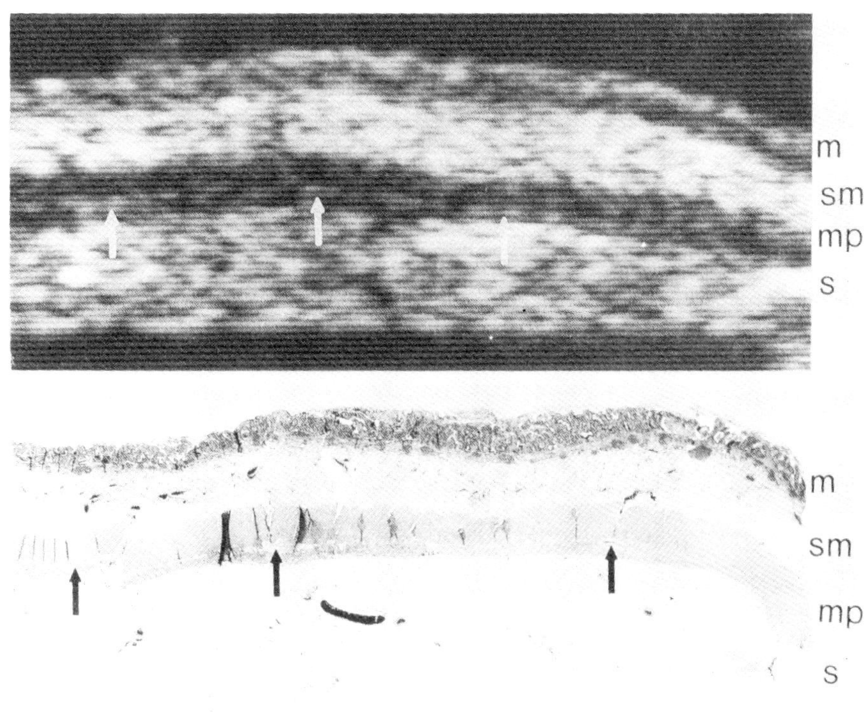

FIG 14–5.
The ultrasound image *(top)* and corresponding histologic section of the segment of rectum from a patient with ulcerative colitis are shown. Mucosa *(m)* submucosa *(sm)*, muscularis propria *(mp)*, connective tissue between the two layers of muscularis propria *(arrows)*, and serosa submucosa *(s)* are shown. (From Kimmey MB, et al: Ultrasound interaction with the intestinal wall: Esophagus, stomach of colon, in Kamar K (ed): *Endoscopic Ultrasonography In Gastroenterology*, ed 1. Tokyo, Igaku-Shoin, 1988, pp 35–44. Used by permission.)

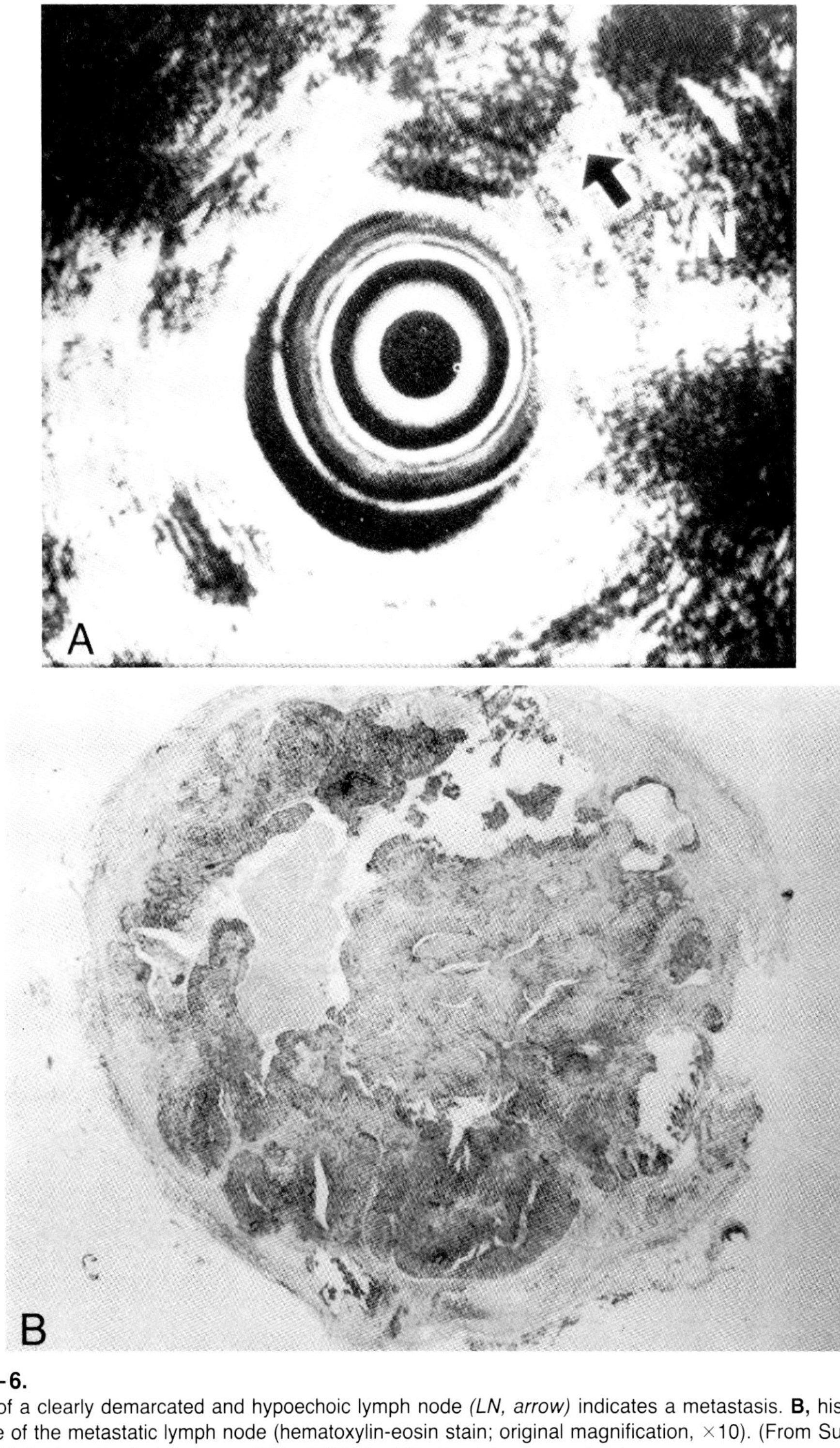

FIG 14–6.
A, EUS of a clearly demarcated and hypoechoic lymph node *(LN, arrow)* indicates a metastasis. **B,** histologic appearance of the metastatic lymph node (hematoxylin-eosin stain; original magnification, ×10). (From Sugimachi K, Ohno S, Fujishima H, et al: *Surgery* 1991; 107:366–371. Used by permission.)

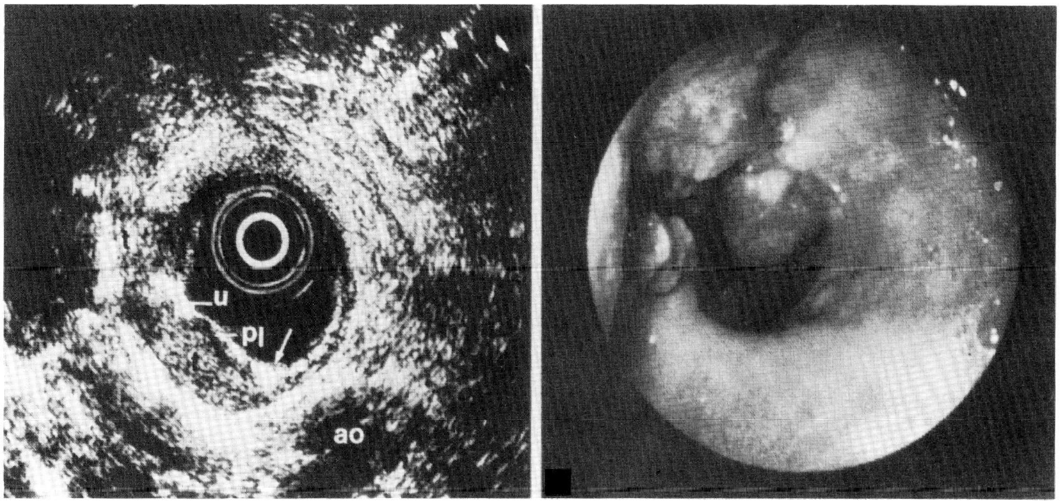

FIG 14–7.
A, EUS shows an ulcerative hypoechoic tumor mass *(t)* with polypoid margins *(pl)* penetrating into the adventitia and periesophageal fat tissue bordering the aorta *(ao)*. Note the clear transition between the normal and pathologic wall structure *(arrow)*. **B,** corresponding picture of the polypoid esophageal carcinoma. (From Tio TL, et al: Evaluation of resectability of gastrointestinal tumors, in Kamar K (ed): *Endoscopic Ultrasonography In Gastroenterology,* ed 1. Tokyo, Igaku-Shoin, 1988, p 106. Used by permission.)

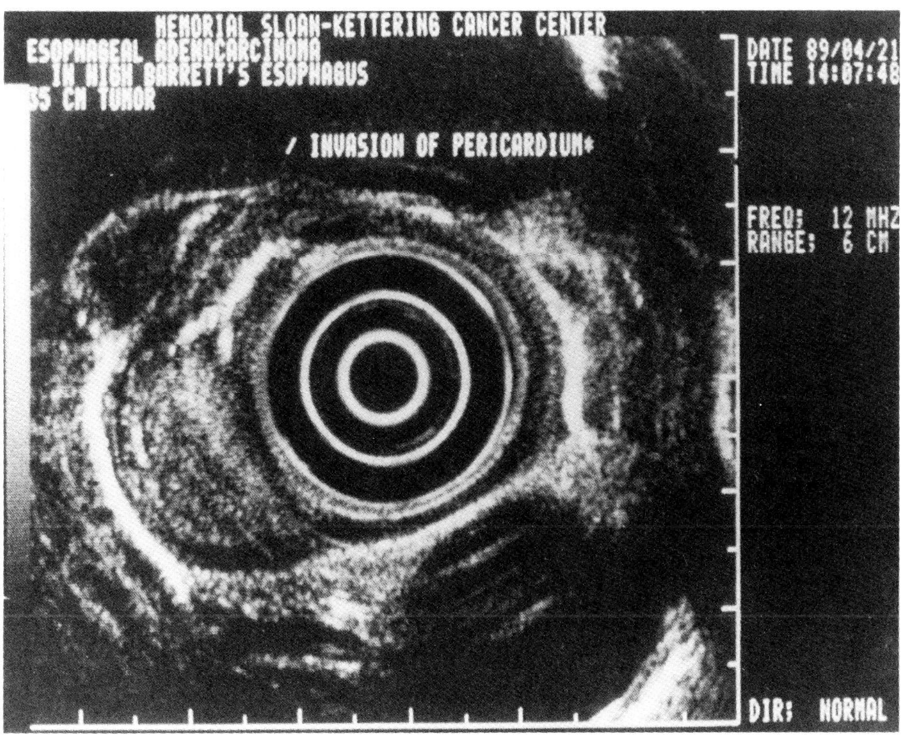

FIG 14–8.
A large esophageal tumor mass is evident as it extends through the adventitia; the pericardium is eroded as indicated by the shaggy, irregular surface (stage 4). (From Lightdale CJ, Botet JF: *Gastrointest Endosc Suppl* 1990; 36:11–16. Used by permission.)

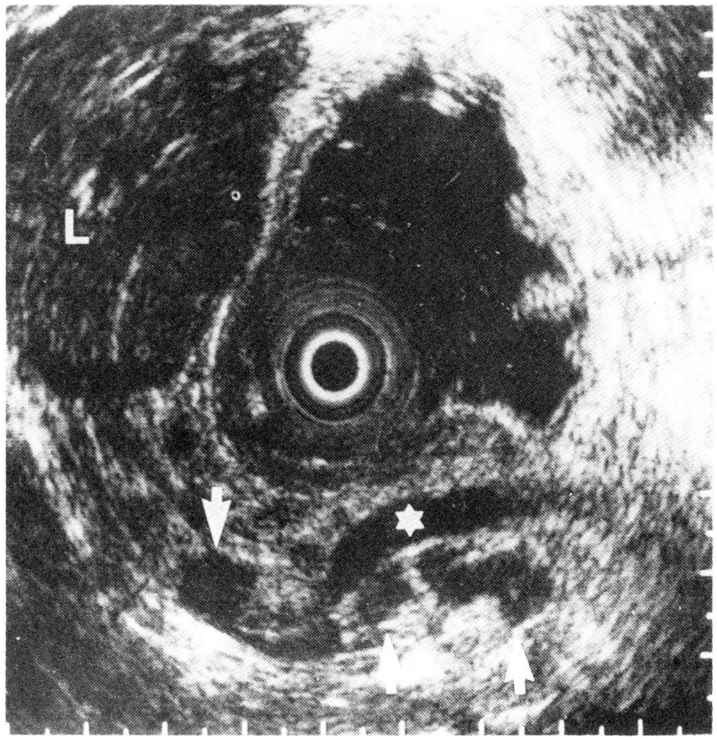

FIG 14–9.
Pancreatic carcinoma *(arrows)* with a mixed echo pattern and a relatively sharp margin (1, spenic vein). (From Dancygier H, Classen M: Pancreatic cancer, In Kamar K (ed): *Endoscopic Ultrasonography in Gastroenterology,* ed 1. Tokyo, Igaku-Shoin, 1988, pp 72–78. Used by permission.)

tegrity of the several echo layers is interrupted, thus defining the depth of invasion of the tumor.[17] Accuracy in defining the depth of invasion varies from 70% to 90%; it is 50% to 90% for lymph node involvement.[18, 19] Lymph nodes greater than 5 mm with a hypoechoic pattern and clearly delineated boundaries are suggestive of malignancy (Fig 14–6). Lymph nodes with hyperechoic patterns and indistinctly demarcated boundaries are considered benign. Direct extension of the primary tumor is considered pathognomonic of malignancy (Figs 14–7 and 14–8). EUS can also detect extramural recurrence of upper GI malignancy, which can be missed by endoscopy and CT scanning, with a 80% to 95% accuracy.[20]

PANCREAS

EUS has proved useful in diagnosing pancreatic cancer, especially small cancers[21, 22] (Fig 14–9). Chronic pancreatitis with pseudocyst formation and duct dilatation can also be detected (Fig 14–10).

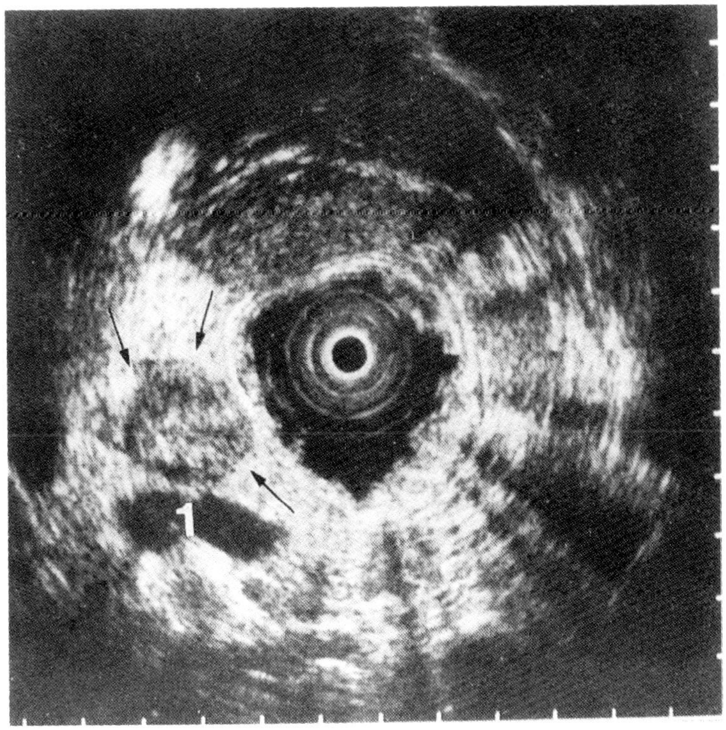

FIG 14–10.
Pseudocysts *(arrows)* in a dilated, but smoothly outlined pancreatic duct *(asterisk)* *L* = liver. (From Dancygier H, Classen M: Pancreatic cancer, in Kamar K (ed): *Endoscopic Ultrasonography In Gastroenterology,* ed 1. Tokyo, Igaku-Shoin, 1988, pp 72–78. Used by permission.)

BILIARY TREE

The biliary tree including the gallbladder, common bile duct, and papilla of Vater can be also imaged. Imaging of the pancreas and the biliary tree is done through the stomach and duodenum (Fig 14–11).[23]

LAPARASCOPIC SONOGRAPHY

Laparascopic sonography of the liver has been investigated. Over 200 procedures have been done, and laparascopic sonography has shown the capability to detect and differentiate occult lesions of the liver, cysts, tumors and various benign focal hyperplasia, and various granulomas.[24]

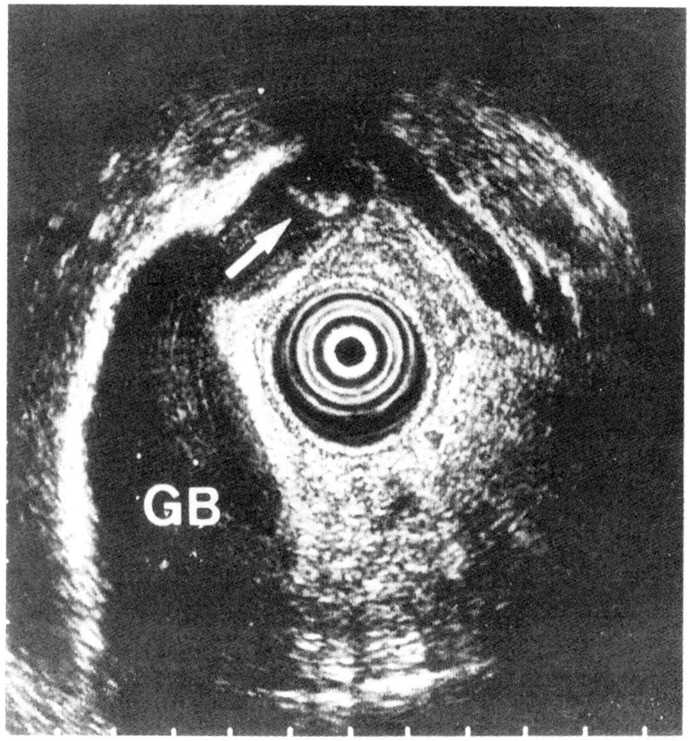

FIG 14–11.
A EUS image of a gallstone *(arrow)* at the neck of the gallbladder *(GB)*. (From Yasuda K, et al: Diseases of the biliary tract and the papilla of Vater, in Kamar K (ed): *Endoscopic Ultrasonography In Gastroenterology,* ed 1. Tokyo, Igaku-Shoin, 1988, p 96. Used by permission.)

FUTURE PROSPECTS

Ultrasound probes are being developed as alternatives to dedicated ultrasound endoscopes. They are designed to pass through the instrument channel of ordinary fiber-optic endoscopes and can achieve frequencies up to 20 MHz. They are best suited for imaging focal endoscopically visible lesions but do not scan large areas of tissue because of the limited depth of penetration.[25]

REFERENCES

1. Straim WH: Gastrointestinal contrast media, in Parez Z, Moncada R, Slovak M (eds): *Contrast Media: Biologic Effects and Clinical Application,* vol 1. Boca Raton, Fla, CRC Press Inc, 1987, pp 9–13.
2. Dagradi AE: History, in: *Gastrointestinal Endoscopy: Technique and Interpretation,* ed 1. Tokyo, Igaku-Shoin, 1983, pp 4–11.
3. Quint LE, Glazer GM, Orringer MB: Esophageal imaging by MR and CT: Study of normal anatomy and neoplasms. *Radiology* 1985; 156:727–731.
4. Picus D, Balfe DM, Koehler RE, et al: Computed tomography in the staging of esophageal carcinoma. *Radiology* 1983; 146:433–438.

5. Hodgman CG, MacCarty RL, Wolff FG, et al: Preoperative staging of rectal carcinoma by computed tomography and the 0.15T magnetic resonance imaging. *Dis Colon Rectum* 1986; 29:446–450.
6. Thompson WM, Halvorsen RA, Foster WL Jr, et al: Preoperative and postoperative CT staging of rectosigmoid carcinoma. *AJR* 1986; 146:703–710.
7. Tio TL, Cohn P, Coene PP, et al: Endosongraphy and computed tomography of esophageal carcinoma. *Gastroenterology* 1989; 96:1478–1486.
8. Sasai T: Development of ultrasonic endoscope, in Kawai K (ed): *Endoscopic Ultrasonography in Gastroenterology,* ed 1. Tokyo, Igaku-Shoin, 1988, pp 18–34.
9. Tio TL, Coene PP, Luiken GL, et al: Endosonography in the clinical staging of esophagogastric carcinoma. *Gastroenterol Endosc Suppl* 1990; 36:2–10.
10. White RA: Indications for fiberoptic angioscopy and intraluminal ultrasound. *Compre Ther* 1990; 16:23–30.
11. West AL: Endovascular ultrasound, in Moore WS, Ahn SS (eds): *Endovascular Surgery.* Philadelphia, WB Saunders Co, 1989, pp 518–523.
12. Jochem RJ, Reading CC, Dozois RR, et al: Endorectal ultrasonographic staging of rectal carcinoma. *Mayo Clin Proc* 1990; 65:1571–1577.
13. Yasuda K, Cho E, Nakajima M, et al: Diagnosis of submucosal lesions of the upper gastrointestinal tract by endoscopic ultrasonography. *Gastroenterol Endosc Suppl* 1990; 36:17–20.
14. Caletti G, Brocchi E, Baraldini M, et al: Assessment of portal hypertension by endoscopic ultrasonography *Gastroenterol Endosc Suppl* 1990; 36:21–27.
15. Rosch T, Lorenz R, Classen M: Endoscopic ultrasonography in the evaluation of colon and rectal disease. *Gastroenterol Endosc Suppl* 1990; 36:33–39.
16. Tsuyoshi A, Tadayoshi T: Benign lesions of the gastrointestinal tract, in Kawai K (ed): *Endoscopic Ultrasonography in Gastroenterology,* ed 1. Tokyo, Igaku-Shoin, 1988, pp 44–55.
17. Yasuda K, Nakajima M, Kawai K: Malignant lesions of the gastrointestinal tract, in Kawai K (ed): *Endoscopic Ultrasonography in Gastroenterology,* ed 1. Tokyo, Igaku-Shoin, 1988, pp 56–71.
18. Sugimachi K, Ohno S, Fujishima H, et al: Endoscopic ultrasonographic detection of carcinomatous invasion of lymph nodes in the thoracic esophagus. *Surgery* 1990; 107:366–371.
19. Glaser F, Schlag P, Herfarth CH: Endorectal ultrasonography for the assessment of invasion of rectal tumors and lymph node involvement. *Br J Surg* 1990; 77:883–887.
20. Lightdale CJ, Botet JF: Esophageal carcinoma: Pre-operative staging and evaluation of anastomotic recurrence. *Gastroenterol Endosc Suppl* 1990; 36:11–16.
21. Dancygier H, Classen M: Pancreatic cancer, in Kawai K (ed): *Endoscopic Ultrasonography in Gastroenterology,* ed 1. Tokyo, Igaku-Shoin, 1988, pp 72–78.
22. Boyce GA, Sivak MV: Endoscopic ultrasonography in the diagnosis of pancreatic tumors. *Gastroenterol Endosc Suppl* 1990; 36:28–32.
23. Morita K, Nakazawa S, Kimoto E, et al: Gallbladder diseases, in Kawai K (ed): *Endoscopic Ultrasonography in Gastroenterology,* ed 1. Tokyo, Igaku-Shoin, 1988, pp 87–95.
24. Fukuda M, Mima S: Laparoscopic sonography in differential diagnosis of liver diseases, in Kawai K (ed): *Endoscopic Ultrasonography in Gastroenterology,* ed 1. Tokyo, Igaku-Shoin, 1988, pp 119–131.
25. Kimmey MB, Martin RW, Silverstein FE: Endoscopic ultrasound probes. *Gastroenterol Endosc Suppl* 1990; 36:40–46.

Chapter 15

Endoscopic Surgery; Controversies in Credentialing and Rational Use of New Devices

Samuel E. Wilson, M.D.

The surgeon seeking to implement a new technique or device into his practice faces a set of three challenges. First, he must be able to evaluate the stage of development of the technology and assess its impact, whether transient or lasting. Then he must undertake training in the new procedure or instrument so that he can safely and competently operate in the clinical arena. When this has been accomplished, the next responsibility is to develop guidelines for the credentialing of surgeons in the new procedures, participate in fair proctoring of other surgeons on the staff, and most importantly, ensure a satisfactory outcome in standard of care. Teaching institutions have a further obligation to integrate the new operation or technology into residency training. This chapter will review methods for the evaluation of new techniques and describe procedures for implementing these techniques into regular practice.

CLINICAL INVESTIGATION OF NEW DEVICES

Before uncritically embracing a new technique or device, the prudent surgeon should have data available for review from at least the first three stages of laboratory and clinical investigation, (Table 15–1). Basic feasibility of a new device will have been tested by in vitro phase I studies. Valuable data can be obtained on the physical limits of the instrumentation, destruction of harvested tissues and organs, and ease of manipulation of the instrument. Phase II in vivo experiments should provide reassuring information on toxicity or hazards of the device, results of animal surgery, and short-term follow-up. For example, when investigating vascular or endovascular instrumentation, results from animal models that have been followed for months to years can provide useful information on vessel or graft patency, susceptibility to infection, neointimalization, and incorporation and durability of prosthetic materials. Lasers used in atherosclerotic animal models can be evaluated for the likelihood of vessel wall perforation, changes in the intimal surface, thrombogenicity, embolization, and short-term patency.

TABLE 15–1.
Phases of Laboratory and Clinical Investigation of a New Device

Phase I	In vitro feasibility testing; collection of physical data
Phase II	In vivo investigation in animal models; patency data, susceptibility to infection; toxicity
Phase III	"Open" clinical trial in carefully selected human subjects
Phase IV	Randomized trial comparing new device with standard methods in large study population, usually multicenter; patients stratified for severity of disease

Now the surgeon should turn to examination of data from the third stage of development—open clinical trials. Even when in vitro feasibility and animal experimentation may appear promising, the limitations of these investigations may result in new therapeutic techniques finding their way into clinical trials with questions remaining about efficacy. A carefully designed clinical trial in patients that uses a protocol approved by a competent research committee and a knowledgeable human subjects review board can answer these questions. Only if the trial is carried out under the formal regulations of an institutional review board can one assume that the data will be relevant to clinical practice. It is essential that patients have given an informed consent that specifically states in lay terms the nature of the study and the potential benefits and disadvantages. Open trials conducted within an academic or other clinical institutional setting helps ensure sufficient numbers of patients with the disease under study and provides an atmosphere of ongoing critical review. Further, research and human subjects committees scrutinize data on a regular basis to ensure that the trial is conducted within the limits of the protocol and that the data are sufficiently good for the study to be renewed. Reports of such open trials should be carefully assessed for the indications for the device or technique and for clear-cut end points in study data. Symptomatic relief alone can be misleading. For example, results based on the patient's evaluation of a symptomatic improvement after laser endovascular therapy showed a 75% success rate, whereas objective hemodynamic measurements showed only 22% patency of the vessel.[1] In the evaluation of treatment of vascular disease, objective end points, in addition to relief of symptoms, may include improvement in the ankle/brachial index and arterial patency demonstrated on repeat arteriography or duplex scanning. Treadmill walking distance or other such test is likely to be more accurate than the patient's report of walking distance. Patients studied should have significant, symptomatic disease that would have required treatment by other conventional methods. Mean follow-up periods should be at 3- to 6-month intervals for no less than 24 months in most cases.

Open clinical trials are often conducted to seek Food and Drug Administration (FDA) approval of drugs or instrumentation. Clinical data from these studies may be compared, albeit imperfectly from a statistical point of view, with historical controls. The key to comparability is stratification of patients' presenting symptoms. The goal in the open clinical trial is primarily to confirm safety and show feasibility of the treatment in patients. Definition of the appropriate clinical role will be further defined by a comparison of the new technique with standard methods. If the data show promise, either in better outcome or similar outcome with less morbidity and patient expense, further trials (phase IV) may be conducted.

At this stage, when data from phase III open trials are released, the surgeon is most likely to consider acquisition of a new skill or instrument. Ideally, it would be best to wait for the phase IV controlled clinical trial evaluation, but this may be impractical. These trials will often take as long as 5 years and require participation of multiple centers and major funding. During this research time, modifications in equipment and techniques can occur to such an extent that the procedure has changed significantly. Consequently, delay in large-scale cooperative studies is furthered because investigators are reluctant to undertake the study of a device unless it has become standardized to the point where it is unlikely to undergo major change during the 3 to 5 years necessary for a comparative trial. Surgeons often feel pressured to learn the new technology before definitive studies are available rather than risk being "left out" in the competitive clinical world. Few waited to see whether laparoscopic cholecystectomy would be safer than an open operation on the basis of controlled trials, and perhaps the answer is obvious in this instance. Yet many invested in expensive laser equipment or gallstone lithotripsy equipment that goes unused.

A cooperative clinical trial is designed to compare a new technique or device with standard methods. For example, percutaneous transluminal angioplasty is compared with a surgical bypass operation, or laser-assisted balloon angioplasty is compared with balloon angioplasty alone. Sufficient patients should have been studied to allow a statistical analysis of the outcome data. Data should be provided on patient demographics, symptomatology, and site and severity of disease according to treatment assigned so that one can ensure equal randomization of patients. Clinical trial data should uncover enough information to ensure that the patients studied were a a representative sample, that is, a true cross section of the patients generally treated by the surgeon for the condition. For example, endoscopic laparotomy for lysis of adhesions in patients without a small-bowel obstruction provides few data of use to the surgeon considering this technique for symptomatic patients.

Data from a clinical trial may be examined from three points of view: first, evaluation of the trial results as to comparability with expected results from standard treatment; second, deciding by inference if the results obtained on the type of disease in patients in the trial would be applicable to one's future patients; and third, deciding among competing treatments.

It is important to differentiate investigation of new devices and new methods from simple modifications of current techniques. Whether one removes the gallbladder through a midline incision, paramedian incision, subcostal incision, or even laparoscopic technique does not alter the basic worth of the procedure. Rather, investigation here would be to determine safety, patient morbidity, later complications, and cost analyses. It is not necessary to conduct a clinical trial to show that patients undergoing laparoscopic cholecystectomy successfully will generally have a much shorter hospital stay, less pain, and less morbidity than by open technique. What does need to be studied is the incidence of postoperative hemorrhages, bile leak, resurgery, retained common duct stones, etc., in patients undergoing the procedures for similar indications.[2]

The spread of new technological devices is so rapid today that often university medical centers are not involved in their evaluation. For example, techniques today may be explored rapidly in the greater surgical community and tried and adopted or abandoned before any type of comparative trial is possible. For example, laparoscopic cholecystectomy first gained widespread use in France between 1987 and 1988.[3] The procedure enjoyed immediate success in community hospitals in the United States. Numerous training programs specific for the procedure were instituted, and within the course of a year, many surgeons in the United States had undertaken a course, and the technique was extended to the majority of hospitals. This all occurred with relatively little input from the academic environment. Patients demanded the procedure, which required only a 1- to 2-day hospitalization, and third party payers appreciated decreased inpatient costs. The morbidity was considerably less and a major scar avoided. Still, with some exceptions,[4] there are few reports of the incidence of operative complications and retained common duct stones. Further, the indications for the operation to date have been primarily for minimally symptomatic patients. The laparoscopic general surgeon would proceed cautiously until these data are at hand. Other examples of early widespread enthusiasm for a technique have not been so favorable. Types of endovascular laser equipment were purchased before adequate clinical data were available only to find that the clinical results did not live up to the in vitro or animal experimentation data. In some instances, large investments in equipment were lost and manufacturers failed financially. The careful approach is to be continually aware of new developments, attend postgraduate courses, review outcome data critically, and adapt technology only when data are satisfactory.

CREDENTIALING

The medical staff bylaws of hospitals and the Joint Commission on Hospital Accreditation require that privileges be extended to surgeons through evaluation of their training and proctoring and ongoing monitoring of quality assurance. Introducing a new technique to hospital practice can be controversial. How should the innovator's clinical and course experience be evaluated and who should proctor him? Which specialty should do a new procedure? Is it appropriate for cardiologists who are quite skilled in dilatation of the coronary arteries to dilate femoral arteries or other vessels? In some instances, such as laser surgery, there are safety issues for both patients and staff.

One workable technique is for the department chairman or the hospital executive committee to establish a subcommittee on credentialing for a new procedure. For example, this may be a laser committee or a committee on laparoscopic intraperitoneal procedures. Guidelines should be established for course training as well as practical clinical experience and proctoring requirements. Individuals applying for privileges should demonstrate attendance at a CME category I course, which ideally includes experience in the animal laboratory. The applicant for new privileges should ideally have observed the procedure performed on patients and perhaps have been a first assistant if possible. Requirements should be reasonable and take into account the fact that that many hospitals have rules against observers in the operating room and legal considerations preclude non–staff members from participating in an operation. Accordingly, the only direct experience obtained may be through the use of video tapes and other visual aids.

When the new technique is introduced into hospital practice, careful records should be kept of results and complications. Periodic review should ensure that the technique is safe and at least comparable with existing methods. Surgeons who have mastered the new procedure should willingly share their experience with others and proctor their colleagues' procedures. Surgeons concerned about being "locked out" of a particular procedure should realize that good ideas and reliable knowledge spread rapidly. There are no secrets in modern medicine.

The national specialty organizations can offer direction in some instances. For example, the American College of Surgeons issued a statement delineating the experience and qualifications necessary for performing a laparoscopic cholecystectomy. They state that "For optimal quality patient care laparoscopic cholecystectomy should be performed by surgeons who are qualified to perform open cholecystectomy." Only such surgeons possess the skills to perform biliary tract surgery procedures, such surgeons are able to determine the best method of cholecystectomy, and only such surgeons can treat complications consequent to laparoscopic cholecystectomy. The Society for Surgery of the Alimentary Tract issued a statement addressing training and credentialing for laparoscopic cholecystectomy in which they recommended that hospital privileges for this procedure be granted to

> Surgeons who are trained general surgeons, competent in open cholecystectomy and in the complications thereof, have expertise in laparoscopic cholecystectomy through previous clinical experience or through instruction, have completed an experience in supervised laparoscopic cholecystectomy including instruction and practice on animals.

They also recommend that surgeons notify patients of their experience with the particular procedure. When these guidelines are followed, the qualifications for the procedure would seem to be clear.

Controversy arises where a particular procedure can be performed by several overlapping specialties. For example, percutaneous transluminal angioplasty may be performed by surgeons, radiologists, and cardiologists. In general, collaboration rather than competition should be encouraged. Opportunists should be discouraged from undertaking treatment of a disease with which they had no former experience simply because new instrumentation and economic incentive is available. For example, performance of a cholecystectomy by any technique clearly involves knowledge of the biliary tree and should be performed by a general surgeon, even though a gynecologist may have more experience with technical details of laparoscopic technique. Peripheral vascular disease is best managed by the general vascular surgeon rather than the cardiologist treating peripheral lesions *en passant.* In some instances it may be appropriate for different specialties to carry out the same operation. For example, it makes little difference whether the surgeon performing a renal transplant is a urologist or a general surgeon in background training as long as he has had specialized experience in transplantation surgery.

RESIDENCY CONSIDERATIONS

Integration of new surgical techniques into residency training should be accomplished as part of the regular training program. A residency program should have access to an animal surgical facility where techniques can be practiced before the procedures are carried out in the operating room under staff supervision.

REFERENCES

1. DeWeese JA in discussion of White RA, White GA, Mehringer MC, Chiang FL, Wilson SE: A clinical trial of laser thermal angioplasty in patients with advanced peripheral vascular disease. *Ann Surg* 1990; 212:257–265.
2. Ebert PA: As I see it (editorial). *Am Coll Surgeons Bull* 1990; 75:2–3.
3. Tompkins RK: Laparoscopic cholecystectomy: Threat or opportunity? *Arch Surg* 1990; 125:1245.
4. Phillips E, Daykhovsky L, Caroll B, et al: Laparoscopic cholecystectomy instrumentation and technique. *J Laparosc Surg,* 1990; 1:3–16.

Index

B

C

D

E

H

I

J

K

L

M